ESSENTIALS OF CLINICAL GERIATRICS

NOTICE

Medicine is an ever-changing science. As new research and clinical experience broaden our knowledge, changes in treatment and drug therapy are required. The authors and the publisher of this work have checked with sources believed to be reliable in their efforts to provide information that is complete and generally in accord with the standards accepted at the time of publication. However, in view of the possibility of human error or changes in medical sciences, neither the authors nor the publisher nor any other party who has been involved in the preparation or publication of this work warrants that the information contained herein is in every respect accurate or complete, and they disclaim all responsibility for any errors or omissions or for the results obtained from use of the information contained in this work. Readers are encouraged to confirm the information contained herein with other sources. For example and in particular, readers are advised to check the product information sheet included in the package of each drug they plan to administer to be certain that the information contained in this work is accurate and that changes have not been made in the recommended dose or in the contraindications for administration. This recommendation is of particular importance in connection with new or infrequently used drugs.

ESSENTIALS OF CLINICAL GERIATRICS

FIFTH EDITION

ROBERT L. KANE, MD

Professor and Minnesota Endowed Chair in Long-Term Care and Aging
School of Public Health
University of Minnesota
Minneapolis, Minnesota

JOSEPH G. OUSLANDER, MD

Professor of Medicine and Nursing
Director, Division of Geriatric Medicine and Gerontology
Chief Medical Officer, Wesley Woods Center
Director, Center for Health in Aging
Emory University
Research Scientist, Birmingham/Atlanta VA GRECC
Atlanta, Georgia

ITAMAR B. ABRASS, MD

Professor and Head, Division of Gerontology and Geriatric Medicine
University of Washington
Seattle, Washington

McGRAW-HILL
Medical Publishing Division

NEW YORK / CHICAGO / SAN FRANCISCO / LISBON / LONDON
MADRID / MEXICO CITY / MILAN / NEW DELHI / SAN JUAN
SEOUL / SINGAPORE / SYDNEY / TORONTO

The McGraw·Hill Companies

ESSENTIALS OF CLINICAL GERIATRICS
FIFTH EDITION

1 2 3 4 5 6 7 8 9 0   DOC/DOC   0 9 8 7 6 5 4 3

ISBN 0-07-140920-3

This book was set in Times Roman by Joanne Morbit of McGraw-Hill's Hightstown, N.J., Professional Book Group composition unit.
The editors were Jim Shanahan, Kitty McCullough, and Mary Bele.
The production supervisor was Catherine Saggese.
The text was designed by Marsha Cohen/Parallelogram.
The cover designer was Kelly Parr.
The index was prepared by Andover Publishing Services.
RR Donnelley was printer and binder.

This book is printed on acid-free paper.

Library of Congress Cataloging-in-Publication Data

Kane, Robert L., 1940-
    Essentials of clinical geriatrics / Robert L. Kane, Joseph G. Ouslander, Itamar B. Abrass.—5th ed.
      p. ; cm.
    Includes bibliographical references and index.
    ISBN 0-07-140920-3
    1. Geriatrics. 2. Aging. 3. Aged—Health and hygiene. I. Ouslander, Joseph G. II. Abrass, Itamar B. III. Title.
    [DNLM: 1. Geriatrics. 2. Aging—physiology. 3. Aging—psychology. 4. Diagnosis, Differential—Aged. 5. Geriatric Assessment. WT 100 K16e 2003]
    RC952.K36   2003

2003051214

CONTENTS

TABLES AND FIGURES

CHAPTER FOUR

CHAPTER FIVE

CHAPTER SIX

CHAPTER SEVEN

CHAPTER EIGHT

CHAPTER ELEVEN

CHAPTER TWELVE

CHAPTER THIRTEEN

CHAPTER FOURTEEN

CHAPTER SEVENTEEN

PREFACE

When this book was originally conceived, geriatrics was still in its developmental phase. It was unclear then whether geriatrics would emerge as a subspecialty on its own or as a basis for educating others in the elements of caring for frail older persons. Much has happened in the intervening two decades. It now appears that the majority of care for older persons will remain in the hands of primary care practitioners; but those ranks have changed. Nurse practitioners are much more evident. At the same time, the importance of chronic disease care in general is more widely appreciated. Many of the principles of good geriatrics care can apply as readily to this larger topic; they are captured within this text.

We continue to view this book as a practical guide, designed for use by a wide variety of present and future practitioners. It presumes a good basic working knowledge of medicine and stresses those aspects of care that are important in helping older persons to live more comfortable lives.

Each new edition provides the opportunity (indeed the need) to look back over the time since its predecessor to determine just how much has changed. The past 5 years or so saw some important developments our understanding of aging, including the emergence of genetics as a potentially potent clinical process. Some new drugs emerged. Some concepts, such as the role of hormone replacement therapy, were reexamined. Medical practice now endorses concepts such as evidence-based medicine and is still struggling to produce the evidence on which to base it, but some well-established practice guidelines are still not widely adopted. But the largest changes seem to have occurred in the way health care is organized and financed. Prospective payment has been extended to many forms of care beyond the hospital. Managed care continues to evolve.

We hope that when we look back on the next 5 years, they will be viewed as period of great mastery of geriatric principles and active incorporation of new and more effective methods of providing care. As we draw ever closer to that demographic horizon when the aging population will demand more-efficient methods to provide necessary and affordable care, we will certainly need a medical work force that is well versed in geriatrics. If this book helps to achieve that goal, we will have accomplished something of value.

PART I

THE AGING PATIENT AND GERIATRIC ASSESSMENT

CHAPTER 1

CLINICAL IMPLICATIONS OF THE AGING PROCESS

The care of older patients differs from that of younger patients for a number of reasons. Some of these can be traced to the changes that occur in the process of aging, some are caused by the plethora of diseases and disruptions that accompany seniority, and still others result from the way old people are treated. Several terms are used by gerontologists to describe the phenomena of aging (Bengston et al., 1999). *The aged* refers to populations who are characterized as having achieved a certain length of life or expected life span. *Aging* relates to the developmental process of growth and senescence over time. *Age-related* refers to how age is taken into account in health and social systems.

Perhaps one of the most intriguing challenges in medicine is to unravel the process of aging. Although we may be able to see pure aging in a cellular culture, it is very hard to visualize in the intact organism. Discussions about aging seem to imply accumulation of chronic diseases. How then does one separate the changes caused solely by aging from the sequelae of disease? Would a group of disease-free older persons be the appropriate models to help us understand the aging process? The prospect sounds uncomfortably like describing life on the basis of a colony of germ-free mice.

Nonetheless, the distinction between so-called normal aging and pathologic changes is critical to the care of older people. We wish to avoid both dismissing treatable pathology as simply a concomitant of old age and treating natural aging processes as though they were diseases. The latter is particularly dangerous because older adults are so vulnerable to iatrogenic effects.

There is growing appreciation that everyone does not age in the same way or at the same rate. The changing composition of today's older adults compared with that of a generation ago may actually reflect a bimodal shift wherein there are both more disabled people and more healthy older people. As described in a recent systematic review, several measures of old age disability and limitations have shown improvements in the last decade (Freedman et al., 2002). Attention has become focused on the variations in aging, with great interest directed toward those described as aging successfully—that is, showing the least decline in function with time (Rowe and Kahn, 1987).

CHANGES ASSOCIATED WITH "NORMAL" AGING

We have already noted the critical and difficult distinction a clinician must make to attribute a finding to either the expected course of aging or the result of pathologic changes. This distinction perplexes the researcher as well. We currently lack precise knowledge of what constitutes normal aging. Much of our information comes from cross-sectional studies, which compare findings from a group of younger persons with those from a group of older individuals. Such data may reflect differences other than simply the effects of age. The older group grew up in a different environment, perhaps with different diet and activities. They represent a cohort of survivors. We have come to appreciate that what we see in the older patient is largely a result of what is brought to old age. For example, the decrease in the frequency of osteoporosis today has been related to the observation that women entering the high-risk period (postmenopause) have stronger bones with thicker cortices.

Many of the changes associated with aging result from gradual loss. These losses may often begin in early adulthood, but—thanks to the redundancy of most organ systems—the decrement does not become functionally significant until the loss is fairly extensive.

Based on cross-sectional comparisons of groups at different ages, most organ systems seem to lose function at about 1 percent a year beginning around age 30 years. Other data suggest that the changes in people followed longitudinally are much less dramatic and certainly begin well after age 70 years.

In some organ systems, such as the kidney, a subgroup of persons appear to experience gradually declining function over time, whereas others' function remains constant. These findings suggest that the earlier theory of gradual loss must be reassessed as reflecting disease rather than aging.

Given a pattern of gradual deterioration—whether from aging or disease or both—we are best advised to think in terms of thresholds.

The loss of function does not become significant until it crosses a given level. Thus the functional performance of an organ in an older person depends on two principal factors: (1) the rate of deterioration and (2) the level of performance needed. It is not surprising then to learn that most older persons will have normal laboratory values. The critical difference—in fact, the hallmark of aging—lies not in the resting level of performance but in how the organ (or organism) adapts to external stress. For example, an older person may have a normal fasting blood sugar but be unable to handle a glucose load within the normal parameters for younger subjects.

The same pattern of decreased response to stress can be seen in the performance of other endocrine systems or the cardiovascular system. An older individual may have a normal resting pulse and cardiac output but be unable to achieve an adequate increase in either with exercise.

Sometimes the changes of aging work together to produce apparently normal resting values in other ways. For example, although both glomerular filtration and renal blood flow decrease with age, many elderly persons have normal serum creatinine levels because of the concomitant decreases in lean muscle mass and creatinine production.

Thus serum creatinine is not as good an indicator of renal function in the elderly as in younger persons. Because knowledge of kidney function is so critical in drug therapy, it is important to get some measure of this parameter. A useful formula for estimating creatinine clearance on the basis of serum creatinine values in the elderly has been developed (Cockcroft and Gault, 1976). (The actual formula is provided in Chap. 14.) Table 1-1 summarizes some of the pertinent changes that occur with aging. For many items, the changes begin in adulthood and proceed gradually; others may not manifest themselves until well into seniority. Readers interested in a more detailed discussion of the changes associated with aging should consult the several excellent reviews on the subject (Birren and Schaie, 2001; Masoro and Austad, 2001).

BIOLOGICAL AGING

It is now a commonly accepted notion that aging is a multifactorial process. Extended longevity is frequently associated with enhanced metabolic capacity and response to stress. The importance of genetics in the regulation of biological aging is demonstrated by the characteristic longevity of each animal species. However, heritability of life span accounts for ≤35 percent of its variance, whereas environmental factors account for >65 percent of the variance (Finch and Tanzi, 1997), and genes specifically selected to promote aging are unlikely to exist.

Several theories of aging have been promulgated and recently reviewed (Vijg and Wei, 1995; Kirkwood and Austad, 2000). These theories fall into either of two general categories: (1) accumulation of damage to informational molecules or (2) the regulation of specific genes (Table 1-2).

DNA undergoes continuous change both in response to exogenous agents and intrinsic processes. Stability is maintained by the double-strandedness of DNA and by specific repair enzymes. It has been proposed that somatic mutagenesis, either owing to greater susceptibility to mutagenesis or deficits in repair mechanisms, is a factor in biological aging. In fact, there is a positive correlation of species longevity with DNA repair enzymes. In humans, the spontaneous mutagenesis rate is not adequate to account for the number of changes that would be

TABLE 1-1   CHANGES ASSOCIATED WITH AGING

ITEM	MORPHOLOGY	FUNCTION
Overall	Decreased height (vertebral compression and stooped posture secondary to increased kyphosis) Decreased weight (after age 80 in longitudinal studies) Increased fat-to-lean body mass ratio Decreased total body water	
Skin	Increased wrinkling Atrophy of sweat glands	
Cardiovascular system	Elongation and tortuosity of arteries, including aorta Increased intimal thickening of arteries Increased fibrosis of media of arteries Sclerosis of heart valves	Decreased cardiac output during exercise Decreased heart rate response to stress Decreased compliance of peripheral blood vessels
Kidney	Increased number of abnormal glomeruli Interstitial fibrosis	Decreased creatinine clearance Decreased renal blood flow Decreased maximum urine osmolality
Lung	Decreased elasticity Decreased activity of cilia	Decreased forced vital capacity and forced expiratory volume Decreased maximal oxygen uptake Decreased cough reflex
Gastrointestinal tract	Decreased hydrochloric acid Fewer taste buds	Slowed intestinal motility
Skeleton	Osteoarthritis Loss of bone structure	
Eyes	Arcus senilis Decreased pupil size Growth of lens	Deceased accommodation Hyperopia Decreased acuity Decreased color sensitivity Decreased depth perception

TABLE 1-1 CHANGES ASSOCIATED WITH AGING (*Continued*)

ITEM	MORPHOLOGY	FUNCTION
Hearing	Degenerative changes of ossicles Increased obstruction of eustachian tube Atrophy of external auditory meatus Atrophy of cochlear hair cells Loss of auditory neurons	Decreased perception in high frequencies Decreased pitch discrimination
Immune system		Decreased T-cell activity
Nervous system	Decreased brain weight Decreased cortical cell count	Increased motor response time Slower psychomotor performance Decreased intellectual performance Decreased complex learning Decreased hours of sleep Decreased hours of rapid eye movement (REM) sleep
Endocrine		Decreased triiodo-thyronine (T_3) Decreased free (unbound) testosterone Increased insulin Increased norepinephrine Increased parathormone Increased vasopressin

necessary, and there is no evidence that a general failure in repair systems causes aging. However, limited maintenance and repair may lead to accumulation of somatic damage.

A related theory, the error catastrophe theory, proposes that errors occur in DNA, RNA, and protein synthesis, each augmenting the other and finally culminating in an error catastrophe. Translation was considered the most likely source for age-dependent errors because it was the final common pathway. However,

TABLE 1-2   MAJOR THEORIES ON AGING

THEORY	MECHANISMS	MANIFESTATIONS
Accumulation of damage to informational molecules	Spontaneous mutagenesis	Copying errors
	Failure in DNA repair systems	
	Errors in DNA, RNA, and protein synthesis	Error catastrophe
	Superoxide radicals and loss of scavenging enzymes	Oxidative cellular damage
Regulation of specific genes	Appearance of specific protein(s)	Genetically programmed senescence

increased translational errors have not been found in either in vivo or in vitro aging. Amino acid substitutions do not increase with age, although some enzyme activities may be altered by changes in posttranslational modification, such as glycosylation.

The major by-products of oxidative metabolism include superoxide radicals that can react with DNA, RNA, proteins, and lipids, leading to cellular damage and aging. There are several scavenging enzymes and some small molecules, such as vitamins C and E, that protect the cell from oxidative damage. There is no significant loss of scavenging enzymes in aging, and vitamins C and E do not increase longevity in experimental animals. However, interest in this hypothesis persists, because overexpression of antioxidative enzymes retards the age-related accrual of oxidative damage and extends the maximum life span of transgenic fruit flies; moreover, caloric restriction lowers levels of oxidative stress and damage and extends the maximum life span of rodents (Finkel and Holbrook, 2000; Masoro, 2000).

One hypothesis of aging is that it is regulated by specific genes. Support for such a hypothesis has been gained mainly from yeast, nematodes, fruit flies, and models of in vitro aging. Several genes in yeast, nematodes, and fruit flies have been found to extend the species life span. They appear to reinforce the importance of metabolic capacity and stress responses in aging. By DNA microarrays, relatively few genes changed in human fibroblasts with aging, and downregulation of genes involved in control of mitosis was proposed as a possible general cause of aging (Ly et al., 2000). However, others have not shown the same gene pattern changes in other aging tissues, suggesting that different changes underlie aging in different tissues.

In adulthood, cells can be placed into one of three categories based on their replicative capacity: continuously replicating, replicating in response to a challenge, and nonreplicating. Epidermal, gastrointestinal, and hematopoietic cells are continuously renewed; liver can regenerate in response to injury; while neurons and cardiac and skeletal muscle do not regenerate.

In vitro replication is closely related to in vivo proliferation. Neurons and cardiac myocytes from adults can be maintained in culture but do not divide, whereas hepatocytes, marrow cells, endothelial cells, and fibroblasts replicate in vitro. Because they are easily obtained from skin, fibroblasts have been the most extensively studied. Although some cells continuously replicate in vivo, they have a finite replicative life. For fibroblasts in vitro, this is about 50 doublings (Hayflick, 1979). Replicative life in vitro correlates with the age of the donor, such that the older the donor, the fewer the doublings in vitro. With time in culture, doubling time decreases and ultimately stops. Several lines of evidence suggest that replicative senescence evolved to protect higher organisms from developing cancer (Campisi, 2000).

With each cell division, a portion of the terminal end of chromosomes (the telomere) is not replicated and therefore shortens. It is proposed that telomere shortening is the clock that results in the shift to a senescent pattern of gene expression and ultimately cell senescence (Fossel, 1998). Telomerase is an enzyme that acts by adding DNA bases to telomeres. Transfection of the catalytic component of this enzyme into senescent cells extends their telomeres as well as the replicative life span of the cells and induces a pattern of gene expression typical of young cells. It is now possible to explore the role of replicative senescence in aging and associated chronic disease processes.

These experiments help define the finite life span of cells in vitro but do not themselves explain in vivo aging. However, factors associated with finite cell replication may more directly influence in vivo aging. Fibroblasts aged in vitro or obtained from older adult donors are less sensitive to a host of growth factors. Such changes occur at both the receptor and postreceptor levels. A decrease in such growth factors, a change in sensitivity to growth factors, and/or a slowing of the cell cycle may slow wound healing and thus place the older individual at greater risk for infection.

For tissues with nonreplicating cells, cell loss may lead to a permanent deficit. With aging, dopaminergic neurons are lost, thus influencing gait and balance and the susceptibility to drug side effects. With further decrements such as ischemia or viral infection, Parkinson's disease may develop. Similar cell loss and/or functional deficits may occur in other neurotransmitter systems and lead to autonomic dysfunction as well as alteration in mental function and neuroendocrine control.

The immune system demonstrates similar phenomena. Lymphocytes from older adults have a diminished proliferative response to a host of mitogens. This appears to be a result of both a decrease in lymphokines and a decrease in response to extracellular signals. As the thymus involutes after puberty, levels of thymic hormones (thymosins) decrease.

Basal and stimulated interleukin-2 (IL-2) production and IL-2 responsiveness also diminish with age. The latter appears to be due, at least in part, to a decreased expression of IL-2 receptors. Some immune functions can be restored by the addition of these hormones to lymphocytes in vitro, or, in vivo, by their administration to aged animals. The proliferative defect can also be reversed in vitro by calcium ionophores and activators of protein kinase C, suggesting that the T-cell defect may be in transduction of extracellular signals to intracellular function.

In vivo, molecular mechanisms such as those described above contribute to physiologic deficits and altered homeostatic mechanisms that predispose older individuals to dysfunction in the face of stress and disease.

The gene for Werner's syndrome, a progeric syndrome associated with early onset of age-related changes—such as gray hair, balding, atherosclerosis, insulin resistance, and cataracts, but not Alzheimer's disease—was recently cloned. The gene codes for a helicase involved in DNA replication. There is great interest in understanding how a defect in just this one gene leads to the multiple abnormalities of this syndrome.

Molecular geneticists have also cloned several genes related to early onset familial Alzheimer's disease and identified susceptibility genes for the late-onset form of the disease (Tanzi et al., 1996).

A small number of families have mutations in the amyloid precursor protein located on chromosome 21. The largest number of families with early onset familial Alzheimer's disease have a mutation in a gene on chromosome 14. This gene has been named presenilin 1. A similar gene has been identified on chromosome 1 and labeled presenilin 2. The role of the presenilins in Alzheimer's disease pathology is not yet known, but the identification of the three loci mentioned above has led to much excitement for the potential understanding of pathophysiologic mechanisms in this devastating disease. Similarly, the identification of apo E alleles as risk factors for late-onset Alzheimer's disease has raised interest in both the diagnosis and pathology of this disease.

Stem cells offer hope to greatly extend the numbers and range of patients who could benefit from cell replacement therapy to treat debilitating diseases such as diabetes, Parkinson's, Huntington's, and Alzheimer's. There is a long way to go in basic research before new therapies will be established, but clinical trials in some diseases are underway (Lovell-Badge, 2001).

CLINICAL IMPLICATIONS

As we try to understand aging, we appreciate the limitations of available information. As noted earlier, most of the data cited to document changes with age come from cross-sectional studies in which individuals of different ages are compared in terms of group averages. Such an approach generally reveals a gradual decline in organ function with age, beginning in early middle life. A few studies have followed cohorts of people longitudinally as they age. Their conclusions are quite different. In several parameters, performance actually increases with age. For example, cognitive function can improve over time among older persons. Similarly, cardiac function in subjects free of heart disease does not show inevitable decline with age (Lakatta, 1999).

The physician must be able to take data derived from group studies and apply them to the individual. It is essential to keep in mind the principle of individual variation. The best predictor of a given patient's performance now is that person's earlier performance rather than an average age-related decline documented in cross-sectional studies. Thus, an 80-year-old runner may well have better cardiovascular function than a 50-year-old sedentary doctor.

Aging is not simply a series of biological changes. That is, when one looks in the mirror and confronts an old person, the noted changes are associated with a variety of alterations in life. Aging is a time of losses: loss of social role (usually through retirement), loss of income, loss of friends and relatives (through death and mobility). It can also be a time of fear: fear for personal safety, fear of financial insecurity, fear of dependency.

In the face of these enormous threats, we should pause to rethink our views about older adults. Rather than being victims, they are the survivors. Most elderly persons have developed mechanisms to cope with multiple limitations. Most nevertheless continue to function. The physician's role is to enhance this coping ability by identifying and treating remediable problems and facilitating changes in the environment to maximize function in the face of those problems that remain.

In some instances, the patient's coping skills may make the physician's task more difficult. The elderly patient has often adapted to problems by denying or ignoring them. In such cases, it will be difficult to obtain a good history. Other patients cope with their disabilities by employing adaptive techniques. For example, a person who is hard of hearing may talk a great deal to hide a hearing deficit. A particularly troublesome problem is the skillful compensation for cognitive losses.

At least once in every physician's career, the physician will encounter a patient who carries on a perfectly lucid conversation, only to discover on closer examination that the patient is completely disoriented to time, place, and person. Because it is easy to miss these cognitive deficits, we recommend that an evaluation of older persons include a formal screening for mental status. A simple method for doing this is described in Chap. 6.

One of the hallmarks of aging is the reduced response to stress, including the stress of disease. Thus, the symptom intensity may be dampened by the aged body's decreased responsiveness. The presentation of illness in the geriatric patient can be thought of as a combination of dampened primary sound in the presence of background noise.

In treating an older adult, it is useful to keep in mind that an individual's ability to function depends on a combination of his or her characteristics (e.g., innate capacity, motivation, pain tolerance) and the setting in which that person is expected to function. The same individual may be functional in one setting and dependent in another.

The physician's first responsibility is to treat the patient, to remedy the remediable by searching for and dealing with those conditions that are treatable. Having improved the patient's ability (physiologically and psychologically) as much as possible, the physician's next task is to structure an environment that will facilitate the patient's functioning with maximum autonomy. This latter mandate should not rest exclusively on the doctor's shoulders. A variety of health-related professionals are available in most situations to play major roles in locating and utilizing supportive environments. But the physician must not abrogate this task. To ignore the environment of a disabled individual is tantamount to prescribing drugs and ignoring the patient's compliance with the treatment regimen.

Conversely, the environment can produce dysfunction. At the simplest level, it may produce hazards that lead to falls (see Chap. 9). At a more subtle level, it may necessitate a level of effort that produces decompensation. For example, an elderly person with dyspnea on exertion may get along reasonably well in a ground-floor apartment but become unmanageable in an apartment on the second floor of a building with no elevator. Similarly, patients with compromised pulmonary or cardiac function will show increased morbidity and mortality as air pollution levels increase. Finally, the environment may create disability by fostering dependency.

At a somewhat more subtle level, physicians must be aware of the forces among caregivers that foster dependency. Patients may be immobile because of the care they get. One important factor is risk aversion. Nursing personnel may be reluctant to mobilize patients for fear that they will fall and sustain injuries. We must provide assurance to staff that they will not be penalized for activating patients appropriately.

Nor is risk aversion confined to professionals. Families may be equally protective, insisting on limiting an older relative's activities or moving him or her to a more closely supervised situation. Such fears are often infused with guilt and may manifest as anger. Families can be helped to see the dangers of such restricted activity.

CLASSIFYING GERIATRIC PROBLEMS

Because diagnoses often do not tell the whole story in geriatrics, it is more helpful to think in terms of presenting problems. One aid to recalling some of the common problems of geriatrics uses a series of I's:

- Immobility
- Instability

- Incontinence
- Intellectual impairment
- Infection
- Impairment of vision and hearing
- Irritable colon
- Isolation (depression)
- Inanition (malnutrition)
- Impecunity
- Iatrogenesis
- Insomnia
- Immune deficiency
- Impotence

The list is important for several reasons. Especially with older patients, the expression of the problem may not be a good clue to the etiology. Conversely, a problem may occur for a variety of reasons.

For example, an individual may be immobilized by a broken hip, by severe angina, or by arthritis. But the patient may also be immobilized by fear. The elderly patient with a successfully repaired hip fracture may be unwilling to walk again for fear of falling and sustaining another fracture. An elderly person living in a deteriorated neighborhood may be confined to the home not by physical limitations but because of a fear of being molested. Such an individual may decide to enter a long-term-care institution to seek a safer environment. In each instance, the physician and coworkers must obtain a sufficient history to understand the true etiology of the problem if they are to develop a successful approach to remedying the condition.

Another factor in generating dependency is cost. It is often much easier and cheaper to do things *for* people with functional limitations than to invest the effort needed to encourage them to do for themselves.

Unfortunately such savings are short-ranged; they will increase the level of dependency and ultimately the amount of care needed.

Among the list of I's is iatrogenesis. The least desirable outcome of medical care is a decrease in the patient's health as a result of contact with the care system. In some cases, there is a real risk that untoward consequences of treatment may worsen a patient's health. The risk:benefit calculation as a basis for urging intervention must be performed carefully for each elderly patient in the context of the patient's condition. Many risks are within the ordinary bounds of medicine.

We are concerned here with those events that result from indifferent or superficial care. The physician who casually adds another drug to the patient's polypharmacy portfolio is playing with a living chemistry set. The reduced rate of drug metabolism and excretion in many elderly persons exacerbates the problem of drug interactions (Chap. 5). Even more dangerous is the careless, hasty application of clinical labels. The patient who becomes confused and disoriented in the hospital may not be suffering from dementia. The individual who has an occasional urinary accident is not necessarily incontinent. Labeling patients as demented or incontinent is too often the first step toward their placement in a nursing home, a setting that can make such labels self-fulfilling prophecies. We must exercise great caution in applying these potent labels. They should be reserved for patients who have been carefully evaluated, lest we unnecessarily condemn countless persons to lifetimes of institutionalization.

DIAGNOSIS VERSUS FUNCTIONAL STATUS

One of the persistent problems surrounding growing discussions about care of the elderly has arisen from the emphasis on functioning. This emphasis on the need to direct clinical attention to the patient's functional status as well as to specific medical conditions has occasionally been misinterpreted. The point is not that functional status is more important or more useful than diagnosis but that both are needed. One is incomplete without the other. Functioning is the result of the innate abilities of the patient and the environment that supports those abilities.

Clearly, the optimal management of an elderly patient involves identifying a correctable problem and correcting it. The first and principal task of the physician is to do precisely that. No amount of rehabilitation, compassionate care, or environmental manipulation will compensate for missing a remediable diagnosis. However, diagnoses alone are usually insufficient. The elderly are the repositories of chronic disease more often cared for than cured.

The process of geriatrics is thus twofold: (1) careful clinical assessment and management to identify remediable problems and (2) equally careful and competent functional assessment to ascertain how the patient's autonomy can be maximized by appropriate human and mechanical assistance and environmental manipulations.

Our goal in orienting primary care providers is to raise their consciousness about the need to consider the whole patient and the patient's environment, but never at the cost of neglecting the search for correctable causes for the patient's problems. In that search for causes, the a priori probabilities will often differ substantially from those of younger patients. For this reason, a problem-focused approach, like that of the I's, outlined above, may prove useful.

References

Bengston VL, Rice CJ, Johnson ML: Are theories of aging important? Models and explanations in gerontology at the turn of the century, in Bengston VC, Schaie KW (eds): *Handbook of Theories of Aging.* New York, Springer, 1999.

Birren JE, Schaie KW (eds): *Handbook of the Psychology of Aging,* 5th ed. San Diego, Academic Press, 2001.

Campisi J: Cancer, aging and cellular senescence. *In Vivo* 14:183–188, 2000.

Cockcroft DW, Gault MH: Prediction of creatinine clearance from serum creatinine. *Nephron* 16:31–41, 1976.

Finch CE, Tanzi RE: Genetics of aging. *Science* 278:407–411, 1997.

Finkel T, Holbrook NJ: Oxidants, oxidative stress and the biology of ageing. *Nature* 408:239–247, 2000.

Fossel M: Telomerase and the aging cell. *JAMA* 279:1732–1735, 1998.

Freedman VA, Martin LG, Schoeni RF: Recent trends in disability and functioning among older adults in the United States. *JAMA* 288:3137-3146, 2002.

Hayflick L: Cell biology of aging. *Fed Proc* 38:1847–1850, 1979.

Kirkwood TBL, Austad SN: Why do we age? *Nature* 408:233–238, 2000.

Ly DH, Lockhart DJ, Lerner RA, et al: Mitotic misregulation and human aging. *Science* 287:2486–2492, 2000.

Lakatta EG: Circulatory function in younger and older humans in health, in WR Hazzard, JP Blass, EL Bierman (eds) : *Principles of Geriatric Medicine and Gerontology* 4th ed New York, McGraw-Hill, 1999.

Lovell-Badge R: The future for stem cell research. *Nature* 414:88–91, 2001.

Masoro EJ: Caloric restriction and aging: an update. *Exp Gerontol* 35:299–305, 2000.

Masoro EJ, Austad SN (eds): *Handbook of the Biology of Aging,* 5th ed. San Diego, Academic Press, 2001.

Rowe JW, Kahn RL: Human aging: usual and successful. *Science* 237:143–149, 1987.

Tanzi RE, Kovacs DM, Kim T-W, et al: The gene defects responsible for familial Alzheimer's disease. *Neurobiol Dis* 3(16):159–168, 1996.

Vijg J, Wei JY: Understanding the biology of aging: the key to prevention and therapy. *J Am Geriatr Soc* 43:426–434, 1995.

Suggested Readings

Bengston VL, Schaie KW (eds): *Handbook of Theories of Aging.* New York, Springer, 1999.

Binstock RH, et al. (eds): *Handbook of Aging and the Social Sciences,* 5th ed. San Diego, Academic Press, 2001.

Fossel M: Cell senescence in human aging: a review of the theory. *In Vivo* 14:29–34, 2000.

Fries J: Compression of morbidity in the elderly. *Vaccine* 18:1584–1589, 2000.

Hayflick L: How and why we age. *Exp Gerontol* 33:639–653, 1998.

Holloszy JO: The biology of aging. *Mayo Clin Proc* 75(Suppl):S3–S9, 2000.

Hornsby PJ: Cellular senescence and tissue aging in vivo. *J Gerontol* 57A:B251–B256, 2002.

Jazwinski SM: Longevity, genes, and aging. *Science* 273:54–59, 1996.

Johnson FB, Sinclair DA, Guarente L: Molecular biology of aging. *Cell* 96:291–302, 1999.

Levy-Lahad E, Bird TD: Genetic factors in Alzheimer's disease: a review of recent advances. *Ann Neurol* 40:829–840, 1996.

Marcotte R, Wong E: Replicative senescence revisited. *J Gerontol* 57A:B257–B269, 2002.

Olshansky SJ, Hayflick L, Carnes BA: Position statement on human aging. *J Gerontol* 57A:B292–B297, 2002.

CHAPTER 2

THE GERIATRIC PATIENT: DEMOGRAPHY, EPIDEMIOLOGY, AND HEALTH SERVICES UTILIZATION

From the physician's perspective, the demographic curve strongly argues that medical practice in the future will include a great many geriatrics. Persons aged 65 years and older currently represent a little more than one-third of the patients seen by a primary care physician. In 40 years, we can safely predict that at least every other adult patient will be an older person (i.e., age 65 or older).

The concern so often heard about the epidemic of aging stems primarily from two factors: numbers and dollars. We hear a great deal of talk about the incipient demise of Social Security, the bankrupt status of Medicare, the death of the family, and dire predictions of demographic cataclysms. There is, indeed, cause for concern but not necessarily for alarm. The message of the numbers is straightforward: we cannot go on as we have; new approaches are needed. The shape of those approaches to meeting the needs of growing numbers of elderly persons in this society will reflect societal values. The costs associated with an aging society have already stimulated major changes in the way we provide care.

There is actually some basis for optimism. Data from the National Long-term Care Survey show a decline in the rate of disability among older people. The number of disabled persons aged 65 years and older in 1982 was 6.4 million. The projected level of disability applied to population projections called for about

9.3 million in 1999. Instead, the actual number was about 7 million. It remains to be seen if this trend toward lower disability rates can be sustained; but if so, it will greatly offset the effects of an aging population.

However, aging is not the major contributor to the rapidly escalating costs of care. Although older people use a disproportionately large amount of medical care, most of the growth in costs is traceable to tremendous expansion in medical technology, both diagnostic and therapeutic. We have potent, but often expensive, tools at our disposal. In some ways, we can be said to be reaping the fruits of our success. While a substantial number of older people live to enjoy many active years, some persons who might not have survived in earlier times are now living into old age and bringing with them the chronic disease burden that would have been avoided by death. Overall, however, the rate of disability among older persons has decreased by 1 percent or more annually for last several decades.

The press for dramatic responses to the growth in the older population and its concurrent medical costs has led in two directions. Programs like managed care have been launched to serve Medicare beneficiaries in the hopes that such approaches might constrain costs. To date, this promise has not been achieved. Managed care programs face strong disincentives to enroll sick people and thus are not motivated to create programs that might attract such a clientele. Nonetheless, the hope persists that some variant of risk-based care could create incentives for greater efficiencies if more appropriate risk-adjusted capitation rates were developed. The second strategy has promoted rationing through the back door, by emphasizing the avoidance of futile care at the end of life. The technique for implementing this objective has been the use of advance directives. Rather than overtly limiting the availability of treatment, advance directives empower patients to authorize less care. However, as discussed in Chap. 17, advance directives may not appeal to many older persons. If such directives fail to stem the tide of end-of-life care, will more draconian strategies be employed?

GROWTH IN NUMBERS

A look at a few trends will help to focus the problem. The numbers of older people in this country (and in the world) have been growing in both absolute and relative terms. The growth in numbers can be traced to two phenomena: (1) the advances in medical science that have improved survival rates from specific diseases and (2) the birth rate. The relative numbers of older persons is primarily the result of two birth rates: (1) the one that occurred 65 or more years ago and the current one. The first one provides the people, most of whom will survive to become old. The second means that the proportion of those who are old depends on how many were born subsequently. This ratio is critical in estimating the size of the work force available to support an elderly population. The looming demographic crisis is based on the forecast of a large number of older persons increasing through the first half of the next century as a result of the post–World War II baby boom. That group of people, born in the late 1940s and early 1950s, will begin to reach seniority by 2010. The relative rate of growth increases with each decade over age 75 years. Indeed, many older persons are now surviving longer. It is no longer rare to encounter a centenarian. Hallmark even makes "Happy 100th Birthday" greeting cards.

The impact of this projection can be better appreciated by looking at Table 2-1, which expresses the growth as a percentage of the total population. Although these forecasts can vary with the future birth and death rates, they are likely to be reasonably accurate. Thus, since the turn of the twentieth century, we have gone from a situation in which 4 percent of the population was 65 or older to a time when more than 12 percent has reached 65 years. By the year 2030, that older population will have almost doubled. Put another way, in 2030 there will be as many people older than 75 years as there are today who are older than 65 years. When that observation is combined with the reduction in births in the cohort behind the baby boomers, then social implications become more obvious. There will be many fewer workers to support the larger older population. This demographic observation has led to several urgent recommendations: (1) redefine retirement age to recognize the increase in life expectancy and thereby reduce the ratio of retirees to workers; (2) encourage younger persons to personally save more for their retirement to avoid excessive dependency on public funds; and (3) change public programs to accrue surpluses to meet these projected drains.

Because older people use more health care services than do younger people, there will be an even greater demand on the health care system and a concomitant rise in total health care costs. Because Medicare beneficiaries use more insti-

TABLE 2-1   THE ELDERLY POPULATION OF THE UNITED STATES: TRENDS 1900–2050

AGE (YEARS)	PERCENT OF THE TOTAL POPULATION						
	1900	1940	1960	1990	2010	2030	2050
65–74	2.9	4.8	6.1	7.3	7.4	12.0	10.5
75–84	1.0	1.7	2.6	4.0	4.3	7.1	7.2
85+	0.2	0.3	0.5	1.3	2.2	2.7	5.1
65+	4.0	6.8	9.2	12.6	13.9	21.8	22.9

Source: U.S. Senate, 1991.

tutional services (i.e., hospital and nursing home care), their health care costs are higher than those for younger groups. Only 12 percent of the population, those age 65 years and older, account for over one-third of health expenditures.

Data from the 1997 National Medical Expenditure Survey indicate that the annual per capita cost of health care for older persons was $5947, as compared with $3226 for those aged 45 to 64 years and $1666 for those aged 18 to 44 years.

The increased number of older persons has been accompanied by a number of changes in the way medical care is financed. Although these programs are discussed in more detail in Chap. 15, we note here that the appearance of programs such as Medicare and Medicaid, with all their shortcomings, has been associated with a growing expenditure on health care for older people and an increasing role in this area for public dollars. It is important to bear in mind that even in the face of greatly increased public financing, the elderly person still must bear a considerable share of the financial burden. In fact, in 1995, elderly persons' out-of-pocket costs for health care represented approximately 21 percent of their income, a figure comparable to that before the passage of Medicare.

The growing number of older persons has created great consternation among forecasters. There is a sense of doom about a future in which all resources will go to support the elderly members of our society. To counter this ageist misimpression, two facts should be borne in mind: (1) The effects of technology on medical care costs dwarf the impact of an aging population. (2) The increasing numbers of older persons will be accompanied by a decrease in the proportion of those younger than 18 years. It is important to consider the overall dependency ratio. This index compares the proportion of the population younger than 18 and older than 65 years with that of persons between the ages of 18 and 64 years (the group presumed to be working to support the rest). While the relative contribution of the older population will increase impressively, the total will never be as high as it was in the mid-1960s.

The growth in the number of aged persons results from improvements in both social living conditions and medical care. Over the course of this century, we have moved from a preponderance of acute diseases (especially infections) to an era of chronic illnesses. Today at least two-thirds of all the money spent on health care goes toward chronic disease. (For older people that proportion is closer to 95 percent.) Medical care can be criticized for continuing to practice in a mode more suited to acute illness than chronic care. Information systems have not yet arisen in common practice to channel clinicians' attention to the problems associated with chronic care.

Table 2-2 reflects the changes in the common causes of death from 1900 to the present. Many of those common at the turn of the twentieth century are no longer even listed. Today, the pattern of death in old age is generally similar to that of the population as a whole. The leading causes are basically the same, but there are some differences in the rankings. The leading causes of death are heart disease, cancer, stroke, chronic obstructive pulmonary disease (COPD), and influenza/pneumonia. Alzheimer's disease features prominently.

TABLE 2-2 CHANGES IN COMMONEST CAUSES OF DEATH, 1900–2000, ALL AGES AND THOSE 65 YEARS AND OLDER

	RATE PER 100,000					
	ALL AGES				AGE 65+	
	1900	RANK	2000	RANK	2000	RANK
Diseases of heart	13.8	4	257.9	1	1712.2	1
Malignant neoplasms	6.4	8	200.5	2	1127.4	2
Cerebrovascular diseases	10.7	5	60.3	3	421.9	3
Chronic lower respiratory diseases	4.5	9	44.9	4	310.2	4
Influenza and pneumonia	22.9	1	24.3	7	173.3	5
Diabetes mellitus	1.1		24.9	6	149.8	6
Alzheimer's disease			17.8	8	139.4	7
Senility	5.0	10				
Nephritis, nephritic syndrome, and nephrosis	8.9	6	13.7	9	90.8	8
Accidents	7.2	7	34.0	5	90.1	9
Septicemia			11.5	10	72.3	10
Tuberculosis	19.4	2				
Diarrhea and enteritis	14.3	3				

Source: Data for 1900 from Linder and Grove, 1947; 2000 data from National Vital Statistics Report, vol 49, No. 12, October 9, 2001.

Although the most dramatic reduction of mortality has occurred in infants and mothers, there has been a perceptible increase in survival even after age 65. Our stereotypes of what to expect from older people may therefore need reexamination. The average 65-year-old woman can expect to live another 19.2 years, and a 65-year-old man another 16.3 years. Even at age 85, there is an expectation of more than 5 years.

However, this gain in survival includes both active and dependent years. Indeed, one of the great controversies of modern gerontological epidemiology is whether the gain in life expectancy brings with it equivalent gains in years free of dependency. The answer lies somewhere between. Although increased survival may be associated with more disability, the overall effect has been a pattern of decreasing disability (Cutler, 2001). Moreover, not all disability is permanent. Some older people experience transient episodes.

Some analysts have used disability as the basis for defining quality of life. They have then seized on the concept of active life expectancy to create a concept of quality-adjusted life years (QALYs). Under this formulation, which is especially popular with economists who are seeking a common denominator against which to weigh all interventions, the goal of health care is to maximize individuals' periods of disability-free time. However, such a formulation immediately raises concerns about the care of all those who are already frail; they would derive no benefit from any actions on their behalf unless they could convert them to a disability-free state.

DISABILITY

The World Health Organization distinguishes between impairments, disabilities, and handicaps. A disease may create an impairment in organ function. That failure can eventually lead to a reduced ability to perform certain tasks. This inability to perform may become a handicap when those tasks are necessary to carry out social activities.

Hence, a handicap is the result of external demands and may be mitigated by environmental alterations. The distinction can provide a useful framework within which to consider the care of older persons.

There is a general pattern of increased impairment in the senses and in orthopedic problems with age. Because they tend to accumulate over time, the prevalence of chronic conditions increases with age. However, the nature of survivorship produces the occasional twist. The association between prevalence and age is not absolute. Those afflicted with diabetes and those with chronic lung disease, for example, do not survive as readily to age 85 and above. Despite having more chronic conditions and impairments, older people tend to report their health as generally good; 40 percent of those aged 65 and older rate their health as very good or excellent, and another 32 percent rate it as good. This contrast highlights the coping abilities of elderly persons discussed in Chap. 1.

Because physicians tend to see the sick, they may form a distorted picture of the senior citizens. Most older persons are indeed self-sufficient and able to function on their own or with minimal assistance.

Those who need help are likely to be the very old. Functioning can be measured in a variety of ways. Commonly, we use the ability to perform specific tasks as a reflection of independence. These are grouped into two classes of measures. The term *instrumental activities of daily living* (IADL) refers to tasks required to maintain an independent household. IADL include such tasks as using the telephone, managing money, shopping, preparing meals, doing light housework, and getting around the community. They generally demand a combination of both physical and cognitive performance. Even among those at age 85 and above, more than half the population living in the community can still perform these tasks independently.

The ability to carry out basic self-care activities is reflected in the so-called *activities of daily living* (ADL). Dependencies in terms of ADL—which include such tasks as eating, using the toilet, dressing, transferring, walking, and bathing—are less common than IADL losses. As shown in Table 2-3, even among the oldest groups, the prevalence of ADL dependency is quite low. Forty percent of females aged 85 or more living in the community needed no assistance with any IADL, and more than 60 percent needed no help with ADL. Overall, among those aged 85 or more of both sexes living in the community, 16 percent needed help with one ADL, 10 percent with two or three ADL, and 9 percent with four or more ADLs.

SOCIAL SUPPORT

An important feature in determining an older person's ability to live in the community is the extent of support available. The family is the heart of long-term

TABLE 2-3   EXTENT OF ADL AND IADL LIMITATIONS AND PERCEIVED HEALTH STATUS BY AGE GROUP

	PERCENT			
	18–44 YEARS	45–64 YEARS	65–74 YEARS	75+ YEARS
Persons experiencing limitations in ADL for which the help of another person is needed	0.5	1.1	3.4	10.7
Persons experiencing limitations in IADL for which the help of another person is needed	1.2	3.3	7.1	21.9
Perceived health status excellent/very good	73.5	68.7	42.2	33.6
Perceived health status fair/poor	5.4	14.3	23.0	31.5

Source: 1997 National Health Interview Survey.

Abbreviations: ADL = activities of daily living (bathing, eating, dressing, getting in and out of bed or chair, using the toilet, or getting around inside the house); IADL = instrumental activities of daily living (everyday household chores, doing necessary business, or shopping).

care (LTC). Family and friends provide the bulk of services in each category with, or more often without, the help of formal caregivers. Informal care is largely provided by women.

Because women are both the major givers and receivers of long-term care, a natural coalition has formed between those advocating for improved LTC and women's organizations. Even as women are entering the work force in large numbers, they continue to bear the majority of the caregiving load. Largely because they outlive men, over twice as many older women, as compared with men, live alone (Fig. 2-1), but the gap narrows by age 85. Wives and daughters are the most important source of family support for older persons.

Survey data suggest that more than 70 percent of persons aged 65 and older have surviving children. (Remember that the children of persons age 85 and older may themselves be aged 65 or older.) These "children" provide more than a third of the informal care.

The difference between needing and not needing a nursing home can depend on the availability of such support. Extrapolating from available data, we estimate that for every person older than age 65 in a nursing home, there are from one to three people equally disabled living in the community. The importance of social support must be kept continuously in mind. Formal community supports will continue to rely heavily on family and friends to see that adequate amounts of care are provided to maintain an elderly individual in the community. Efforts to reduce the burden of caregiving include encouraging respite care and providing direct assistance to the caregivers, both formal care to share the burden and pragmatic instruction about how to cope with the behavioral problems of demented patients. The physician must work diligently to maintain and bolster such support so as to avoid nursing home placement.

USE OF SERVICES

In general, the use of health care services increases with age. Table 2-4 and Fig. 2-2 summarize some of these differences. The exception to the pattern of age-related increase is seen with dental care; it is not clear whether this reflects the lack of coverage under Medicare or a loss of teeth, but probably is at least greatly influenced by the former. Older people are more likely to see physicians because of chronic problems.

The introduction of the new prospective payment system (PPS) for hospitals under Medicare in 1984, was associated with shorter lengths of stay and decreased admission rates. Table 2-5 shows the most common discharge diagnoses and surgical procedures in 1999. Heart disease, cancer, stroke and pneumonia continue to dominate the scene. The growth of technology can be seen in the frequent use of procedures, especially catheterization and endoscopy.

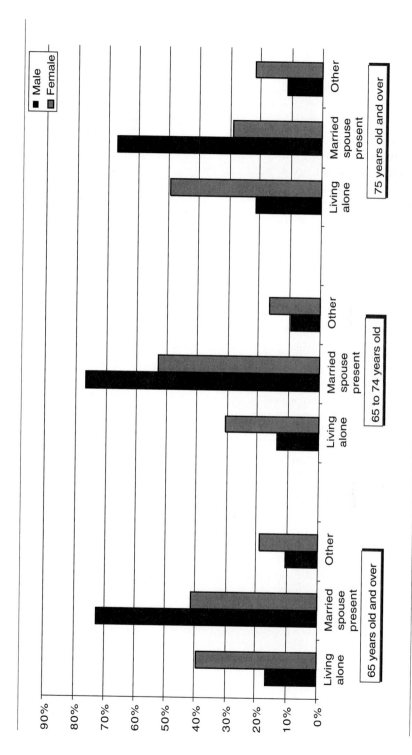

— FIGURE 2-1 — *Living arrangements of older adults.* (Source: US Census Bureau data March 2000.)

TABLE 2-4   USE OF MEDICAL SERVICES BY AGE GROUP

	PERCENT		
	18–44 YEARS	45–64 YEARS	65+ YEARS
Hospitalization	7	8	18
Ambulatory care	69	79	90
Home care	1	3	14 (65–74) 48 (75+)
Prescription medicine	58	72	87
Dental care	41	49	41

Source: 1996 Medical Expenditure Panel Survey; 1997 National Health Interview Survey.

The introduction of PPS greatly spurred the use of postacute care. Patients discharged earlier from hospitals often needed someplace to recuperate. As a result, Medicare began paying twice for hospital care. It paid a fixed amount for shorter stays and then often paid again for the posthospital care. Indeed, postacute care has been the fastest growing segment of Medicare. In reaction, the 1997 Balanced Budget Act imposed separate prospective payment methods on each of the predominate modes of postacute care (home health care, skilled nursing facilities, and inpatient rehabilitation). Table 2-6 shows the effects of the 1997 Balanced Budget Act on postacute care use for several conditions commonly associated with postacute care. For those often requiring active rehabilitation, the overall effects were minimal although there was shift away from home health care use, but for the more medical conditions there was a decrease in postacute care use, especially in home health care.

Table 2-7 describes the patterns for ambulatory visits at various ages. Despite the general principle that bad things are more common with increasing age after age 75, not all diagnoses increase with age.

NURSING HOME USE

The nursing home has traditionally been used as the touchstone for long-term care, but its role has changed with the changes in hospital payment under Medicare. The fixed-payment approach and the consequent shortening of hospital stays have spawned a new industry of posthospital care, sometimes called subacute care. In effect, care that was formerly rendered in a hospital is now

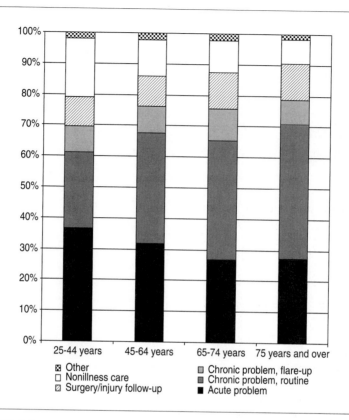

— FIGURE 2-2 — *Distribution of office visits by age group.* (Source: 1999 National Ambulatory Medical Care Survey.)

provided in other settings, including the nursing home and the home of the patient.

Some nursing homes have sought to increase their capacity to support such care by upgrading their nursing staffs, but others have adopted the new title without changing their modus operandi. Thus, the distinction between long-stay and short-stay nursing home residents has become more exaggerated. Some residents are there for chronic care, whereas others are just visiting for a brief spell of recuperation and rehabilitation.

While nursing homes have increased their Medicare business dramatically, their long-stay business has been threatened by a growing disinclination to use such facilities. New forms of care, like assisted living, have provided other options, especially for those who can pay for such care.

We are prone to cite a figure of 5 percent for the proportion of those aged 65 years and older who are in nursing homes at any moment. Such a figure is a

TABLE 2-5   HOSPITAL DISCHARGE DIAGNOSES AND PROCEDURES FOR
PERSONS AGE 65 YEARS AND OLDER

Diagnoses	Rate per 10,000 Population
Pneumonia	236.5
Congestive heart failure	221.1
Malignant neoplasms	212.8
Cerebrovascular disease	205.5
Coronary atherosclerosis	189.2
Acute myocardial infarction	148.6
Cardiac dysrhythmias	143.5
Chronic bronchitis	107.8
Osteoarthritis	88.6
Fracture, neck of femur	85.2
Volume depletion	72.2
Psychoses	62.0
Diabetes mellitus	58.0

Procedures	
Arteriography and angiography using contrast material	1006
Cardiac catheterization	618
Endoscopy of small intestine	552
Diagnostic ultrasound	551
Respiratory therapy	509
Removal of coronary artery obstruction and insertion of stent	504
Computerized axial tomography	453
Endoscopy of large intestine	357
Coronary artery bypass graft	322
Insertion, removal, replacement, or revision of pacemaker	285
Insertion of endotracheal tube	244
Hemodialysis	226
Open reduction of fracture with internal fixation	203
Total knee replacement	182
Cholecystectomy	158
Partial excision of large intestine	146
Prostatectomy	140
Bronchoscopy	138
Débridement of wound, infection, or burn	121
Total hip replacement	102
Cystoscopy	100

Source: 1999 National Hospital Discharge Survey.

TABLE 2-6 POSTACUTE CARE USED WITHIN 30 DAYS, 1996 AND 2000

	ANY PAC	SNF	REH	HHA	COMBINATION
Stroke, DRG 14					
1996	70%	37%	16%	33 %	16%
2000	66%	37%	18%	26.7%	16%
Hip procedure, DRG 209					
1996	86%	43%	20%	57%	34%
2000	85%	43%	25%	51%	33%
Hip fracture, DRG 210 and 211					
1996	89%	68%	14%	33%	26%
2000	89%	70%	16%	29%	25%
COPD, DRG 88					
1996	42%	12%	NA	33%	4%
2000	36%	15%	NA	24%	5%
Pneumonia, DRG 89 and 90					
1996	46%	21%	NA	29%	5%
2000	42%	24%	NA	22%	5%
CHF, DRG 127					
1996	50%	15%	NA	39%	5%
2000	44%	18%	NA	29%	6%

Abbreviations: DRG = diagnosis-related group; HHA = home health agency; NA = not applicable; PAC = postacute care; REH = inpatient rehabilitation unit; SNF = skilled nursing facility.

TABLE 2-7   PERCENT OF OFFICE VISITS BY SELECTED MEDICAL
CONDITIONS, 1996

	45–64 YEARS	65–74 YEARS	75+ YEARS
Arthritis	11.9	23.6	33.4
Atherosclerosis	3.4	9.9	15.1
Chronic obstructive pulmonary disease	3.4	7.5	8.5
Depression	8.9	5.2	5.2
Diabetes	9.8	13.9	11.6
Hypertension	24.5	35.9	36.9
Obesity	11.4	7.3	4.7

Source: From Woodwell DA: *National Ambulatory Medical Cen. Survey: 1996 Summary. Advance Data from Vital and Health Statistics* (295). Hyattsville, MD, National Center for Health Stattistics, 1997.

potentially misleading generalization in two respects. As Fig. 2-3 suggests, age is a very important factor. Among those age 65 to 74 years old, the rate is less than 2 percent. It rises to approximately 7 percent for those age 75 to 84, and then jumps to 20 percent for those age 85 and older. Moreover, what were formerly considered permanent stays have increasingly become transient visits. Thus, it is important to distinguish between these prevalence rates and the lifetime probability of entering a nursing home. Longitudinal studies suggest that persons age 65 have better than a 40 percent chance of spending some time in a nursing home before they die. Of those who enter a nursing home, 55 percent will spend at least 1 year there and 21 percent will spend 5 years or more (Kemper and Murtaugh, 1991). The proportion of persons spending at least some time in a nursing home is likely to increase if nursing homes continue to play a role in subacute care.

Nursing homes are needed not only because of the presence of diseases or even functional disabilities, but also as a result of a lack of social support. Often the family becomes exhausted after caring for an elderly patient for a long period. Family fatigue is especially a problem when the patient has symptoms that are very disruptive.

Among the most disturbing are incontinence and behavior problems that involve wandering or disruptive behavior. Table 2-8 summarizes the factors associated with increased likelihood of nursing home placement.

Approximately three-fourths of nursing home admissions come from hospitals. A 3-day hospital stay is a prerequisite for nursing home coverage available

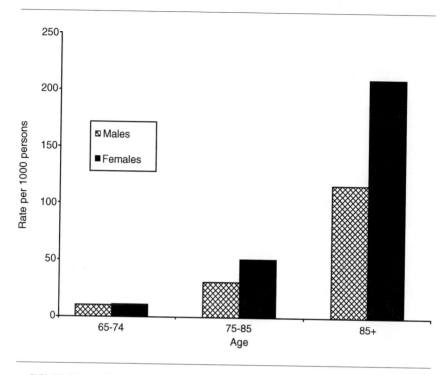

— FIGURE 2-3 — *Nursing Home Utilization, 1999.* (Source: National Center for Health Statistics. Hyattsville, MD, 2002.)

under Medicare (unless the patient is covered under a managed care plan). The hospitalization often represents the last step in a series of steps involving the deterioration of the patient and the patient's social supports. For others, the hospitalization results from an acute event, for example, a broken hip or a stroke, which then necessitates long-term care.

In 1997, almost 15 percent of hospital patients aged 65 and older were discharged to nursing homes. As with those from the community, the rate of nursing home placement increases with age and is greater for females than for males. Table 2-7 summarizes some of the factors that can identify those older patients in hospitals at risk of nursing home placement. The most significant single factor predicting discharge to a nursing home is being admitted from one. Effectively all of the nursing home residents who survive their hospital stay will be returned to a nursing home. For those patients originating from the community, the most important factors are associated with dependency and cognitive status. Compared with those going home or to a rehabilitation unit, nursing home admissions are likely to have worse functional status and more confusion (Kane et al., 1996).

TABLE 2-8   FACTORS AFFECTING THE NEED FOR NURSING HOME ADMISSION

Characteristics of the individual
  Age, sex, race
  Marital status
  Living arrangements
  Degree of mobility
  Activities of daily living
  Instrumental activities of daily living
  Clinical prognosis
  Level of function prior to hospitalization
  Urinary continence
  Behavior problems
  Mental status/memory impairment
  Mood disturbance
  Ability to distinguish both sides of body
  Vertigo and falls
  Ability to manage medication
  Income
  Payment eligibility
  Need for special services
Characteristics of the support system
  Family capability
    For married respondents, age of spouse
    Presence of responsible relative (usually adult child)
    Family structure of responsible relative
    Employment status of responsible relative
  Physician availability
  Amount of care currently received from family and others
Community resources
  Formal community resources
  Informal support systems
  Presence of long-term-care institutions
  Characteristics of long-term-care institutions

Models have been developed to predict the time to nursing home admission for persons with Alzheimer's disease (Stern et al., 1997).

Especially now that nursing home care includes both subacute and long-term care, any analysis of nursing home residents must carefully distinguish between data based on a study of those who reside in a facility at a given time and those entering or leaving the facility. The conclusions reached about the nursing home population may be quite different depending on which groups are examined.

Short-stay and long-stay residents have distinct characteristics. The former tend to be younger, have more physical problems, and enter from the hospital. The long-term residents are more likely to be older, confused, and incontinent.

Nursing home data can be very confusing. Not only must one distinguish between admissions and residents but one must also look at the time course of former residents to appreciate the true nature of such long-term care. On the one hand, the picture is much more dynamic than is usually suspected. The majority of persons admitted to a nursing home are discharged within 3 months. On the other hand, many of these people die in the nursing home, and many of the discharges are really transfers to hospitals. From there a majority of patients either return to the nursing home or die in a hospital. It is more accurate to talk about long-term care "careers" than to think in terms of discrete episodes.

As we enter an era of more aged persons with chronic disease, physicians will find themselves working increasingly in institutions such as nursing homes. They will be challenged to provide leadership in upgrading the care available in such settings. They will need to be familiar with the array of resources available to meet the needs of their patients and the factors determining access to these resources. A guide to long-term-care resources is presented in Chap. 15.

References

Cutler DM: Declining disability among the elderly. *Health Aff (Millwood)* 20(6):11–27, 2001.

Kane RL, Finch M, Blewett L, et al: Use of post-hospital care by Medicare patients. *J Am Geriatr Soc* 44:242–250, 1996.

Kemper P, Murtaugh CM: Lifetime use of nursing home care. *N Engl J Med* 324:595–600, 1991.

Linder FE, Grove RD: Vital Statistics Rates in the United States 1900–1940. Washington, DC. *US Government Printing Office*, 1947.

Stern Y, Tang MX, Albert MS, et al: Predicting time to nursing home care and death in individuals with Alzheimer disease. *JAMA* 277(10):806–812, 1997.

Suggested Readings

Fries JF: Aging, natural death, and the compression of morbidity. *N Engl J Med* 303:130–136, 1980.

Gill TM, Williams CS, Tinetti ME: Assessing the risk for the onset of functional dependence among older adults: the role of physical performance. *J Am Geriatr Soc* 43:603–609, 1995.

Moon M: What Medicare has meant to older Americans. *Health Care Fin Rev* 18(2):49–59, 1996.

Vita AJ, Terry RB, Hubert HB, et al: Aging, health risks, and cumulative disability. *N Engl J Med* 338:1035–1041, 1998.

CHAPTER 3

EVALUATING THE GERIATRIC PATIENT

Comprehensive evaluation of an older individual's health status is one of the most challenging aspects of clinical geriatrics. It requires a sensitivity to the concerns of people, an awareness of the many unique aspects of their medical problems, an ability to interact effectively with a variety of health professionals, and often a great deal of patience. Most importantly, it requires a perspective different from that used in the evaluation of younger individuals. Not only are the a priori probabilities of diagnoses different, but one must be attuned to more subtle findings. Progress may be measured on a finer scale. Special tools are needed to ascertain relatively small improvements in chronic conditions and overall function compared with the more dramatic cures of acute illnesses often possible in younger patients. Creativity is essential in order to incorporate these tools efficiently in a busy clinical practice.

The purposes of the evaluation and the setting in which it takes place will determine its focus and extent. Considerations important in admitting a geriatric patient with a fractured hip and pneumonia to an acute care hospital during the middle of the night are obviously different from those in the evaluation of an older demented patient exhibiting disruptive behavior in a nursing home. Elements included in screening for treatable conditions in an ambulatory clinic are different from those in assessment of older individuals in their own homes or in long-term-care facilities.

Despite the differences dictated by the purpose and setting of the evaluation, several essential aspects of evaluating older patients are common to all purposes and settings. Figure 3-1 depicts these aspects. Several comments on addressing them are in order:

1. Physical, psychological, and socioeconomic factors interact in complex ways to influence the health and functional status of the geriatric population.
2. Comprehensive evaluation of an older individual's health status requires an assessment of each of these domains. The coordinated efforts of several

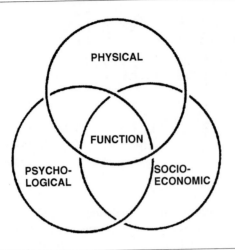

– FIGURE 3-1 – *Components of assessment of older patients.*

different health care professionals functioning as an interdisciplinary team are needed.

3. Functional abilities should be a central focus of the comprehensive evaluation of geriatric patients. Other more traditional measures of health status (such as diagnoses and physical and laboratory findings) are useful in dealing with underlying etiologies and detecting treatable conditions, but in the geriatric population, measures of function are often essential in determining overall health, well being, and the need for health and social services.

Just as function is the common language of geriatrics, assessment lies at the heart of its practice. Special techniques that address multiple problems and their functional consequences offer a way to structure the approach to complicated geriatric patients. Geriatric assessment has been tested in a variety of forms. Table 3-1 summarizes the findings from a number of randomized, controlled trials of different approaches to geriatric assessment (Rubenstein, 1991). A randomized trial of annual in-home comprehensive geriatric assessment demonstrated the potential to delay the development of disability and reduce permanent nursing home stays (Stuck et al., 1995; Bula et al., 1999). More recent controlled trials of approaches to hospitalized geriatric patients suggest comprehensive geriatric assessment by a consultation team with limited follow-up does not improve health or survival of selected geriatric patients (Reuben et al., 1995), but that a special acute geriatric unit can improve function and reduce discharges to institutional care (Landefeld et al., 1995). A controlled multisite VA trial of inpatient geriatric evaluation and management demonstrated significant reductions in func-

TABLE 3-1   EXAMPLES OF RANDOMIZED CONTROLLED TRIALS OF GERIATRIC ASSESSMENT

SETTING	EXAMPLES OF ASSESSMENT STRATEGIES	SELECTED OUTCOMES*
Community/outpatients	Social worker assessment and referral Nursing assessment and referral Annual in-home assessment by nurse practitioner Multidisciplinary clinic assessment	Reduced mortality Reduced hospital use Reduced permanent nursing home use Delayed development of disability
Hospital inpatient (specialized units)	Interdisciplinary teams with focus on function, geriatric syndromes, rehabilitation	Reduced mortality Improved function Reduced acute hospital and nursing home use
Hospital inpatient consultation	Geriatric consultation teams	Mixed results Some studies improved function and lower short-term mortality Other studies show no effects

* Not all studies show improvements in all outcomes. See text and Rubenstein et al., 1991.

tional decline without increased costs (Cohen et al., 2002). Results of outpatient geriatric assessment have been mixed and less compelling (Cohen et al., 2002). However, a randomized trial of outpatient geriatric assessment with an intervention to improve adherence to the recommendations prevented functional decline (Reuben et al., 1999).

There is considerable variation in approaches to the comprehensive assessment of geriatric patients. Various screening and targeting strategies have been used to identify appropriate patients for more comprehensive assessment. These strategies range from selection based on age to targeting patients with a certain number of impairments or specific conditions. Sites of assessment vary as well, and include the clinic, the home, the hospital, and different levels of long-term care. Geriatric assessment also varies in terms of which discipline carries out the different components of the assessment as well as in the specific assessment tools used. Despite the dramatic variation in approach to targeting, personnel used, and measures employed, a clear pattern of effectiveness has emerged. Taken together, these results are both heartening and cautioning. Systematic approaches to patient care are obviously desirable. The issue is more how formalized these assessments should be. Research data suggest that the specifics of the assessment process seem to be less important than the very act of systematically approaching older people with the belief that improvement is possible.

Because of the multidimensional nature of geriatric patients' problems and the frequent presence of multiple interacting medical conditions, comprehensive evaluation of the geriatric patient can be time-consuming and thus costly. Strategies that can make the evaluation process more efficient include the following:

1. The development of a closely-knit interdisciplinary team with minimal redundancy in the assessments performed.
2. Use of carefully designed questionnaires that reliable patients and/or caregivers can complete before an appointment.
3. Incorporation of screening tools that target the need for further, more in-depth assessment.
4. Use of assessment forms that can be readily incorporated into a computerized relational data base.
5. Integration of the evaluation process with case management activities that target services based on the results of the assessment.

This chapter focuses on the general aspects of assessing geriatric patients. Sections on geriatric consultation, preoperative evaluation, and environmental assessments are included at the end of the chapter.

Chapter 15 includes information on case management and other health services, and Chap. 16 is devoted to the assessment and management of geriatric patients in the nursing home setting.

THE HISTORY

Sir William Osler's aphorism, "Listen to the patient, he'll give you the diagnosis," is as true in older patients as it is in younger patients. In the geriatric population, however, several factors make taking histories more challenging, difficult, and time-consuming.

Table 3-2 lists difficulties commonly encountered in taking histories from geriatric patients, the factors involved, and some suggestions for overcoming these difficulties. Impaired hearing and vision (despite corrective devices) are common and can interfere with effective communication.

TABLE 3-2   POTENTIAL DIFFICULTIES IN TAKING GERIATRIC HISTORIES

DIFFICULTY	FACTORS INVOLVED	SUGGESTIONS

Communication	Diminished vision
	Diminshed hearing
		Use well-lit room
		Eliminate extraneous noise
		Speak slowly in a deep tone
		Face patient, allowing
		  patient to see your lips
		Use simple amplification
		  device for severely
		  hearing impaired
		If necessary, write
		  questions in large print

	Slowed psychomotor performance	Leave enough time for the patient to answer

Underreporting of
symptoms
	Health beliefs
	Fear
	Depression
	Altered physical and
	  physiological responses
	  to disease process
	Cognitive impairment
		Ask specific questions
		  about potentially
		  important symptoms (see
		  Table 3-3)
		Use other sources of
		  information (relatives,
		  friends, other caregivers)
		  to complete the history

Vague or non-
specific symptoms
	Altered physical and
	  physiological responses
	  to disease process
	Altered presentation of
	  specifc diseases
	Cognitive impairment
		Evaluate for treatable
		  diseases,even if the
		  symptoms (or signs) are
		  not typical or specific
		  when there has been a
		  rapid change in function
		Use other sources of
		  information to complete
		  history

TABLE 3-2 POTENTIAL DIFFICULTIES IN TAKING GERIATRIC HISTORIES (*Continued*)

DIFFICULTY	FACTORS INVOLVED	SUGGESTIONS
Multiple complaints	Prevalence of multiple coexisting diseases Somatization of emotions— "masked depression" (see Chap. 5)	Attend to all somatic symptoms, ruling out treatable conditions Get to know the patient's complaints; pay special attention to new or changing symptoms Interview the patient on several occasions to complete the history

Techniques such as eliminating extraneous noises, speaking slowly and in deep tones while facing the patient, and providing adequate lighting can be helpful. The use of simple, inexpensive amplification devices with "Walkman"-style earphones can be especially effective, even among the severely hearing impaired. Patience is truly a virtue in obtaining a history; because thought and verbal processes are often slower in older than in younger individuals, patients should be allowed adequate time to answer in order not to miss potentially important information.

Many older individuals underreport potentially important symptoms because of their cultural and educational backgrounds as well as their expectations of illness as a normal concomitant of aging. Fear of illness and disability or depression accompanied by a lack of self-concern may also render the reporting of symptoms less frequent. Altered physical and physiologic responses to disease processes (see Chap. 1) can result in the absence of symptoms (such as painless myocardial infarction or ulcer and pneumonia without cough). Symptoms of many diseases can be vague and nonspecific because of these age-related changes. Impairments of memory and other cognitive functions can result in an imprecise or inadequate history and compound these difficulties. Asking specifically about potentially important symptoms (such as those listed in Table 3-3) and using other sources of information (such as relatives, friends, and other caregivers) can be very helpful in collecting more precise and useful information in these situations.

At the other end of the spectrum, geriatric patients with multiple complaints can frustrate the health care professional who is trying to sort them all out. The

TABLE 3-3 IMPORTANT ASPECTS OF THE GERIATRIC HISTORY

SOCIAL HISTORY

Living arrangements
Relationships with family and friends
Expectations of family or other caregivers
Economic status
Abilities to perform activities of daily living (see Table 3-8)
Social activities and hobbies
Mode of transportation
Advance directives (see Chap. 17)

PAST MEDICAL HISTORY

Previous surgical procedures
Major illnesses and hospitalizations
Previous transfusions

Immunization status
    Influenza, pneumococcal, tetanus

Preventive health measures
    Mammography
    Papanicolaou (Pap) smear
    Flexible sigmoidoscopy
    Antimicrobial prophylaxis
    Estrogen replacement

Tuberculosis history and testing

Medications (use the "brown bag" technique; see text)
    Previous allergies
    Knowledge of current medication regimen
    Compliance

Perceived beneficial or adverse drug effects

SYSTEMS REVIEW

Ask questions about general symptoms that may indicate treatable underlying disease such as fatigue, anorexia, weight loss, insomnia, recent change in functional status

TABLE 3-3   IMPORTANT ASPECTS OF THE GERIATRIC HISTORY
(*Continued*)

SYSTEMS REVIEW

Attempt to elicit key symptoms in each organ system, including the following:

SYSTEM	KEY SYMPTOMS
Respiratory	Increasing dyspnea Persistent cough
Cardiovascular	Orthopnea Edema Angina Claudication Palpitations Dizziness Syncope
Gastrointestinal	Difficulty chewing Dysphagia Abdomnal pain Change in bowel habit
Genitourinary	Frequency Urgency Nocturia Hesitancy, intermittent stream, straining to void Incontinence Hematuria Vaginal bleeding
Musculoskeletal	Focal or diffuse pain Focal or diffuse weakness
Neurological	Visual disturbances (transient or progressive) Progressive hearing loss Unsteadiness and/or falls Transient focal symptoms
Psychological	Depression Anxiety and/or agitation Paranoia Forgetfulness and/or confusion

multiplicity of complaints can relate to the prevalence of coexisting chronic and acute conditions in many geriatric patients. These complaints may, however, be deceiving. Somatic symptoms may be manifestations of underlying emotional distress rather than symptoms of a physical illness, and symptoms of physical conditions may be exaggerated by emotional distress (see Chap. 7). Getting to know patients and their complaints and paying particular attention to new or changing symptoms are helpful in detecting potentially treatable conditions.

Table 3-3 lists aspects of the history that are especially important in geriatric patients. It is often not feasible to gather all information in one session; shorter interviews in a few separate sessions may prove more effective in gathering these data from some geriatric patients.

Often shortchanged in medical evaluations, the social history is a critical component. Understanding the patient's socioeconomic environment and ability to function within it is crucial in determining the potential impact of an illness on an individual's overall health and need for health services. Especially important is the assessment of the family's feelings and expectations. Many family caregivers of frail geriatric patients have feelings of both anger (at having to care for a dependent family member) and guilt (over not being able or willing to do enough), and have unrealistic expectations. Such unrealistic expectations are often based on a lack of information and can interfere with care if not discussed. Unlike younger patients, older patients often have had multiple prior illnesses. The past medical history is, therefore, important in putting the patient's current problems in perspective; this can also be diagnostically important. For example, vomiting in an elderly patient who has had previous intraabdominal surgery should raise the suspicion of intestinal obstruction from adhesions; nonspecific constitutional symptoms (such as fatigue, anorexia, and weight loss) in a patient with a history of depression should prompt consideration of a relapse. Because older individuals are often treated with multiple medications, they are at increased risk of noncompliance and adverse effects (see Chap. 14). A detailed medication history (including both prescribed and over-the-counter drugs) is essential.

The "brown bag" technique is very helpful in this regard; have the patient or caregiver empty the patient's medicine cabinet into a brown paper bag and bring it at each visit. More often than not, one or more of these medications can, at least in theory, contribute to geriatric patient's symptoms.

A complete systems review, focusing on potentially important and prevalent symptoms in the elderly, can help overcome many of the difficulties described above. Although not intended to be all-inclusive, Table 3-3 lists several of these symptoms.

General symptoms can be especially difficult to interpret. Fatigue can result from a number of common conditions such as depression, congestive heart failure, anemia, and hypothyroidism. Anorexia and weight loss can be symptoms of an underlying malignancy, depression, or poorly fitting dentures and diminished taste sensation. Age-related changes in sleep patterns, anxiety, gastroesophageal reflux, congestive heart failure with orthopnea, or nocturia can underlie complaints of insomnia. Because many frail geriatric patients limit their activity, some important symptoms may be missed. For example, such patients may deny angina and dyspnea but restrict their activity to avoid the symptoms. Questions such as "How far do you walk in a typical day?" and "What is the most activity you carry out in a typical day?" can be helpful in patients suspected of limiting their activities to avoid certain symptoms.

THE PHYSICAL EXAMINATION

The common occurrence of multiple pathologic physical findings superimposed on age-related physical changes complicates interpretation of the physical examination. Table 3-4 lists common physical findings and their potential significance in the geriatric population.

TABLE 3-4   COMMON PHYSICAL FINDINGS AND THEIR POTENTIAL
              SIGNIFICANCE IN GERIATRICS

PHYSICAL FINDINGS	POTENTIAL SIGNIFICANCE
VITAL SIGNS	
Elevated blood pressure	Increased risk for cardiovascular morbidity; therapy should be considered if repeated measurements are high (see Chap. 11)
Postural changes in blood pressure	May be asymptomatic and occur in the absence of volume depletion
	Aging changes, deconditioning, and drugs may play a role
	Can be exaggerated after meals
	Can be worsened and become symptomatic with antihypertensive, vasodilator, and tricyclic antidepressant therapy
Irregular pulse	Arrhythmias are relatively common in otherwise asymptomatic elderly; seldom need specific evaluation or treatment (see Chap. 11)

TABLE 3-4   COMMON PHYSICAL FINDINGS AND THEIR POTENTIAL
SIGNIFICANCE IN GERIATRICS (*Continued*)

PHYSICAL FINDINGS	POTENTIAL SIGNIFICANCE
VITAL SIGNS	
Tachypnea	Baseline rate should be accurately recorded to help assess future complaints (such as dyspnea) or conditions (such as pneumonia or heart failure)
Weight changes	Weight gain should prompt search for edema or ascites Gradual loss of small amounts of weight common; losses in excess of 5% of usual body weight over 12 months or less should prompt search of underlying disease
GENERAL APPEARANCE AND BEHAVIOR	
Poor personal grooming and hygiene (e.g., poorly shaven, unkempt hair, soiled clothing)	Can be signs of poor overall function, caregiver neglect, and/or depression; often indicates a need for intervention
Slow thought processes and speech	Usually represents an aging change; Parkinson's disease and depression can also cause these signs
Ulcerations	Lower extremity vascular and neuropathic ulcers common Pressure ulcers common and easily overlooked in immobile patients
Diminished turgor	Often results from atrophy of subcutaneous tissues rather than volume depletion; when dehydration suspected, skin turgor over chest and abdomen most reliable

TABLE 3-4   COMMON PHYSICAL FINDINGS AND THEIR POTENTIAL SIGNIFICANCE IN GERIATRICS (*Continued*)

PHYSICAL FINDINGS	POTENTIAL SIGNIFICANCE
EARS (SEE CHAP. 13)	
Diminished hearing	High-frequency hearing loss common; patients with difficulty hearing normal conversation or a whispered phrase next to the ear should be evaluated further Portable audioscopes can be helpful in screening for impairment
EYES (SEE CHAP. 13)	
Decreased visual acuity (often despite corrective lenses)	May have multiple causes, all patients should have thorough optometric or ophthalmologic examination Hemianopsia is easily overlooked and can usually be ruled out by simple confrontation testing
Cataracts and other abnormalities	Fundoscopic examination often difficult and limited; if retinal pathology suspected, thorough ophthalmologic examination necessary
MOUTH	
Missing teeth	Dentures often present; they should be removed to check for evidence of poor fit and other pathology in oral cavity Area under the tongue is a common site for early malignancies
SKIN	
Multiple lesions	Actinic keratoses and basal cell carcinomas common; most other lesions benign

TABLE 3-4   COMMON PHYSICAL FINDINGS AND THEIR POTENTIAL SIGNIFICANCE IN GERIATRICS (*Continued*)

PHYSICAL FINDINGS	POTENTIAL SIGNIFICANCE
CHEST	
Abnormal lung sounds	Crackles can be heard in the absence of pulmonary disease and heart failure; often indicate atelectasis
CARDIOVASCULAR (SEE CHAP. 11)	
Irregular rhythms	See vital signs, above
Systolic murmurs	Common and most often benign; clinical history and bedside maneuvers can help to differentiate those needing further evaluation Carotid bruits may need further evaluation
Vascular bruits	Femoral bruits often present in patients with symptomatic peripheral vascular disease
Diminished distal pulses	Presence or absence should be recorded as this information may be diagnostically useful at a later time (e.g., if symptoms of claudication or an embolism develop)
ABDOMEN	
Prominent aortic pulsation	Suspected abdominal aneurysms should be evaluated by ultrasound
GENITOURINARY (SEE CHAP. 8)	
Atrophy	Testicular atrophy normal; atrophic vaginal tissue may cause symptoms (such as dyspareunia and dysuria) and treatment may be beneficial

TABLE 3-4   COMMON PHYSICAL FINDINGS AND THEIR POTENTIAL
SIGNIFICANCE IN GERIATRICS (*Continued*)

PHYSICAL FINDINGS	POTENTIAL SIGNIFICANCE
GENITOURINARY (SEE CHAP. 8)	
Pelvic prolapse (cystocele, rectocele)	Common and may be unrelated to symptoms; gynecologic evaluation helpful if patient has bothersome, potentially related symptoms
EXTREMITIES	
Periarticular pain	Can result from a variety of causes and is not always the result of degenerative joint disease; each area of pain should be carefully evaluated and treated (see Chap. 10)
Limited range of motion	Often caused by pain resulting from active inflammation, scarring from old injury, or neurologic disease; if limitations impair function, a rehabilitation therapist could be consulted
Edema	Can result from venous insufficiency and/or heart failure; mild edema often a cosmetic problem; treatment necessary if impairing ambulation, contributing to nocturia, predisposing to skin breakdown, or causing discomfort Unilateral edema should prompt search for a proximal obstructive process
NEUROLOGIC	
Abnormal mental status (i.e., confusion, depressed affect)	See Chaps. 6 and 7
Weakness	Arm drift may be the only sign of residual weakness from a stroke Proximal muscle weakness (e.g., inability to get out of chair) should be further evaluated; physical therapy may be appropriate

An awareness of age-related physical changes is important to the interpretation of many physical findings and therefore subsequent decision making. For example, age-related changes in the skin and postural reflexes can influence the evaluation of hydration and volume status; age-related changes in the lung and lower-extremity edema secondary to venous insufficiency can complicate the evaluation of symptoms of heart failure.

Certain aspects of the physical examination are of particular importance in the geriatric population. Detection and further evaluation of impairments of vision and hearing can lead to improvements in quality of life. Evaluation of gait may uncover correctable causes of unsteadiness and thereby prevent potentially devastating falls (see Chap. 9). Careful palpation of the abdomen may reveal an aortic aneurysm, which, if large enough, might warrant consideration of surgical removal. The mental status examination is especially important; this aspect of the physical examination is discussed further below and in Chap. 6.

LABORATORY ASSESSMENT

Abnormal laboratory findings are often attributed to "old age." While it is true that abnormal findings are common in geriatric patients, few are true aging changes. Misinterpretation of an abnormal laboratory value as an aging change may result in underdiagnosis and undertreatment of conditions such as anemia.

Table 3-5 lists those laboratory parameters unchanged in the elderly and those commonly abnormal. Abnormalities in the former group should prompt further evaluation; abnormalities in the latter group should be interpreted carefully. Table 3-5 also notes important considerations in interpreting commonly abnormal laboratory values.

FUNCTIONAL ASSESSMENT

General Concepts

Ability to function should be a central focus of the evaluation of geriatric patients (see Fig. 3-1). Medical history, physical examination, and laboratory findings are all of obvious importance in diagnosing and managing acute and chronic medical conditions in older people, as they are in all age groups. But once the dust settles, functional abilities are just as, if not more, important to the overall health, well being, and potential need for services of older individuals. For example, in a patient with hemiparesis, the nature, location, and extent of the lesion may be important in the management, but whether the patient is continent and can climb the steps to an apartment makes the difference between going home to live or going to a nursing home.

TABLE 3-5   LABORATORY ASSESSMENT OF GERIATRIC PATIENTS

LABORATORY PARAMETERS UNCHANGED*

Hemoglobin and hematocrit

White blood cell count

Platelet count

Electrolytes (sodium, potassium, chloride, bicarbonate)

Blood urea nitrogen

Liver function tests (transaminases, bilirubin, prothrombin time)

Free thyroxine index

Thyroid-stimulating hormone

Calcium

Phosphorus

COMMON ABNORMAL LABORATORY PARAMETERS†

PARAMETER	CLINICAL SIGNIFICANCE
Sedimentation rate	Mild elevations (10–20 mm) may be an age-related change.
Glucose	Glucose tolerance decreases (see Chap. 12); elevations during acute illness are common.
Creatinine	Because lean body mass and daily endogenous creatinine production decline, high-normal and minimally elevated values may indicate substantially reduced renal function.
Albumin	Average values decline (<0.5 g/mL) with age, especially in acutely ill, but generally indicate undernutrition.
Alkaline phosphatase	Mild asymptomatic elevations common; liver and Paget's disease should be considered if moderately elevated.
Serum iron, iron-binding capacity, ferritin	Decreased values are not an aging change and usually indicate undernutrition and/or gastrointestinal blood loss.

TABLE 3-5 LABORATORY ASSESSMENT OF GERIATRIC PATIENTS
(*Continued*)

COMMON ABNORMAL LABORATORY PARAMETERS†	
PARAMETER	CLINICAL SIGNIFICANCE
Prostate-specific antigen	May be elevated in patients with benign prostatic hyerplasia. Marked elevation or increasing values when followed over time should prompt consideration of further evaluation in patients for whom specific therapy for prostate cancer would be undertaken if cancer were diagnosed.
Urinalysis	Asymptomatic pyuria and bacteriuria are common and rarely warrant treatment; hematuria is abnormal and needs further evaluation (see Chap. 8).
Chest radiographs	Interstitial changes are a common age-related finding; diffusely diminished bone density generally indicates advanced osteoporosis (see Chap. 12).
Electrocardiogram	ST-segment and T-wave changes, atrial and ventricular arrhythmias, and various blocks are common in asymptomatic elderly and may not need specific evaluation or treatment (see Chap. 11).

*Aging changes do not occur in these parameters; abnormal values should prompt further evaluation.
†Includes normal aging and other age-related changes.

The concern about function as a core component of geriatrics deserves special comment. Functioning is the end result of the various efforts of the geriatric approach to care. Optimizing function necessitates integrating efforts on several fronts. It is helpful to think of functioning as an equation:

$$\text{Function} = \frac{\text{physical capabilities} \times \text{medical management} \times \text{motivation}}{\text{social, psychological, and physical environment}}$$

This admitted oversimplification is meant as a reminder that function can be influenced on at least three levels. The clinician's first task is to remediate the remediable. Careful medical diagnosis and appropriate treatment are essential in good geriatric care. Adequate medical management, however, is necessary but not sufficient. Once those conditions amenable to treatment have been addressed, the next step is to develop the environment that will best support the patient's autonomous function.

Environmental barriers can be both physical and psychological. It is easier to recognize the physical barriers: stairs for the person with dyspnea, inaccessible cabinets for the wheelchair-bound, and so on. Psychological barriers refer especially to the dangers of risk aversion. Those most concerned about the patient may restrict activity in the name of protecting the patient or the institution. For example, hospitals are notoriously averse to risk; older patients will be restricted to a wheelchair rather than risk them falling when walking.

This risk-averse behavior may be compounded by concerns about efficiency. Personal care is personnel intensive. It takes much more time and patience to work with patients to encourage them to do things for themselves than to step in and do the task. But that pseudoefficiency breeds dependence.

The third factor relates to the concept of motivation. If the care providers believe that the patient cannot improve, they will likely induce despair and discouragement in their charges. The tendency toward functional decline may become a self-fulfilling prophecy. Indeed, the opposite belief—that improvement is quite likely with appropriate intervention—may be the critical element in the success of geriatric evaluation units. Belief in the possibility of improvement can play another critical role in geriatric care. Psychologists have developed a useful paradigm referred to as "the innocent victim." The basic concept is that caregivers respond in a hostile manner to those they feel impotent to help. If given a sense of empowerment, perhaps by using assessment tools and intervention strategies such as the ones provided in this book, for approaching the complex problems of older persons, care providers are likely to feel more positive toward those individuals and be more willing to work with them rather than avoiding them. The more an information system can provide feedback on accomplishments and progress toward improved function, the more the provider will feel positively about the older patient.

Table 3-6 summarizes several other important concepts about comprehensive functional assessment in the geriatric population, which were identified in a Consensus Development Conference at the National Institutes of Health (NIH, 1988). To a large extent the purpose, setting, and timing of the assessment dictate the nature of the assessment process. Table 3-7 lists the different purposes and objectives of functional status measures. Generally, functional assessment begins with a case-finding or screening approach in order to identify individuals for whom more in-depth and interdisciplinary assessment might be of benefit. Assessment is often carried out at points of transition, such as a threatened or actual decline in health status or impending change in living situation. Without this type of targeting, the assessment of older people may be time-consuming and

TABLE 3-6   IMPORTANT CONCEPTS FOR GERIATRIC FUNCTIONAL ASSESSMENT

1. The nature of the assessment should be dictated by its purpose, setting, and timing (see Table 3-7).

2. Input from multiple disciplines is often helpful, but routine multidisciplinary assessment is not cost-effective.

3. Assessments should be targeted:
   a. Initial screening to identify disciplines needed.
   b. Times of threatened or actual decline in status, impending change in living situation, and other stressful situations.

4. Standard instruments are useful, but there are numerous potential pitfalls:
   a. Instruments should be reliable, sensitive, and valid for the purposes and setting of the assessment.
   b. How questions are asked can be critically important (e.g., performance vs. capability).
   c. Discrepancies can arise between different informants (e.g., self-report vs. caregiver's report).
   d. Self- or caregiver report of performance, or direct observation of performance may not reflect what the individual does in everyday life.
   e. Many standard instruments have not been adequately tested for reliability and sensitivity to changes over time.

5. Open-ended questions are helpful in complementing information from standardized instruments.

6. The family's expectations, capabilities, and willingness to provide care must be explored.

7. The patient's preferences and expectations should be elicited and considered paramount in planning services.

8. A strong link must exist between the assessment process and follow-up in the provision of services.

not cost-effective. Numerous standardized instruments are available to assist in the assessment process.

There are numerous potential pitfalls in the use of standardized assessment instruments (Kane and Kane, 2000; see Table 3-6). The critical concept in using standardized instruments is that they should fit the purposes and setting for which they are intended, and there must be a solid link between the assessment process and the follow-up provision of services. In addition, the assessment process

TABLE 3-7   PURPOSES AND OBJECTIVES OF FUNCTIONAL STATUS
            MEASURES

PURPOSE	OBJECTIVES
Description	Develop normative data Depict geriatric population along selected parameters Assess needs Describe outcomes associated with various interventions
Screening	Identify from among population at risk those individuals who should receive further assessment and by whom
Assessment	Make diagnosis Assign treatment
Monitoring	Observe changes in untreated conditions Review progress of those receiving treatment
Prediction	Permit scientifically based clinical interventions Make prognostic statements of expected outcomes on the basis of given conditions

should include a clear discussion of the patient's preferences and expectations, as well as the family's expectations and willingness to provide care. The importance of functional status assessment has been highlighted by data documenting the ability of functional status measures to predict mortality in older hospitalized patients (Inouye et al., 1998).

Assessment Tools for Functional Status

This chapter focuses on the assessment of physical and mental function. Mental function is also discussed in Chap. 6. Table 3-8 lists examples of measures of physical functioning. Physical functioning is measured along a spectrum. For disabled persons, one may focus on the ability to perform basic self-care tasks, often referred to as *activities of daily living* (ADL). The patient is assessed on ability to conduct each of a series of basic activities. Data usually come from the patient or from a caregiver (e.g., a nurse or family member) who has had a sufficient opportunity to observe the patient. In some cases, it may be more useful to have the patient actually demonstrate the ability to perform key tasks. Grading of performance is usually divided into three levels of dependency: (1) ability to perform the task without human assistance (one may wish to distinguish

TABLE 3-8   EXAMPLES OF MEASURES OF PHYSICAL FUNCTIONING

Basic activities of daily living (ADL)
Feeding
Dressing
Ambulation
Toileting
Bathing
Transfer (from bed and toilet)
Continence
Grooming
Communication
Instrumental activities of daily living (IADL)
Writing
Reading
Cooking
Cleaning
Shopping
Doing laundry
Climbing stairs
Using telephone
Managing medication
Managing money
Ability to perform paid employment duties or outside work (e.g., gardening)
Ability to travel (use public transportation, go out of town)

those persons who need mechanical aids like a walker but are still independent); (2) ability to perform the task with some human assistance; and (3) inability to perform, even with assistance. Distinguishing "independent without difficulty" from "independent *with* difficulty" may provide complementing prognostic information (Gill et al., 1998).

Commonly used tools for assessing physical function are included in the Appendix. There may be discrepancies between patient or caregiver reports and what the individuals actually do in their everyday life. Moreover, there may be differences between reported physical functional status and actual measures of physical performance. Reuben's Physical Performance Test is one example of a practical assessment that provides insights into actual performance and prognostic information (Reuben et al., 1992). (The Physical Performance Test is included in the Appendix.) Other performance-based assessments of gait and balance are discussed in Chap. 9.

In addition to these general geriatric measures of functional status, other functional assessment tools are commonly used in different settings. Examples include the following:

1. The Short Form 36—a global measure of function and well-being that is increasingly being used in outpatient settings. This measure has a disadvantage in the frail geriatric population because of a ceiling effect—that is, it does not distinguish well between sick and very sick older people.
2. The Minimum Data Set (MDS)—a comprehensive assessment mandated on admission with quarterly updates in Medicare/Medicaid certified nursing facilities.
3. The Functional Independence Measure (FIM)—a detailed assessment tool commonly used to monitor functional status progress in rehabilitation settings.

A structured assessment of cognitive function should be part of every complete geriatric functional assessment. Because of the high prevalence of cognitive impairment, the potential impact of such impairment on overall function and safety and the ability of patients with early impairments to mask their deficits, clinicians must specifically attend to this aspect of functional assessment. At a minimum, assessment should include a test for orientation and memory. A standardized geriatric mental status test is included in the Appendix (the Folstein Mini-Mental State Examination). Although these tests do not probe the variety of intellectual functions appropriate for a more detailed assessment, they are quick, easy, scorable, and reliable. More detailed assessment of cognitive function is discussed in Chap. 6.

ENVIRONMENTAL ASSESSMENT

We emphasized earlier that patient function is the result of innate ability and environment. The clinician must, therefore, be particularly concerned with the older patient's environment. For many patients, an assessment should include an evaluation of the available and potential resources to maintain functioning. Just as physicians comfortably prescribe drugs, they should also be prepared to prescribe environmental interventions when necessary.

Rehabilitation therapists (i.e., physical, occupational, speech) are especially skilled at functional assessment, developing and implementing rehabilitative plans of care targeted at potentially remediable functional impairments, and making specific recommendations about environmental modifications that can enhance safety and functional ability. An environmental prescription may include alterations in the physical environment (e.g., ramps, grab bars, and elevated toilet seats), special services (e.g., "meals on wheels," homemaking, home nursing), increased social contact (e.g., friendly visiting, telephone reassurance, participation in recreational activities), or provision of critical elements (e.g., food or money).

The ability to identify the environmental interventions and function supports needed to maintain in the community may be the essential difference between enabling an older person to remain at home versus transferring that person to an institution. Although identifying the need is not tantamount to providing the resource, it is an important first step.

ASSESSMENT FOR PAIN

Recent guidelines published by the American Geriatrics Society recommend that on initial presentation or admission of an older person to any healthcare service, the patient should be assessed for evidence of persistent pain (AGS Panel on Persistent Pain in Older Persons, 2002). Patients with persistent pain that may affect physical function, psychosocial function, or other aspect of quality of life should undergo a comprehensive pain assessment. Tables 3-9 and 3-10 list important aspects of the history and physical examination in assessment of pain, respectively. For patients who are cognitively intact assessment of pain should be by direct questioning of the patient. Quantitative assessment of pain should be recorded by use of a standard pain scale. A verbal scale of zero to ten, with zero meaning no pain and ten meaning the worst pain possible, is frequently used. Other scales, pain thermometer and faces, studied in older populations, are illustrated in Figure 3-2. In cognitively impaired and nonverbal patients pain assessment should be by direct observation or history from caregivers. Patients should be observed for pain-related behaviors during movement. Unusual behavior in a patient with severe dementia should trigger assessment for pain as a potential cause.

TABLE 3-9   IMPORTANT ASPECTS OF THE HISTORY IN ASSESSMENT
OF PAIN

1. Characteristics of the pain
2. Relation of pain to impairments in physical and social function
3. Analgesic history (present, previous, prescribed, over-the-counter, alternative remedies, alcohol use, side effects)
4. Patient's attitudes and beliefs about pain and its management
5. Effectiveness of treatments
6. Satisfaction with current pain management
7. Social support and health care accessibility

TABLE 3-10   IMPORTANT ASPECTS OF THE PHYSICAL EXAMINATION IN ASSESSMENT OF PAIN

1. Careful examination of the site of pain, and common sites for pain referral
2. Focus on the musculoskeletal system
3. Focus on the neurological system including weakness and dysesthesia
4. Observation of physical function
5. Psychological function
6. Cognitive function

NUTRITIONAL ASSESSMENT

Several parameters are used in assessing nutritional status in older adults. Some anthropometric variables are probably effective estimators of major aspects of body composition (Table 3-11). They cannot provide a complete description of the nutritional status of an individual and are not highly correlated with biochemical or hematologic indicators of nutritional status.

Although weight is a global measure, it can be obtained easily from adults and is useful in the absence of edema. Body mass index (BMI = kg/m^2) is best correlated with total body fat. Triceps and subscapular skin folds are highly correlated with the percentage of body fat in older adults. Waist:hip ratio is a parameter of central adiposity. Upper arm circumference is correlated with lean body mass and may be particularly helpful in edematous patients in whom weight is misleading. The effect of the aging process on lean body mass is so great that it remains a poor reflection of nutritional status in older adults.

Serum albumin is a practical indicator of malnutrition in older adults. However, liver disease, proteinuria, and protein-losing enteropathies must be excluded. A low serum albumin may be indicative of malnutrition, but a normal or increased serum albumin concentration does not necessarily indicate normality. Thyroxine-binding prealbumin and/or retinol-binding protein are more sensitive indices than are albumin and transferrin.

In animals, dietary deprivation of protein results in anemia. Because anemia is one of the earliest manifestations of protein-calorie malnutrition, its presence should alert the physician to the possibility of malnutrition. Total lymphocyte count may be a very good marker for nutritional problems.

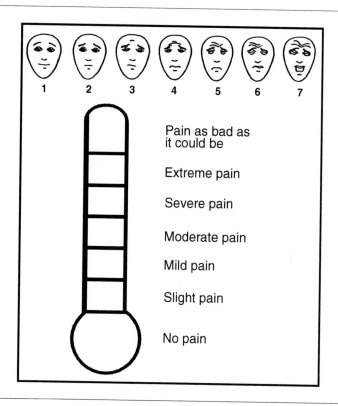

— FIGURE 3-2 — *Samples of two pain intensity scales that have been studied in older persons. Directions: Patients should view the figure without numbers. After the patient indicates the best representation of their pain, the appropriate numerical value can be assigned to facilitate clinical documentation and follow-up.* (From AGS Panel, 2002).

Some important factors need to be considered in evaluating a given patient. Table 3-12 presents some factors that put older patients at risk for malnutrition. Individuals with such problems should have an evaluation of nutritional status. Some patients may have several concurrent diseases that impair nutritional status (Table 3-13). Protein-energy malnutrition may ensue and is associated with poor prognosis. The Mini Nutritional Assessment (MNA) and Subjective Global Assessment (SGA) predict mortality in geriatric patients (Persson et al., 2002), and are valuable tools for the assessment of nutritional status in older adults. The Short-Form Mini Nutritional Assessment (MNA-SF) can be used in a two step screening process in which persons identified as "at risk" on the MNA-SF would receive additional assessment (Rubenstein et al., 2001; Table 3-14). The MNA

TABLE 3-11   ASSESSMENT OF BODY COMPOSITION

ASSESSMENT	COMPONENT
Weight	Global
Body mass index	Total fat
Skin fold	Percent fat
Waist:hip ratio	Central adiposity
Upper arm circumference	Lean body mass

TABLE 3-12   CRITICAL QUESTIONS IN ASSESSING A PATIENT FOR
MALNUTRITION

Is there any reason to suspect malnutrition?

If so, of which nutrient(s) and to what extent?

What are the pathophysiological mechanisms (e.g., alteration in nutrient intake, digestion and absorption, metabolism, excretion, or requirements)?

What etiology underlies the pathophysiological mechanism(s)?

TABLE 3-13   FACTORS THAT PLACE OLDER ADULTS AT RISK FOR
MALNUTRITION

Drugs (e.g., reserpine, digoxin, antitumor agents)

Chronic disease (e.g., congestive heart failure, renal insufficiency, chronic gastrointestinal disease)

Depression

Dental and periodontal disease

Decreased taste and smell

Low socioeconomic level

Physical weakness

Isolation

Food fads

TABLE 3-14 MINI NUTRITION ASSESSMENT

A. Has food intake declined over the past three months due to loss of appetite, digestive problems, chewing or swallowing difficulties?
0 = severe loss of appetite
1 = moderate loss of appetite
2 = no loss of appetite

☐

B. Weight loss during last three months
0 = weight loss greater than 3 kg (6.6 lbs)
1 = does not know
2 = weight loss between 1 and 3 kg (2.2 and 6.6 lbs)
3 = no weight loss

☐

C. Mobility
0 = bed or chair bound
1 = able to get out of bed/chair but does not go out
2 = goes out

☐

D. Has suffered psychological stress or acute disease in the past three months
0 = yes
2 = no

☐

E. Neuropsychological problems
0 = severe dementia or depression
1 = mild dementia
2 = no psychological problems

☐

F. Body Mass Index (BMI) (weight in kg)/(height in m)^2
0 = BMI less than 19
1 = BMI 19 to less than 21
2 = BMI 21 to less than 23
3 = BMI 23 or greater

☐

Screening score (subtotal max. 14 points)
12 points or greater: Normal–no need for further assessment
11 points or below: Possible malnutrition–continue assessment

☐☐

Note: if greater specificity is desired consider 10 points or below as possible malnutrition.
Alternative height calculations using knee to heel measurements:
with knee at 90° angle (foot flexed or flat on floor or bed board), measure from bottom of heel to top of knee.
Men = (2.02 × knee height, cm) × (0.04 × age) + 64.19
Women = (1.83 × knee height, cm) × (0.24 × age) + 84.88
Body weight calculations in amputees:
For amputations, increase weight by the percentage below for contribution of individual body parts to obtain the weight to use to determine Body Mass Index.
Single below knee 6.0% Single at knee 9.0%
Single above knee 15.0% Single arm 6.5%
Single arm below elbow 3.6%
Source: From Rubenstein et al., 2001, with permission.

(Guigoz et al., 1996) may be advantageous for the latter since it classified fewer patients than the SGA as well-nourished and those identified as well-nourished on the MNA had a better 3-year survival than those well-nourished by the SGA (Persson et al., 2002).

GERIATRIC CONSULTATION

Geriatric consultation may be requested to address specific clinical issues (e.g., confusion, incontinence, recurrent falling), to perform a comprehensive geriatric assessment (often in the context of determining the need for placement in a difficult living setting), or to perform a preoperative evaluation of a high-risk geriatric patient. In this chapter, we discuss the latter two types of consultation.

Comprehensive Geriatric Consultation

A comprehensive geriatric consultation includes the following:

1. A geriatric-oriented history and physical examination attending to the issues reviewed earlier in this chapter.
2. Medication review; in addition, geriatric patients should be questioned about alcohol abuse.
3. Functional assessment.
4. Environmental and social assessment, focusing especially on caregiver support and other resources available to meet the patient's needs.
5. Discussion of advance directives.
6. A complete list of the patient's medical, functional, and psychosocial problems.
7. Specific recommendations in each domain.

A systematic screening process to identify potentially remediable geriatric problems may be a useful tool for the comprehensive consultation.

One such screening strategy is illustrated in Table 3-15 (Moore and Siu, 1996). It may also be useful, especially in capitated systems, to use a tool that identifies risk for crises and expensive health care utilization. The Pra instrument is one such tool (Table 3-16; Pacala et al., 1997). Among frail, dependent, geriatric patients, screening for risk factors and elder abuse is important. Elder abuse is more common among older people who are in poor health and who are physically and cognitively impaired. Additional risk factors include shared living arrangements with a relative or friend suspected of alcohol or substance abuse, mental illness, or a history of violence.

Frequent emergency room visits for injury or exacerbations of chronic illness should also raise suspicion for abuse. Table 3-17 illustrates an example of an

TABLE 3-15 EXAMPLE OF A SCREENING TOOL TO IDENTIFY POTENTIALLY REMEDIABLE GERIATRIC PROBLEMS

PROBLEM	SCREENING MEASURE	POSITIVE RESULT
Poor vision	Ask, "Do you have difficulty driving, watching television, reading, or doing any of your daily activities because of your eyesight?" If yes, then test acuity with Snellen chart, with corrective lenses	Inability to read better than 20/40 on Snellen chart
Poor hearing	With audioscope set at 40 dB, test hearing at 1000 and 2000 Hz	Inability to hear 1000 or 2000 Hz in both ears or either frequency in one ear
Poor leg mobility	Time the patient after asking, "Rise from the chair. Walk 20 feet briskly, turn, walk back to the chair, and sit down."	Unable to complete task in 15 s
Urinary incontinence	Ask, "In the past year, have you ever lost your urine and gotten wet?" If yes, then ask, "Have you lost urine on at least 6 separate days?"	Yes to both questions
Malnutrition and weight loss	Ask, "Have you lost 10 pounds over the past 6 months without trying to do so?" and then weigh the patient	Yes to the question or weight <100 lb
Memory loss	Three-item recall	Unable to remember all three items after 1 min
Depression	Ask, "Do you often feel sad or depressed?"	Yes to the question

TABLE 3-15   EXAMPLE OF A SCREENING TOOL TO IDENTIFY POTENTIALLY
REMEDIABLE GERIATRIC PROBLEMS (*Continued*)

PROBLEM	SCREENING MEASURE	POSITIVE RESULT
Physical disability	Ask six questions: "Are you able to: • Do strenuous activities such as fast walking or bicycling? • Do heavy work around the house like washing windows, walls, or floors? • Go shopping for groceries or clothes? • Get to places that are out of walking distance? • Bathe: either a sponge bath, tub bath, or shower? • Dress, including putting on a shirt, buttoning and zipping, and putting on shoes?"	No to any question

Source: From Moore and Siu, 1996, with permission.

effective format for documenting the results of the consultation, listing the problems and recommendations first.

PREOPERATIVE EVALUATION

Geriatricians are often called upon by surgeons and anesthesiologists to assess elderly patients before surgical procedures. Table 3-18 lists several of the key factors involved in the preoperative evaluation of geriatric patients. Although older patients (age >70 years) have higher rates of major perioperative complications and mortality after nonemergent major noncardiac surgical procedures than do younger patients, mortality is low, even in patients 80 years of age or older (Polanczyk et al., 2001). Morbidity and mortality, however, are influenced to a greater extent by the presence and severity of systemic illnesses and whether the procedure is elective versus emergent. Thus, evaluating a geri-

TABLE 3-16 QUESTIONS ON THE PRA INSTRUMENT FOR IDENTIFYING
GERIATRIC PATIENTS AT RISK FOR HEALTH SERVICE USE

1. In general, would you say your health is:
   (excellent; very good; good; fair; poor)

2. In the previous 12 months, have you stayed overnight as a patient in a
   hospital?
   (not at all; one time; two or three times; more than three times)

3. In the previous 12 months, how many times did you visit a physician or
   clinic?
   (not at all; one time; two or three times; four to six times; more than six
   times)

4. In the previous 12 months, did you have diabetes?
   (yes; no)

5. Have you ever had: Coronary heart disease? (yes; no)
   Angina pectoris? (yes; no)
   A myocardial infarction? (yes; no)
   Any other heart attack? (yes; no)

6. Your sex?
   (male; female)

7. Is there a friend, relative, or neighbor who would take care of you for a
   few days if necessary?
   (yes; no)

8. Your date of birth?
   (month   ; day   ; year   )

Source: From Pacala et al., 1997, with permission. Copyright Regents of the University of
Minnesota. All rights reserved.

atric patient's preoperative status and risk for surgery necessitates a thorough
assessment of cardiopulmonary and renal function as well as nutritional and
hydration status. Factors that increase the risk of perioperative cardiac complications in patients undergoing noncardiac surgery include ischemic heart disease, congestive heart failure, diabetes mellitus, and renal insufficiency (Lee et al.,
1999). Patients with a recent history of myocardial infarction, active angina, pulmonary edema, and severe aortic stenosis are at especially high risk (Mangano
and Goldman, 1995). Preoperative pulmonary function tests and arterial blood
gases are rarely of prognostic value. Assessment of exercise tolerance may be
helpful, for example, the ability to climb one flight of stairs. In patients with low

TABLE 3-17 SUGGESTED FORMAT FOR SUMMARIZING THE RESULTS OF
A COMPREHENSIVE GERIATRIC CONSULTATION

1. Identifying data, including referring physician
2. Reason(s) for consultation
3. Problems
   a. Medical Problem List
   b. Functional Problem List
   c. Psychosocial Problem List
4. Recommendations
5. Standard documentation
   a. History, including medications, significant past medical
      and surgical history, system review
   b. Social and environmental information
   c. Functional assessment
   d. Advance directive status
   e. Physical exam
   f. Laboratory and other test data

risk for cardiac complications, no beta-blockade is necessary. In patients at increased risk for cardiac complications, modified exercise testing, dipyridamole thallium scanning, or dobutamine echocardiography may be indicated (Palda and Detsky, 1997). Coronary artery bypass grafting or percutaneous coronary revascularization should be limited to patients who have a clearly defined need for the procedure that is independent of the need for noncardiac surgery (Fleisher and Eagle, 2001).

Underlying conditions that are prevalent in the geriatric population, such as hypertension, congestive heart failure, chronic obstructive lung disease, diabetes mellitus, anemia, and undernutrition, need particularly careful management in the preoperative period (Thomas and Ritchie, 1995; Schiff and Emanuele, 1995). Medication regimens should be scrutinized in order to determine whether specific drugs should be continued or withheld. Results from several well-designed clinical trials suggest that use of beta-blockers perioperatively is associated with significant reductions in cardiac morbidity and mortality (Auerbach and Goldman, 2002). High and intermediate cardiac event risk patients with negative noninvasive test results should begin beta-blockade therapy. Those with positive noninvasive test results should have consideration of additional therapies to reduce risk, for example, coronary revascularization. Careful consideration should also be given to perioperative prophylactic measures for the prevention of thromboembolism and infection, many of which have documented efficacy in specific situations (Medical Letter, 1999; Geerts et al., 2001).

TABLE 3-18   KEY FACTORS IN THE PREOPERATIVE EVALUATION OF THE
GERIATRIC PATIENT

1. Age >70 is associated with an increased risk of complications and death
   a. Risk varies with the type of procedure and local complication rates
   b. Emergency procedures are associated with much higher risk
   c. Comorbid conditions, especially cardiovascular, are more important
      risk factors than age per se

2. The appropriateness and risk-benefit ratio of the proposed surgery must
   be carefully considered

3. Underlying conditions must be evaluated and optimally managed before
   nonemergency surgery, e.g.:
   a. Cardiovascular disease, especially heart failure
   b. Pulmonary status
   c. Renal function
   d. Diabetes mellitus
   e. Thyroid disease (which is often occult)
   f. Anemia
   g. Nutrition
   h. Hydration and volume status, especially in patients on diuretics

4. Medication regimens should be carefully planned; some drugs should be
   continued, others should be withheld, and some necessitate dosage
   adjustments

5. Several cardiovascular conditions substantially increase risk, including:
   a. Myocardial infarction within 6 months
   b. Pulmonary edema
   c. Angina (especially if unstable)
   d. Severe aortic stenosis

6. Specific laboratory evaluations may be helpful in some situations, e.g.:
   a. Pulmonary function tests and arterial blood gas with respiratory
      symptoms, obesity, chest deformity (e.g., kyphoscoliosis), abnormal
      chest radiographs, planned thoracic or upper abdominal procedure
   b. Noninvasive cardiac testing in high and intermediate risk for cardiac
      event patients
   c. Creatinine clearance with unstable or borderline renal function, or the
      use of nephrotoxic or renally excreted drugs

7. The documented effectiveness, risks, and benefits of perioperative prophylactic measures should be considered:
   a. Beta-blocker administration*
   b. Antithrombotic prophylaxis†
   c. Antimicrobial prophylaxis ‡

* See Fleisher and Eagle, 2001.
† See Geerts et al., 2001.
‡ See Medical Letter, 1999.

Many surgeons and anesthesiologists tend to favor regional over general anesthesia for geriatric patients. Regional anesthesia (e.g., epidural), however, may have several potential disadvantages. Patients may require added intravenous sedation and/or analgesia, thus increasing the risks of perioperative cardiovascular and mental status changes. Significant cardiovascular changes can, in fact, occur during regional anesthesia; thus invasive monitoring may be required in some patients. Neither the incidence of deep vein thrombosis nor the amount of blood loss seems to be substantially decreased compared to general anesthesia. Thus, decisions about the type of anesthesia should be carefully individualized on the basis of patient factors, the nature of the procedure, and the preferences of the surgical team.

References

AGS Panel on Persistent Pain in Older Persons: The management of persistent pain in older persons. *J Am Geriatr Soc* 50:S205–S224, 2002.

American College of Physicians: Guidelines for assessing and managing the perioperative risk from coronary artery disease associated with major noncardiac surgery. *Ann Intern Med* 127:309–312, 1997.

Auerbach AD, Goldman L: β-Blockers and reduction of cardiac events in noncardiac surgery: scientific review. *JAMA* 287:1435–1444, 2002.

Bula CJ, Berod AC, Stuck AE, et al: Effectiveness of preventive in-home geriatric assessment in well-functioning, community-dwelling older people: secondary analysis of a randomized trial. *J Am Geriatr Soc* 47:389–395, 1999.

Cohen HJ, Feussner JR, Weinberger M, et al: A controlled trial of inpatient and outpatient geriatric evaluation and management. *N Engl J Med* 346:905–912, 2002.

Fleisher LA, Eagle KA: Lowering cardiac risk in noncardiac surgery. *N Engl J Med* 345:1677–1682, 2001.

Geerts WH, Heit JA, Clagett GP, et al: Prevention of venous thromboembolism. *Chest* 119:132S–175S, 2001.

Gill TM, Robison JT, Tinetti ME: Difficulty and dependence: two components of the disability continuum among community-living older persons. *Ann Intern Med* 128:96–101, 1998.

Guigoz Y, Vellas B, Garry PJ: Assessing the nutritional status of the elderly: the Mini Nutritional Assessment as part of the geriatric evaluation. *Nutr Rev* 54:559–565, 1996.

Inouye SK, Peduzzi PN, Robison JT, et al: Importance of functional measures in predicting mortality among older hospitalized patients. *JAMA* 279:1187–1993, 1998.

Kane RL, Kane RA: *Assessing Older Persons: Measures, Meaning, and Practical Applications.* New York, Oxford University Press, 2000.

Katz S, Ford A, Moskowitz R, et al: The index of ADL: a standardized measure of biological and psychosocial function. *JAMA* 185:914–919, 1963.

Landefeld CS, Palmer RM, Kresevic DM, et al: A randomized trial of care in hospital medical unit especially designed to improve the functional outcomes of acutely ill older patients. *N Engl J Med* 332:1338–1344, 1995.

Lee TH, Marcantonio ER, Mangione CM, et al: Derivation and prospective validation of a simple index for prediction of cardiac risk of major noncardiac surgery. *Circulation* 100:1043–1049, 1999.

Mangano DT, Goldman L: Preoperative assessment of patients with known or suspected coronary disease. *N Engl J Med* 333:1750–1756, 1995.

Medical Letter on Drugs and Therapeutics: Antimicrobial prophylaxis in surgery. *Med Lett* 41(1060):75–80, 1999.

Moore AA, Siu AL: Screening for common problems in ambulatory elderly: clinical confirmation of a screening instrument. *Am J Med* 100:438–443, 1996.

NIH Consensus Development Conference Statement: Geriatric assessment methods for clinical decision making. *J Am Geriatr Soc* 36:342–347, 1988.

Pacala JT, Boult C, Reed RL, Aliberti E: Predictive validity of the Pra instrument among older recipients of managed care. *J Am Geriatr Soc* 45:614–617, 1997.

Palda VA, Detsky AS: Perioperative assessment and management of risk from coronary artery disease. *Ann Intern Med* 127:313–328, 1997.

Persson MD, Brismar KE, Katzarski KS, et al: Nutritional status using Mini Nutritional Assessment and Subjective Global Assessment predict mortality in geriatric patients. *J Am Geriatr Soc* 50:1996–2002, 2002.

Polanczyk CA, Marcantonio E, Goldman L, et al: Impact of age on perioperative complications and length of stay in patients undergoing noncardiac surgery. *Ann Intern Med* 134:637–643, 2001.

Reuben DB, Siu A, Kimpau S: The predictive validity of self-report and performance-based measures of function and health. *J Gerontol Med Sci* 47:106–110, 1992.

Reuben DB, Borok GM, Wolde-Tsadik G, et al: A randomized trial of comprehensive geriatric assessment in the care of hospitalized patients. *N Engl J Med* 332:1345–1350, 1995.

Reuben DB, Frank JC, Hirsch SH, et al: A randomized clinical trial of outpatient comprehensive geriatric assessment coupled with an intervention to increase adherence to recommendations. *J Am Geriatr Soc* 47:371–372, 1999.

Rubenstein LZ, Stuck AE, Sill AL, Wieland D: Impacts of geriatric evaluation and management programs on defined outcomes: overview of the evidence. *J Am Geriatr Soc* 39(Suppl):85–165, 1991.

Rubenstein LZ, Harker JO, Salva A, et al: Screening for undernutrition in geriatric practice: developing the Short-Form Mini-Nutritional Assessment (MNA-SF). *J Gerontol A Biol Sci Med Sci* 56A:M366–M372, 2001.

Schiff RL, Emanuele MA: The surgical patient with diabetes mellitus: guidelines for management. *J Gen Intern Med* 10:154–161, 1995.

Stuck AE, Aronow HU, Steiner A, et al: A trial of annual in-home comprehensive geriatric assessments for elderly people living in the community. *N Engl J Med* 333:1184–1189, 1995.

Thomas DR, Ritchie CS: Preoperative assessment of older adults. *J Am Geriatr Soc* 43:811–821, 1995.

Suggested Readings

Applegate WB, Blass JP, Williams TF: Instruments for functional assessment of older patients. *N Engl J Med* 322:1207–1214, 1990.

Crum RM, Anthony SC, Bassett SS, Folstein MF: Population-based norms for the Mini-Mental State Examination by age and educational level. *JAMA* 269:2386–2391, 1993.

Feinstein AR, Josephy BR, Wells CK: Scientific and clinical problems in indexes of functional disability. *Ann Intern Med* 105:413–420, 1986.

Finch M, Kane RL, Philp I: Developing a new metric for ADLs. *J Am Geriatr Soc* 43:877–884, 1995.

Fleming KC, Evans JM, Weber DC, Chutka DS: Practical functional assessment of elderly persons: a primary-care approach. *Mayo Clin Proc* 70:890–910, 1995.

Folstein MF, Folstein S, McHuth PR: Mini-Mental State: a practical method for grading the cognitive state of patients for the clinician. *J Psychiatr Res* 12:189–198, 1975.

Gill TM, Feinstein AR: A critical appraisal of the quality of quality-of-life measurements. *JAMA* 272:619–626, 1994.

Palda VA, Detsky AS: Perioperative assessment and management of risk from coronary artery disease. *Ann Intern Med* 127:313–328, 1997.

Reuben DB, Siu AL: An objective measure of physical function of elderly persons: the physical performance test. *J Am Geriatr Soc* 38:1105–1112, 1990.

Scheitel SM, Fleming KC, Chutka DS, Evans JM: Geriatric health maintenance. *Mayo Clin Proc* 71:289–302, 1996.

Siu A: Screening for dementia and its causes. *Ann Intern Med* 115:122–132, 1991.

Williams ME, Hadler N, Earp JA: Manual ability as a mark of dependency in geriatric women. *J Chronic Dis* 40:481–489, 1987.

CHAPTER 4

DEVELOPING CLINICAL EXPECTATIONS

Health professionals' and informal care providers' attitudes toward older patients can affect their care. As with most chronic disease, the effect of good care is generally slowing the rate of decline rather than a reversal of a clinical course. Thus, it may be harder to discern without information about what would happen in the absence of good care. Moreover, elderly patients are in danger of being dismissed as hopeless or not worth the effort on the basis of their age. Physicians faced with the question of how much time and resources to spend in searching for a diagnosis will want to consider the probability of benefit for the investment. In some cases, older patients are better investments than younger ones. This apparent paradox occurs in the case of some preventive strategies when high risk of susceptibility and the discounted benefits of future health favor older persons. But it also arises in situations where small increments of change can yield dramatic differences.

Perhaps the most striking example of the latter is found in the case of nursing home patients. Very modest changes in their routine—such as introducing a pet, giving them a plant to tend, or increasing their sense of control over their environment—can produce dramatic improvements in mood and morale.

At the same time, the risk:benefit ratio is different with older patients. Treatments that might be easily tolerated in younger patients may pose a much greater risk of producing harmful effects in older patients. As shown in Figure 4-1, the therapeutic window that separates benefit from harm is narrower. In effect, the dosage that will produce a positive effect more closely approaches one that can lead to a toxic effect. As noted earlier, one of the hallmarks of aging is a loss of responsiveness to stress. In this context, treatment may be viewed as a stress.

Those who treat older patients must also consider the theory of competitive risks. Because older persons often suffer from multiple problems, treating one problem may provide an opportunity for more adverse effects from another. In essence, eliminating one cause of death increases the likelihood of death from other causes.

Physicians treating older patients may suffer simultaneously from too much information and too little. A patient with a substantial history of care may come

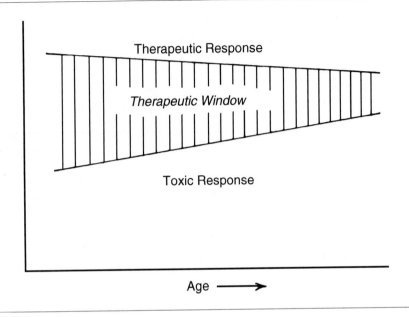

— FIGURE 4-1 — *Narrowing of the therapeutic window. This diagram portrays in a conceptual manner how the space between a therapeutic dose and a toxic dose narrows with age.*

with a multivolume set of charts from which little usable data can be gleaned in the time allotted for an outpatient encounter. Modern laboratory reports often provide more data than is requested, distracting as well as overinforming.

A useful tool for creating a more proactive and focused attitude among those who care for older persons is the flowchart. Focusing on a few clinical parameters that are both significant and most likely to be affected by treatment helps the clinicians focus their attention and recognize changes early. Because the changes are likely to be subtle, it is often helpful to establish treatment goals with time frames for achieving them. Both the health care team and the patient can then agree on expectations and follow progress toward the goal.

It is important that the goals be achievable. Small successes are very important and reinforcing. Thus the units of measurement should be capable of detecting small but meaningful changes. In many instances, small gains can, in fact, make an enormous difference. The stroke patient, for example, who regains the use of hand muscles has a greatly improved ability to function. Being able to change position in bed may mean the difference between getting pressure sores and not. Regaining a method of communication, whether by speech or some other means, can restore social contact.

By introducing gradual, small steps, a functional task may appear more achievable. We have all had some experience in getting a bedridden patient to resume a more active role. For an older person who has been at bed rest for a long period, this task requires overcoming both physiological and psychological problems. Small steps will often ease the transition and provide an opportunity to monitor the effects at each stage to minimize risk.

CLINICAL GLIDE PATHS

In one sense, geriatrics can be thought of as the intersection of chronic disease care and gerontology. The principles of chronic disease care apply in spades here. As noted earlier in this book, care for chronic disease is conceptually different from that for acute disease. To provide effective chronic care, one needs a longitudinally oriented information system that is sensitive to change. Each clinical encounter with a chronically ill patient is essentially a part of a continuing episode of care; it has a history and a future. Caring for a chronically ill patient, especially one with multiple problems, demands an enormous feat of memory as the patient's list of problems is unearthed and the history, treatments, and expectations associated with each are reviewed. Clinicians caring for such patients (often under enormous time pressures) may find themselves either overwhelmed with large volumes of data from which they must quickly extract the most salient facts or, alternatively, relying on inadequate data from which to reconstruct the patient's clinical course. Moreover, because patients live with their disease 24 hours a day, 7 days a week, they are best positioned to make regular observations about its progress. Such constructive patient involvement responds to another principle of chronic care. These goals can be achieved using a simple information system that can focus the clinician's attention on salient parameters.

One approach to help to focus clinicians' attention on the salient parameters of a chronic condition is the clinical glide path. This technique is modeled on the way one lands an airplane. The goal is to establish a flight path that will lead to a safe landing. Information about the plane's position is provided regularly to allow the pilot to make small corrections in order to avoid making drastic adjustments at the last minute or crashing. In a similar vein, one can manage chronic illnesses by establishing the salient parameters, the indications that the patient's clinical course is being achieved. For each chronic problem, the clinician should identify the one or two parameters (physiologic or functional) that will best indicate how things are going. Such information is often symptoms such as shortness of breath, pain, or fatigue; but they can also be simple signs such as weight change, blood pressure or blood sugar. This information is then systematically collected (by the clinician or more likely by the patient) and entered into a flow sheet, which can be converted into a graph. As long as the patient's course is as good as or better than predicted, no adjustments need be made; but indications that the course is beginning to slip below that expected should trigger an early reassessment, in the same way that a pilot is warned when the plane begins to move out of the glide path box. Figure 4-2 shows an example of a glide path.

The choice of the parameters to be tracked for each problem can either be left up to each practitioner or the practitioner can choose from a window of pertinent

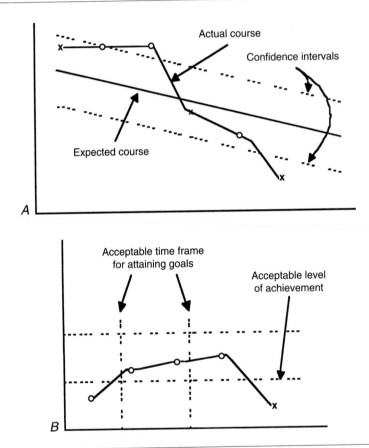

— FIGURE 4-2 — *Clinical glide path models. In this model (A), the expected course (solid line) calls for gradual decline. The confidence intervals are shown as dotted lines. Actual measures that are within or better than the glide path are shown as o. When the patient's course is worse than expected, the o changes to an x. The design shown uses confidence intervals with upper and lower bounds, but actually only the lower bound is pertinent. Any performance above the upper confidence interval boundary is very acceptable. The design of the glide path can also take another form (B). It may be preferable to think in terms of reaching a threshold level within a given time window (e.g., in recuperating from an illness) and then maintaining that level.*

options. In most cases, the latter makes the most sense. It provides some structure but permits an individualized approach.

The clinical glide path approach combines making a prognosis about a patient's expected course with the collection of systematic information on salient parameters. The prognosis can be generated intuitively or derived from statistical data. Unfortunately, we do not yet have systematic data collection from which to generate such statistics.

Implementing a glide path system has to rely on clinical judgment about prognosis. This judgment can be made by each clinician, or one can rely on the systematic judgment of experts. Initially the value of the glide path system will come less from assessing the rate of achieving the expected path than from the systematic attention to patients' courses. Rendering a great deal of complex information more coherently and setting expectations should have a positive effect on chronic care.

It is important to distinguish the clinical glide path approach from clinical pathways. The latter specify an expected course with specific milestones and dictates what care should be provided at specific junctures. This approach works well in very predictable situations such as postoperative recovery and even some instances of rehabilitation, but most of chronic care management is not as predictable. The glide path method specifies what data should be collected, not what actions should be taken. Its underlying premise holds that when clinicians can be aided in focusing their attention on a patient's salient parameters, they will be able to manage the chronic problems better.

DISEASE MANAGEMENT

Focusing attention on the management of specific problems has become a consistent theme in efforts to improve the management of chronic illness. Disease management is most commonly used by health plans, which use the available administrative data from encounters, drug records, and lab tests to identify all enrollees with a given condition. Protocols can then be applied to look for errors of both omission and commission. In some cases, potential complications can be flagged and checks built in to try to avoid untoward events such as drug interactions.

A more active approach to disease management uses case managers for patients who are determined to need special attention, either because they have a diagnosis that suggests high risk of subsequent use or their history indicates problems in controlling their disease(s). These case managers work with the patients to be sure that they understand their regimens. They encourage the patients to raise any questions early. They telephonically monitor the course of the illness using parameters like those described above. They may make home visits to ascertain how the patients are doing and to ensure that they can function effectively in their natural habitats. The positive reports from trials of this approach have encouraged many replications.

Another variation on disease management is being practiced in a few managed care organizations. Here patients with a given disease (sometimes a more heterogeneous cluster of patients is assembled) are brought together for periodic sessions that include health education and group support, as well as individual clinical attention. It has proven more efficient to use groups in this way. The same sessions can draw upon specialists to see problematic cases more efficiently.

Particularly in the context of managed care, there is a strong incentive to try to identify high-risk patients in order to attend to them before they develop into high-cost cases. Various predictive models have been developed to identify such cases. One widely used model is the Pra (probability of repeat admissions).

This tool uses an eight-item questionnaire to flag older patients who are most likely to have two or more hospital admissions in the next several years (Boult et al., 1993; Pacala et al., 1995). A modification of this method has been developed to use administrative data bases as well. A similar approach is being developed to identify those at high risk for needing long-term care. Once these patients have been targeted, an intervention is needed to change the predicted course. The Pra model does not specify what actions should be taken; it was initially developed as a method for identifying those in need of a comprehensive geriatric examination.

Other efforts have sought to target high-risk groups. An analysis of the Medicare Current Beneficiary Survey identified a model that could identify older persons at risk of death or functional decline (Saliba et al., 2001). Another index can identify older adults who have an increased risk of death 1 year after a hospitalization (Walter et al., 2001).

Interventions have also been developed to address those at highest risk. A meta-analysis of geriatric assessment declared it a substantial boon to care, because it was associated reduced mortality and improved function (Stuck et al., 1993). Another meta-analysis suggests that home visits can prevent nursing home admissions and functional decline (Stuck et al., 2002).

Function has proven to be an important predictive risk factor for both subsequent use of expensive services and or outcomes in general. Poor functional status in hospital patients predicts later mortality over and above the effects of burden-of-illness measures.

BENCHMARKS

The clinical glide path system is closely related to another approach that combines a set of prognoses and the criteria for predicted progress. The latter are termed *benchmarks*. Ideally, each physician would evaluate each patient as a unique combination of problems and potential.

However, the time involved may prove prohibitive. An alternative is to use a previously conceived set of basic benchmarks geared to the common problems of geriatrics. The generation of a problem list then leads to the implementation of the appropriate benchmarks. These can be modified to fit the more specific character-istics of a given patient. A great advantage of this approach lies in its capacity to enhance delegation. The benchmarks provide a structure to guide ongoing infor-mation gathering. They target the pertinent information and can even offer general guidelines about what steps to take when the observed results deviate from those expected. (These actions are usually couched in terms of varying stages of urgency for seeking help.) The benchmark system does not preclude gathering additional data or recognizing the development of a new problem.

One setting ideally suited to such an approach is the nursing home. Because the system guides the collection of information and relates each item to one or more specific problems, it has an educational role as well as a clinical one. Nursing home staff who may feel isolated from the infrequently seen physician now have a more effective means of communication. They know what information is being sought and why. They have a format for recording those data, which offers desired information. The benchmark system was, in fact, developed for use in the nursing home and has been used effectively in that setting. Because the general level of lit-eracy among nursing home aides is quite low, the system was specifically designed to require minimal narrative by using symbols in a flowchart format.

Table 4-1 presents a sample set of benchmark criteria for hip fracture. The two scales referred to—independence and behavior—were specially developed for the project but could be replaced by measures of activities of daily living and a standardized mood scale such as that for depression. Other clinicians may choose to add, delete, or modify items to fit their pattern of practice. Figure 4-3 offers a hypothetical chart for recording data pertinent to this problem. Specific narrative notes are made only when an event warrants them. The flowchart format readily shows when a change in pattern occurs and intervention is indicated. This basic approach has been taken a step farther. "Extended care pathways" have been developed, largely in the arena of nursing, whereby specific outcomes are defined and timelines laid out by which they should be met. Charting is done for excep-tions. Treatments and next steps are usually indicated.

The benchmark system was originally developed for use with a nurse practi-tioner as the person giving primary care under supervision of physicians. Nurse practitioners have proved themselves very effective in such roles for nursing home patients, and the care they provide is now covered by Medicare Part B.

Neither the benchmark system nor the extended care pathways fit easily into the current system of regulations for physician attendance to nursing home patients. The present rules are designed to achieve at least a minimal frequency of contact with these patients (usually once a month). Unfortunately, the result is too often superficial attention to the patient's chart. The doctor's signature is the ticket to continued coverage under Medicaid. Particularly when the same system discourages frequent visits, the care of nursing home patients is neglected.

Nursing home care has never attracted a great deal of physician enthusiasm, but this need not continue to be the case. If we can implement a new form of

TABLE 4-1 EXAMPLE OF BENCHMARK INSTRUCTIONS: HIP FRACTURE

OBSERVATION	FREQUENCY	BENCHMARK	ACTION
1. Independence scale score	Every 2 weeks	Decreased score or no change within 6 weeks after therapy is begun	Inform physician
2. Behavioral scale score	Every 2 weeks	Decreased score or no change within 6 weeks after therapy is begun	Inform physician
3. Soreness in either calf (use: R5 right soreness, L5 left soreness)	Daily; check by pushing foot up with knee extended	Present	Place patient on bed rest Notify physician
4. Temperature (°F), pain, malaise	Increased hip pain, calf pain in afternoon	Above 100.8°F (38.2°C) orally for 8–16 h	Notify physician Take temperature every 4–8 h if elevated
5. Contracture or stiff joint, especially foot drop, hip flexion, knee flexion, hip abducted or turned out (+ or −)	Daily	Present	Continue to position properly and give range of motion to tolerance; inform physician; chart location of contracture
6. Distance walked at one time (in yards)	Daily	Decrease over 3 days or no improvement within 1 week after therapy is begun	Inform physician
7. Pain in hip (+ for pain)	Afternoon	No relief by medication after 24 h of administration	Notify physician

Source: From Pepper GA, Jorgonson LB, Kane RL, et al: *Problem-Oriented Process: Nurse's Manual.* Salt Lake City, University of Utah, 1972, with permission.

DATE	8/12	8/13	8/14	8/15	8/16	8/17	8/18	8/19	8/20	8/21	8/22	8/23	8/24	8/25	8/26	8/27
Hip Fracture																
1. Independence Scale Score	20															
2. Behavior Scale Score								40								
3. Soreness In either calf (–, R or L)		–	–	–	–	–	–	*R R	R							
4. Contracture (+ or –)		–	c+	+	+	*+	+	+	–	–	–	–	–	–	–	–
5. Distance Walked (yds.)	10	10	11	12	13	14	15	C 2								
6. Temperature (°F) prn								101° F								

— FIGURE 4-3 — *Hypothetical example of benchmark chart. See nurse's notes in chart, as some appropriate for charting this observation concerning this observation on this day.*

record keeping that provides better information to staff and demands better performance from them, we should see an improvement in morale and hence a more attractive atmosphere in which to practice.

MINIMUM DATA SET FOR NURSING HOMES

The Omnibus Budget Reconciliation Act of 1987 (OBRA 1987) produced many changes in the way nursing homes were regulated. Perhaps none was as influential as the requirement that all nursing home residents covered by federal funds be assessed regularly using a standardized form, the Minimum Data Set for Nursing Home Resident Assessment and Care Screening (MDS). This information is designed to be completed by a nurse, but it draws on data from a number of disciplines.

The MDS summarizes a number of facets about each resident, including functional levels, cognitive and behavioral problems, special care needs, skin condition, nutritional status, and psychosocial well-being (the last not very well).

In addition to serving as a basic data set, problems identified trigger more detailed required documentation, called *Resident Assessment Protocols* (RAPs), in 18 areas. Table 4-2 lists the RAPs.

The MDS is intended to provide a basis for developing better plans of care and for assessing the changes in functional levels over time. A copy of the MDS is shown in the Appendix.

The MDS can also prove a useful tool for physicians. It is a compact source of information about various aspects of each nursing home resident. If the pertinent parameters for goals determined to be achieved in the care plan were systematically charted in a flow sheet, it would be possible to see progress at a glance or to recognize the need for a change in the plan of care. Physicians can

TABLE 4-2   RESIDENT ASSESSMENT PROTOCOL (RAP) TOPICS

Delirium	Cognitive loss/dementia
Visual function	Communication
ADL functional/rehabilitation potential	Urinary incontinence
Psychosocial well-being	Mood state
Behavior problem	Activities
Falls	Nutritional status
Feeding tubes	Dehydration/fluid maintenance
Dental care	Pressure ulcers
Psychotropic drug use	Physical restraints

ADL = activity of daily living.

play a key role in helping nursing home staff to see how such information can be used to improve care, not just to meet external mandates for better documentation.

However, several important shortcomings of the MDS must be acknowledged. The MDS was designed to be a means of recording judgments. These judgments inevitably pass through several hands. The persons with the most direct opportunity to observe behavior are the nurses aides, who then communicate their observations to the nurses completing the forms. The overall reliance on observations means that, in effect, all nursing home residents are being assessed as though they were cognitively impaired. This limitation is especially severe, because the MDS purports to measure critical elements of quality of life. Assuming that one can truly infer another person's emotional state, the degree to which they are engaged in meaningful activities or whether they have real social relationships seems like an act of hubris. Even using observations to determine a person's cognitive capacity seems to require heroic assumptions. It may be possible to detect extremes of behavior, but no one would want to argue that such an approach is the best way to assess many of these critical domains. Nonetheless, the MDS does not use specific questions put to those patients who can respond. Work is currently underway to test methods to assess quality of life among nursing home residents. Many, including those who are cognitively impaired can be interviewed directly. The challenge comes in how to gather information on those who cannot respond reliably. Proxy use works poorly at the individual level, although the mean values correspond well with those obtained from residents and thus can be used to assess the performance of nursing home as a whole.

The MDS has also been used as the basis for assessing the quality of nursing home care. A set of quality indicators has been developed on the basis of MDS information. These are now being nationally normed, although more work is needed on risk adjustment to allow for valid comparisons among nursing homes that may have quite different case mixes.

OASIS

The federal government has also prescribed a data system for home health care. OASIS (Outcome and Assessment Information Set) is intended to play much the same role in this venue that MDS does in the nursing home, providing both a consistent information base for quality assessment and serving as the basis for better care planning.

ROLE OF OUTCOMES IN ASSURING QUALITY OF LONG-TERM CARE

Quality of care remains a critical, if elusive, goal for long-term care. As we consider steps for resource allocation, we might first address the question of whether we are spending our current funds most wisely. There is at once a growing demand for more creativity and more accountability in long-term care. It may be possible to reduce the regulatory burden, increase the meaningful accountability, and make the incentives within the system more rational. Progress in long-term care and chronic care will require more innovation and creativity, but it will also require accountability. Outcomes monitoring (and ultimately outcomes-based rewards) allows both to coexist.

Before we can talk about how to package care or how to buy it cheaper, we need a better understanding of what we are really buying. One hears more and more about the value of shifting attention from the process of care to the actual outcomes achieved in acute care. These arguments apply at least as strongly to long-term care.

Two basic concepts must be kept in mind when discussing outcomes.

1. The term *outcomes* is used to mean the relationship between achieved and expected.
2. Because outcomes relies on probabilities, it is inappropriate to base assessments of outcomes on an individual case. Outcomes are always judged on the basis of group data.

Table 4-3 summarizes the reasons for looking toward outcomes as the way to assess and assure quality.

Clinicians frequently balk at being judged on the basis of outcomes. This discomfort can be traced to several issues.

1. Virtually all of clinical training addresses the process of care. Clinicians are schooled in what to do for whom. They reasonably believe, therefore, that if they do the right thing well, they have provided a quality service. They do not like to discuss clusters of patients, preferring to review their care one patient at a time.
2. Many factors can affect the outcomes of care that are out of the clinicians' control. They have difficulty with the concept of probability and prefer to either be responsible or not.
3. Outcomes are by their nature post hoc. Often, a long period can elapse between the time of an action and the report of its success. It is thus too late to intervene in that case.
4. Outcomes indicate a problem but offer no solution. Outcomes do not often point to specific actions that must be taken to correct the problems.

Hence, introducing outcomes, however rational, has not been easy. Making clinicians comfortable with an outcomes philosophy will require substantial training and new incentives. Physicians need to be trained to think in terms of both condition-specific and generic outcomes. They need access to data systems that can display the outcomes of their care for clinically relevant groups of patients under their care and compare them with what are reasonable outcomes for comparable patients receiving good care. Table 4-4 summarizes the key issues in outcomes measurement and its applications.

TABLE 4-3 RATIONALE FOR USING OUTCOMES

1. Outcomes encourage creativity by avoiding domination by current professional orthodoxies or powerful constituencies.
2. Outcomes permit flexibility in the modality of care.
3. Outcomes permit comparisons of efficacy across modalities of care.
4. Outcomes permit more flexible responses to different levels of performance, and thus avoid the "all-or-none" difficulties of many sanctions. At the same time, outcomes have some limitations.
5. Outcomes necessitate a single point of accountability; all the actors— facility operators, agencies, staff, physicians, patients, and family— contribute to them. Under this approach the role of the provider includes motivating others.
6. Outcomes are largely influenced by the patient's status at the beginning of treatment. The easiest and most direct way to address this issue is to think of the relationship between achieved and expected outcomes as the measure of success.
7. Outcomes must also take cognizance of case mix. Predicting outcomes necessitates information about disease characteristics (e.g., diagnosis, severity, and comorbidity) and patient characteristics (e.g., demographic factors, prior history, and social support).

Outcomes should be used as the basis for quality assurance in long-term care. The outcome approach can be used in several ways.

1. As reflected in the OBRA 1987 regulations (which, in turn, were stimulated by the Institute of Medicine's 1986 report), there is already growing national interest in increasing the emphasis on outcomes in regulatory activities. Outcome measures can be substituted for most of the current structure and process measures. It is appropriate to continue regulation in areas such as life safety. Concomitant with an outcomes emphasis would be the reduction of regulatory burden. It is important to recognize, however, that it is *not* appropriate to dictate structure, process, and outcome at the same time. Such a policy removes all degrees of freedom and stifles creativity at the point when we want to encourage it. Under an outcome-regulated approach, providers whose patients do better than expected are rewarded and are less worried about their style of caregiving, whereas those whose patients do relatively poorly are investigated more closely.
2. Outcomes can be incorporated into the payment structure to link payment with effects of care. Payments, either in the form of bonuses and penalties or

TABLE 4-4   OUTCOMES MEASUREMENT ISSUES

ISSUE	COMMENTS
Need outcome measures that are both clinically meaningful and psychometrically sound.	Use combination of condition-specific and generic measures. Usually better to adapt extant measures than to develop measures de novo.
Outcomes are always post hoc.	Expand outcomes information systems to include data on risk factors. These data should be useful in guiding clinicians to collect information that will identify potential problems. Use these data to create risk warnings to flag high-risk cases.
Every physician has all the tough cases.	Need to include a wide variety of case-mix adjusters for severity and comorbidity. Ask clinicians in advance to identify potential risk adjusters. Collect almost any item that a clinician might want to see. Test the ability of the potential risk factor to predict outcomes and discard if it has little predictive power.
Because no two clinicians see the same cases, comparisons are unfair.	Use risk adjustment. Create clinically homogeneous subgroups; use risk propensities (groups of patients with same a priori likelihood of developing the outcome).
Cannot control for selection bias; patients may receive different treatments because of subtle differences.	Adjust for all clinically identifiable differences. Use statistical methods (e.g., instrumental variables) to adjust for unmeasured differences.

as a more fundamental part of the payment structure, can be used to reward and penalize good and bad outcomes, respectively. (For example, an outcome approach might use a factor reflecting the overall achieved/expected ratio for a patient as a multiplier against the costs of care to develop a total price paid for that period of time; or one might use a similar ratio to weigh the amount of money going to a given provider from a fixed pool of dollars committed to such care.) Such an approach must be viewed carefully within the context of our present case-mix reimbursement scheme for nursing homes, because the latter indirectly rewards deterioration in function. An outcome approach to payment is compatible with a case-mix approach that is used on admission only.

3. An outcomes approach can be incorporated into the basic caring process. Where the information base used in assessing patients and developing care plans is structured, the emphasis on outcomes can become a proactive force to guide care. Optimally, the information used to assess outcomes will come from the clinical records and will be the same information used to guide care. Using available computer technology, it is now feasible to collect such data, translate them into care plans, and aggregate these data for quality assurance at minimal additional cost. The great advantage of such a scheme is its potential both to provide a better information base with which to plan care and to reinforce the creative use of such information to achieve improvements in function. Much of the current efforts going into more traditional regulatory activities might be redirected to this effort, with assessors used to validate the assessment and to focus more intense efforts on the miscreants.

We have generally good consensus on the components of outcomes, which include elements of both quality of care and quality of life; but we are less clear about how to sum them to produce composite scores. The gerontologic literature is consistent in citing the following as outcomes:

- Physiologic function (e.g., blood pressure control, lack of decubiti)
- Functional status (usually a measure of activities of daily living [ADL])
- Pain and discomfort
- Cognition (intellectual activity)
- Affect (emotional activity)
- Social participation (based on preferences)
- Social relations (at least one person who can act as a confidant)
- Satisfaction (with care and living environment)

To these must be added more global outcomes, such as death and admission to hospital.

Work is already available with nursing home residents to show that these factors can be predicted with sufficient accuracy to be used in a regulatory model. There is similar work to show that there is reasonable consensus across a variety of constituencies about the relative weights to be placed on them for different kinds of patients (e.g., different levels of physical and cognitive function at baseline).

The outcomes approach offers significant assistance with a recurrent problem in regulation—the development of standards. This approach may avoid many of these difficulties by relying on empirical standards. Rather than arguing about what is a reasonable expectation, the standard can be empirically determined. Expectations can be derived from the actual outcomes associated with real care given by those felt to represent a reasonable level of practice. This could include the entire field or a designated subset. Under this arrangement, providers would be comparing their achievements to each other's past records, with the possibility that everyone can do better.

TECHNOLOGY FOR QUALITY IMPROVEMENT

Ideally, one would like to see a measurement approach that

- Can cover the spectrum of performance
- Is easy and rapid to administer
- Is sensitive to meaningful change in performance
- Is stable within the same patient over time
- Performs consistently in different hands
- Cannot be manipulated to meet the needs of either the provider or the patient

The solution to this challenge is to create an assessment approach that incorporates the features designed to maximize these elements.

To cover the broad spectrum sought and still be relatively quickly administered, an instrument should have multiple branch points. These permit the user to focus on the area along the continuum where the patient is most likely to function and to expand that part of the scale to measure meaningful levels of performance. Branching can also ensure that the assessment is comprehensive but not burdensome.

By using key questions to screen an area, interviewers can ascertain whether to obtain more detailed information in each relevant domain. Where the initial response is negative, they can go on to the next branch point. Reliability is more likely to be achieved when the items are expressed in a standardized fashion tied closely to explicit behaviors. Whenever possible, performance is preferred over reports of behavior.

One cannot expect to totally avoid the gaming of an assessment. If the patient knows that poor performance is needed to ensure eligibility, he or she may be motivated to achieve the requisite low level. One can use some test of response bias, such as measures of social desirability, but they will not prevent gaming the system or detect all cheating.

COMPUTER TECHNOLOGY

Clinical medicine seems headed inevitably toward electronic medical records. This step could represent a major advance in the care of older people, if the opportunity is properly harnessed. Simply reproducing the current unstructured information set in a more legible and transmissible format will not suffice. Structured information provides the vehicle for assuring a more systematic evaluation and follow-up of cases. By distinguishing between missing and normal values, it can provide the structure to focus clinicians' attention on salient items.

Computer technology can dramatically reduce redundancy. Properly mobilized, computers can provide the structure needed to assure a comprehensive assessment with no duplication of effort. Because they are interactive, they can carry out much of the desired branching and can even use simple algorithms to clarify areas of ambiguity and retest areas where some unreliability is suspected. Similar algorithms can look for inconsistency to screen for cheating.

Data stored on computers can be aggregated to display performance across patients by provider (e.g., physician, nursing home, or agency). Data on a patient can be traced across time to look at changes in function and, in turn, can be aggregated.

The next important step in the progression is to move the focus from a single point of care to the linking of related elements of care. In an ideal system, patient information would be linked to permit tracing changes in status for that individual as he or she moves from one treatment modality to another. Thus, hospital admission and discharge information, long-term care information, and primary care information would be merged into a common, computer-linked record, which allows one to trace the patient's movements and status.

Finally, it would be desirable to have data on the process of care as well as the outcomes. This combination would permit analyses of what elements of care made a difference for which patients.

Such an approach to assuring quality is within our grasp if we are prepared to invest in data systems and to commit ourselves to collecting standardized information. It necessitates a shift in some of our fundamental paradigms from thinking about whether we did the right thing to deciding if it made any difference after all.

Two basic changes in thinking are necessary in order to establish an outcome-based philosophy, both of which are difficult for clinicians:

1. Thinking in the aggregate, using averages instead of examining each case; outcomes do not work well for individual cases because there is always a chance that something will go wrong, and life does not provide a control group.
2. Attributing responsibility to the whole enterprise rather than placing blame on an individual; a pattern of poor outcomes will mandate closer inspection of the process of care, but outcomes per se are a collective responsibility.

Computerized records greatly facilitate the task of monitoring the outcomes of care. Ideally, such a record system should be proactive, directing the collection of clinical information to encourage adequate coverage of relevant material. Long-term care is actually ahead of acute care in this regard, with the federal requirement for computerized versions of the MDS. Unfortunately, most of the systems in use are simply inputting mechanisms. They do not begin to tap the real potential of a computerized information system. Because long-term care depends heavily on poorly educated personnel for so much of its core services, the availability of an information support system, which can provide feedback and direction, is especially appropriate.

The computer can provide both the flexibility and the brevity sought by using branching logic to expand a category when there is reason to explore it more thoroughly. It can avoid duplication by displaying data already collected by others while still permitting the second observer to correct and challenge earlier entries. More important, it can display information to show change over time, thus permitting both the regulators and the caregivers to look at the effects of care.

Once the data are in electronic form, they are easily transmitted and manipulated. It is not hard to envision a large set of data derived from these systematic observations that would permit calculations of expected courses for different types of long-term-care patients. These could then be compared to individual patient's courses to assess the potential impact of care on outcomes.

The computer's ability to compare observed and expected outcomes extends beyond its role as a regulatory device. It could be a major source of assistance to caregivers. One of the great frustrations in long-term care, especially in the trenches, is the difficulty in sensing whether the caregiver is making a difference. Because so many patients enter care when they are already declining, the benefits of care are often best expressed as a slowing of that decline curve. Without some measure of expected course in the absence of good care, those who render care daily may not appreciate how much they are accomplishing and thereby may forgo one of the important rewards of their labors.

To display information about the change in patient condition over time, a simple task for a computer, will assist the long-term caregiver to think more in terms of the overall picture, rather than a series of separate snapshots in time. Given the computer's ability to translate data into graphics, it is a simple procedure to develop pictorial representations of the changes occurring for a given patient or group of patients and to contrast those with what might be reasonably expected.

Again the effort is directed toward changing perceptions about older persons, especially those in long-term care. For too long, long-term care has worked in a negative spiral—a self-fulfilling prophecy that expected patients to deteriorate served to discourage both care providers and patients. Such an attitude is hardly likely to attract the best and the brightest in any of the health professions. As noted earlier in this chapter, nursing home patients are among the most responsive to almost any form of intervention. Any information system that can reinforce a prospective view of long-term care, especially one that can display patient progress, represents an important adjunct to such care.

TERMINAL CARE

The physician's concern with the patient's functioning continues throughout the course of the chronic disease. Elderly patients will die. In many cases, death is not a reflection of medical failure. The approach to the dying patient will often raise difficult dilemmas. No simple answers suffice. Perhaps the best advice is not to take on the whole burden. Too often the dying patient is treated as an object. Ignored and isolated, the patient may be discussed in the third person.

Physicians must come to terms with death if they are to treat elderly patients. Often the patients are more comfortable with the subject than are their physicians. Fleeing from the dying patient is inexcusable. Dying patients need their doctors. At a very basic level, everything should be done to keep the patient as comfortable as possible. One simple step is to identify the pattern of discomforting symptoms and arrange the dosage schedule of palliatives to prevent rather than respond to the symptoms.

Patients need an opportunity to talk about their death. Not everyone will take advantage of that chance, but a surprising number will respond to a genuine offer made without time pressure. Such discussions are not conducted on the run. Often several invitations accompanied by appropriate behavior (e.g., sitting down at the bedside) are necessary.

Some physicians are unable to confront this aspect of practice. For them, the challenge is to recognize their own behavior and get appropriate help. Such help is available at various levels: help for the physician and for the patient. Groups and therapy are readily available to assist doctors to deal with their feelings. Patients of doctors who fear death need the help of other caregivers. Often other professionals—nurses, social workers—who are working with these patients already can play the lead role in helping them work through their feelings. But the active intervention of another caregiver is not justification to ignore the patient.

The rise of the hospice movement has created a growing cadre of persons and settings to help with the dying patient. The lessons coming from this experience suggest that much can be done to facilitate this stage of life, although the formal studies done to evaluate hospice care do not show dramatic benefits.

Patients should be encouraged to be as active as possible and as interactive as they wish. Even more than in other aspects of care, the unique condition of the dying patient necessitates that the physician be prepared to listen carefully to the patient and to share in decision making about how and when to do things.

SUMMARY

In many respects, geriatrics is the epitome of chronic disease care. New paradigms are needed, which recognize the changing role of patients their own care, the need to think differently about the pay-off horizons for investments in care, and how to track the course of disease to identify when intervention is needed. With geriatrics and chronic disease in general the benefits of good care may be hard to discern, because they represent a slowing of decline. This effect is invisible unless there is some basis for forming an expected clinical course against which to compare the actual course.

Physicians caring for older patients need to think in prospective terms. They will enjoy their practices more if they can learn to set reasonable goals for patients, to record progress toward these goals, and to use the failure to achieve progress as an important clinical sign of the need for reevaluation.

References

Beck A, Scott J, Williams P, et al: A randomized trial of group outpatient visits for chronically ill older HMO members: the cooperative health care clinic. *J Am Geriatr Soc* 45:543–549, 1997.

Boult C, Dowd B, McCaffrey D, et al: Screening elders for risk of hospital admission. *J Am Geriatr Soc* 41:811–817, 1993.

Clark F, Azen SP, Zemke R, et al: Occupational therapy for independent-living older adults: a randomized controlled trial. *JAMA* 278:1321–1326, 1997.

Fiatarone MA, O'Neil EF, Ryan ND, et al: Exercise training and nutritional supplementation for physical frailty in very elderly people. *N Engl J Med* 330:1769–1775, 1994.

Kane RL: The chronic care paradox. *J Aging Soc Policy* 11(2/3):107–114, 2000.

Pacala JT, Boult C, Boult L: Predictive validity of a questionnaire that identifies older persons at risk for hospital admission. *J Am Geriatr Soc* 43:374–377, 1995.

Saliba D, Elliott M, Rubenstein LZ, et al: The vulnerable elders survey: a tool for identifying vulnerable older people in the community. *J Am Geriatr Soc* 49:1691–1699, 2001.

Stuck AE, Egger M, Hammer A, Minder CE, Beck JC: Home visits to prevent nursing home admission and functional decline in elderly people: systematic review and meta-regression analysis. *JAMA* 287(8):1022–1028, 2002.

Stuck AE, Siu AL, Wieland GD, et al: Comprehensive geriatric assessment: a meta-analysis of controlled trials. *Lancet* 342:1032–1036, 1993.

Walter LC, Brand RJ, Counsell SR, et al: Development and validation of a prognostic index for 1-year mortality in older adults after hospitalization. *JAMA* 285:2987–2994, 2001.

PART II

DIFFERENTIAL DIAGNOSIS AND MANAGEMENT

CHAPTER 5

PREVENTION

GENERAL PRINCIPLES

The new and emerging generations of older people are increasingly interested in promoting healthy aging. Prevention should play a central role in that pursuit. It is hard to be against prevention, but there exists a fine line between endorsing prevention and excusing poor care. It would be a grave mistake to look to prevention as the primary answer to solving the problems of chronic care, or as an excuse for not actively addressing the need for systematic reform to meet this challenge. We do not want to end up blaming the victims, by suggesting that their disease is their own fault and hence not society's responsibility.

Ageism may lead people to discount the value of prevention in caring for older persons, but the evidence suggests that many preventive strategies are effective in this age group. To some extent, one's enthusiasm for preventive care for older persons may reflect concern about their future and the value of that future. Enthusiasm for prevention is based on beliefs about the following:

1. The efficacy of the intervention in preventing disease or dysfunction in the future. This includes an estimate of the likelihood of the patient's following the preventive regimen.
2. The value of the health gained. In the case of older patients, this includes concerns about the likelihood of other problems reducing the benefit.
3. The cost of the preventive activity. This includes both the direct cost and the indirect costs, such as anxiety, restricted lifestyle, and false-positive results.

Perhaps the most preventable problem connected with caring for older persons is iatrogenic disease. Here some of the major issues and strategies surrounding more conventional preventive activities are discussed. The major thesis here, as with much covered elsewhere in this volume, is that age alone should not be a predominant factor in choosing an approach to a patient. A number of preventive strategies deserve serious consideration in light of their immediate and future benefits for many elderly patients.

Preventive activities can be divided into three types: primary prevention, where some specific action is taken to render the patient more resistant or the environment less harmful; secondary prevention, or screening and early detection for asymptomatic disease or early disease; and tertiary prevention, or efforts to improve care to avoid later complications. All three areas are relevant to geriatric care. Table 5-1

TABLE 5-1   PREVENTIVE STRATEGIES FOR OLDER PERSONS

PRIMARY	SECONDARY	TERTIARY
Immunization	Papanicolaou (Pap) smear	Assessment
Influenza	Breast exam	Foot care
Pneumococcal	Breast self-exam	Dental care
Tetanus	Mammography	Toileting efforts
Blood pressure	Fecal blood	
Smoking	Hypothyroidism	
Exercise	Depression	
Obesity	Vision	
Cholesterol	Hearing	
Sodium	Oral cavity	
Social support	Tuberculosis	
Environment		
Seat belts		

offers examples of activities in each category. Not all the items indicated in Table 5-1 are supported by clear research findings. In some cases—such as seat belts, exercise, and social support—they are based on prudent judgment.

In addressing prevention for older persons, it is important to bear in mind the goals pursued. The World Health Organization has provided a useful continuum, which progresses from disease to impairment to disability to handicap. Preventive efforts for older people can be productively targeted at several points along this spectrum. Efforts can seek to prevent disease, but they can also be designed to minimize its consequences, by reducing the progression to disability. This is, in essence, the heart of geriatrics.

Preventive efforts on behalf of elderly patients are special, beyond the emphasis on function. The narrowing of the therapeutic window, discussed in Chap. 4, means that older persons may be susceptible to the side effects of prevention as well as of treatment. Some risk factors that strongly predict the onset of disease in younger persons may not be appropriate for modification in older persons. Perhaps the condition has already become well established and is resistant to change, or the factor may have already exerted its influence at an earlier stage of life.

Clearly, primary prevention is the most desirable. But the nature of the changes required to achieve this end vary substantially. Some require a single brief contact (e.g., immunization), but others imply sustained change in behaviors. If a brief encounter can confer some form of long-lasting protection at minimal risk, such a strategy will be actively pursued.

Many risk reduction strategies, however, require major changes in behavior, many of which are pursued because they are pleasurable. Enthusiasm for attempting to change major health behaviors, especially those that that are associated with either pleasure or addiction, is limited. Thoughtful geriatricians struggle with the overall benefit of enforcing a major life style change on someone who has both survived and has a finite life expectancy, with limited opportunities for pleasure. The task is made even harder when strong economic interests advertise the very products physicians seek to discourage.

One approach to risk reduction that fits with the predominant medical model is to transform the risk into a disease and treat it as such. For example, high blood pressure becomes hypertension; high cholesterol becomes hypercholesterolemia; thin bones become osteoporosis. When effective medications become available, as is the case in each of these scenarios, the drug companies now become active allies preaching to both the medical profession and the consumers. From a societal perspective the question becomes one of cost-effectiveness. If the medications are expensive (especially over a lifetime), how much should be spent on this prevention? Many of the calculations suggest that those strategies that involve costly medications are not cost-effective, or that the strategy must be carefully targeted to those at highest risk.

Because the number of activities that are both safe and effective is small, we must rely on the other two preventive strategies, each of which comes at a cost. Screening for one or another condition is useful where the disease process can be detected in advance of the condition's clinical appearance, but this may be excessively costly if the number of treatable cases detected is low. Screening is usually judged on the criteria of sensitivity and specificity. The former refers to the proportion of actual cases correctly identified and the latter to the accuracy of labeling of noncases (normal individuals). Alas, the two factors are usually linked, so that an improvement in one comes at the cost of a decrement in the other. The decision about where to set them relative to each other depends on the expected prevalence of the problem and the consequences of a false-positive and a false-negative finding with respect to a given clinical condition.

Tertiary prevention is a central part of good geriatric care, which strives to minimize the progression of disease to disability. It requires a comprehensive effort to address both the physiologic and environmental factors that can create dependency.

While older persons have been traditionally excluded from preventive trials, that situation is changing. As it does, findings suggest that primary prevention is appropriate for older persons as well, but the problems associated with translating the results of clinical trials into practice are at least as great as with younger persons. Active treatment of hypertension (both systolic and diastolic) is associated with reduced cardiovascular complications. Control of systolic blood pressure is associated with preventing heart failure.

Even more broadly, the value of geriatric assessment suggests that important problems in primary care of older persons are being ignored or undertreated. Reports that a yearly visit by a nurse practitioner to unselected persons aged 75 years and older can lead to substantial functional improvement and reduced nursing home admissions raise serious questions about how well the current primary care system is working. The concept of geriatric assessment has given way to a model of geriatric evaluation and management (GEM), which allows for the geriatric team to assume responsibility for the patient's care for a period sufficient to permit stabilization of the patient's condition and, in some instance, therapeutic trials. The problem still remains that when the patient is returned to the care of his or her primary care physician, the benefits of this rehabilitation may be lost unless provision is made to sustain the therapeutic changes. In the absence of this continuity, the investment represented by geriatric assessment may be threatened.

Clinicians' enthusiasm for prevention will be tempered by their ability to be paid for this work. Medicare's coverage of preventive services is modest. Table 5-2 shows the extent of this coverage.

EFFECTIVENESS OF PREVENTION IN OLDER PEOPLE

In evaluating the efficacy of preventive activities for older persons, we must confront a dilemma. Because older people were systematically excluded from many trials of prevention strategies, there are few hard data on which to base judgments. At the same time, there are strong feelings from both sides about the value of prevention. Active advocates for wellness among elderly people urge strenuous efforts to promote major life changes. They are allied with those who view many of the accoutrements of aging as acquired and hence capable of modification. They cite data showing that muscle strength and endurance can be regained with active training even at advanced ages.

Another group argues that older people have already reached a stage in life where they have demonstrated a capacity to cope. They would accept many of the consequences of aging and note that the demonstrated gains are less strongly associated with major improvements in morbidity and function than with values derived from testing.

The US Preventive Services Task Force attempted to assess available scientific information on the efficacy of preventive efforts for persons at all ages (US Preventive Services Task Force, 1996). Table 5-3 summarizes the major recommendations from the Task Force and other sources for screening activities for those age 65 years and older. Many of these recommendations are based on expert judgment in lieu of hard data. For example, in the case of foot care, although there are no formal studies to confirm the effects, clinical experience strongly suggests the benefits of podiatry in improving the ambulation of many elderly patients. Not only diabetics should receive attention to their feet; each elderly person should be carefully asked about foot pain and discomfort and checked for bunions and corns.

Appropriate treatment can do a great deal to keep such patients ambulatory and stable. The US Task Force avoided the debate about false-positive results with regard to screening for glaucoma by recommending that the decision be made by an ophthalmologist, but the importance of vision in the overall functioning of the elderly patient argues strongly for attention to this area. In a similar vein, the potential for improving function by replacing cataracts with implanted lenses mandates greater attention to visual problems as well as concern about the excess use of surgery. However, the functional benefit is not realized by cognitively impaired persons. More recent practice has shifted diabetes care attention from the usual concerns about eyes and feet to a greater appreciation about the importance of cardiovascular disease. Because of the vascular effects of diabetes, close attention should be paid to the lipid profiles of diabetics.

Some preventive interventions seem intuitively worthwhile, but occasionally data raise irksome questions. For example, vaccination against influenza is strongly recommended for older persons. Indeed, over the last several years the rate of such immunization has increased dramatically. However, ironically the rate of hospitalizations among older persons for influenza and pneumonia has also gone up during the same period, raising perplexing questions about the value of this widely lauded preventive measure.

Pneumococcal vaccines are now in widespread use, and many consider them to be useful in the care of elderly persons at risk, especially those in institutions, but there remains an active controversy about their cost-effectiveness. Tuberculosis remains a problem among older people, especially those in institutions. Special care must be taken in interpreting a lack of reaction to tuberculin skin tests in elderly persons because of the risk of anergy.

In addition to specific recommendations for preventive actions, a number of areas can be usefully examined as part of routine care. Table 5-4 offers examples of such geriatric health maintenance activities. It is important to recognize that these recommendations, as well as those from the Task Force, are intended to be carried out as part of regular primary care. No special visits for prevention are implied.

Particularly in our current system, where Medicare Part B does not pay for many preventive services, it is important to appreciate that much can be done in prevention without special visits for that purpose. Most, if not all, of the procedures can be performed by an appropriately trained nonphysician.

In some cases, care must be taken to avoid penalizing older persons on the basis of stereotypes. For example, the US Preventive Services Task Force was skeptical about the usefulness of breast self-examination in elderly women. Moreover, physicians tend to be less enthusiastic about treating older patients with breast cancer.

TABLE 5-2 PREVENTIVE SERVICES COVERED BY THE MEDICARE PROGRAM AS OF JANUARY 2002

SERVICE	YEAR FIRST COVERED	GROUPS COVERED	FREQUENCY OF SERVICE	COST-SHARING REQUIREMENTS [*]
		IMMUNIZATIONS		
Pneumococcal	1981	All beneficiaries	As needed (probably once per lifetime)	None
Hepatitis B	1984	Beneficiaries at intermediate or high risk of contracting hepatitis B	As needed (probably once per lifetime)	Copayment after deductible
Influenza	1993	All beneficiaries	Every year	None
		SCREENING SERVICES		
Cervical cancer—Papanicolaou (Pap) smear	1990	All female beneficiaries	Every 2 years	Copayment with no deductible [†]
Breast cancer—mammography	1991	Female beneficiaries age 35 to 39	One baseline	Copayment with no deductible
		Female beneficiaries age 40 and older	Mammogram this period every year	
Vaginal cancer—pelvic exam	1998	All female beneficiaries	Every 2 years [‡]	Copayment with no deductible [†]
Colorectal cancer—fecal occult blood test	1998	Beneficiaries age 50 and older	Every year	No copayment or deductible

Colorectal cancer—sigmoidoscopy§	1998	Beneficiaries age 50 and older	Every 4 years	Copayment after deductible¶
Colorectal cancer—colonoscopy§	1998	All beneficiaries	Every 10 years**	Copayment after deductible¶
Osteoporosis—bone mass measurement	1998	Estrogen-deficient female beneficiaries at clinical risk for osteoporosis as well as other qualified individuals††	Every 2 years‡‡	Copayment after deductible
Prostate cancer—prostate-specific antigen test and/or digital rectal examination	2000	Men age 50 and older	Every year	Copayment after deductible†
Glaucoma	2002	Beneficiaries medically determined to be at high risk for glaucoma	Every year	Copayment after deductible

*Applicable Medicare cost-sharing requirements generally include a 20 percent copayment after a $100 per year deductible. Each year, beneficiaries are responsible for 100 percent of the payment amount until those payments equal a specified deductible amount, $100 in 2002. Thereafter, beneficiaries are responsible for a copayment that is usually 20 percent of the Medicare approved amount. For certain tests, the copayment may be higher.

†The costs of the laboratory test portion of these services are not subject to copayment or deductible. The beneficiary is subject to a deductible and/or copayment for physician services only.

‡The exam is covered once every 12 months if the beneficiary has had an abnormality within the prior 3 years or is otherwise determined to be a high-risk candidate for cervical cancer.

§The doctor can decide to use a barium enema instead of a sigmoidoscopy or colonoscopy for beneficiaries age 50 and older. The frequency of service is the same as the sigmoidoscopy or colonoscopy it substitutes for.

¶The copayment is increased from 20 to 25 percent for services rendered in an ambulatory surgical center.

**Beneficiaries medically determined to be at high risk may receive a colonoscopy every 2 years.

††The statute defines "other qualified individuals" as those who have vertebral abnormalities or primary hyperparathyroidism, or who are receiving long-term glucocorticoid steroid or osteoporosis drug therapy.

‡‡CMS permits coverage of a bone mass measurement at any time—sooner than 2 years—if the service is medically necessary.

Source: GAO Report: GAO-02-422 *Medicare Beneficiary Use of Clinical Preventive Services,* April 2002.

TABLE 5-3   SUMMARY OF PREVENTIVE RECOMMENDATIONS FOR
             OLDER ADULTS

MANEUVER	RECOMMENDATION (SOURCE)
Screening*	
Blood pressure	Every exam, at least every 1–2 years (USPSTF, AHA)
Physician breast exam	Annually >40 (ACS, USPSTF)
Mammogram	Annually >40 (ACS) or every 1–2 years, age 50–69 (USPSTF, ACP); Continue every 1–3 years, age 70–85, in willing/appropriate patients (AGS, USPSTF)
Pelvic exam/Papanicoloau (Pap) smear	Every 2–3 years after three negative annual exams; can then ↓ or discontinue after age 65–69 (ACS, USPSTF, CTF, AGS)
Cholesterol	Adults every 5 years (NCEP, ACP, USPSTF)
Rectal exam/fecal occult blood test	Annually >50 (ACS, AHCPR, Win)
Sigmoidoscopy	Every 5 years >50 years of age or colonoscopy/BE every 10 years (ACS)
Visual acuity test	Periodically in older adults (various)
Test/inquire for hearing impairment	Periodically in older adults (various)
Mouth, nodes, testes, skin, heart, lung exams	Annually (ACS, AHA)
Glucose	Periodic in high-risk groups (USPSTF); every 3 years (ADA)
Thyroid function	Clinically prudent for elderly, especially women (USPSTF)
Electrocardiogram	Periodically > age 40–50 (AHA)
Glaucoma screening	Periodically by eye specialist > age 65 (USPSTF)
Mental/functional status	As needed; be alert for decline (USPSTF)
Osteoporosis (bone densitometry)	If needed for treatment decision (USPSTF)
Prostate exam/prostate-specific antigen	Annually > age 50 (ACS); NR [†] especially > age 70 (USPSTF, ACP)
Chest x-ray	NR/as needed (USPSTF)

TABLE 5-3   SUMMARY OF PREVENTIVE RECOMMENDATIONS FOR
OLDER ADULTS (Continued)

MANEUVER	RECOMMENDATION (SOURCE)
Prophylaxis/counseling	
Exercise	Encourage aerobic and resistance exercise as tolerated (AHA)
Tetanus-diphtheria vaccine	1° series then booster every 10 years (ACP, USPSTF)
Influenza vaccine	Annually > age 65 or chronically ill (ACP, USPSTF)
Pneumovax	23-Valent at least once > age 65 years (ACP, USPSTF)
Calcium	800–1500 mg/d (various)
Aspirin	Men > age 50, 80–325 mg/d or on alternate days (various)
Vitamin E, red wine	?

*Screening recommendations apply only to asymptomatic individuals; specific clinical circumstances may necessitate different testing and treatment schedules. Where no upper age limits are listed, screening should continue until approximately age 85 or when the patient is not a treatment candidate because of limited active life expectancy/quality.

†NR = Not recommended for routine screening in asymptomatic individuals, though may be useful when clinically indicated.

Source: From Goldberg and Chavin, 1997. Reproduced with permission of the author and updated by the author on the Internet (URL: http/members.aol.com/ TGoldberg/prevrecs.htm). Based on recommendations from American College of Physicians (ACP), American Cancer Society (ACS), American Geriatrics Society (AGS), American Heart Association (AHA), Canadian Task Force on the Periodic Health Examination (CTF), National Cholesterol Education Program (NCEP), U.S. Preventive Services Task Force (USPSTF), American Diabetes Association (ADA), Winawer SJ, Fletcher RH, Miller L: Colorectal screening clinical guidelines and rationale. Gastroenterology 112: 59–62, 1997 (Win); and the authors' interpretations of the literature.

The value of screening depends on the availability of an effective intervention and the likelihood that the intervention will change the clinical course. There is reason to believe that some cancers may perform differently in older persons. Although the incidence (and certainly the prevalence) increases with age, the rate of growth may be slower. Thus there is great controversy around the efficacy of active screening for prostate and breast cancer in older persons. The recent reanalysis of data from clinical trials of mammography illustrates

TABLE 5-4   GERIATRIC HEALTH MAINTENANCE ITEMS WORTH
                     INCLUDING IN A ROUTINE SCREENING PROGRAM

Historical information
    Tobacco

Physical examination
    Height and weight
    Blood pressure
    Hearing and vision
    Gait and fall assessment

Diagnostic tests
    Mammography
    Papanicolaou smear in underscreened women
    Flexible sigmoidoscopy

Interventions
    Aspirin therapy to prevent coronary artery disease (CAD)

Immunizations
    Influenza
    Tetanus

Source: Modified from Scheitel et al., 1996, with permission.

just how confusing this literature can be. One analysis suggested that screening with mammography after age 69 leads to a small gain in life expectancy and is modestly cost-effective (Kerlikowske et al., 1999).

At the same time, some areas are well served by increased clinical attention. Greater physician sensitivity to identifying depression in older persons can detect an often remediable condition. Detection of mental problems is greatly enhanced by structured screening data. Awareness of the likelihood of alcoholism can lead to recognizing a problem that can be corrected.

There is more controversy about the desirability of increasing the recognition of cognitive deficiency. Although standardized testing can detect cases that might otherwise be masked in older persons who have skillfully compensated for their loss, it is not immediately clear that there is great benefit in such early uncovering. Given the relatively small proportion of dementia cases that have reversible etiologies, screening for dementia would not seem to pass the first test of screening. However, some geriatricians suggest that the modest benefits of anticholinesterase therapy can gain at least months of function and postpone institutionalization, thus justifying an aggressive approach to screening. Others suggest that increasing the period of time when a person knows they have dementia may be a mixed blessing at best.

Routine screening for geriatric populations tends to uncover problems that are already known. Among a group of elderly persons coming for a health screening, 95 percent had at least one positive finding. Approximately 55 percent were referred to a physician for further evaluation and 15 percent were treated for the finding. Routine annual laboratory testing of nursing home residents has received mixed reviews. A modest panel—including a complete blood count, electrolytes, renal and thyroid function tests, and a urinalysis—may be useful.

Behavior change represents at once the most promising and the most frustrating component of prevention. While some may argue that "you can't teach an old dog new tricks" or that ingrained habit patterns are hard to break, there is no evidence to support such pessimism. Quite to the contrary, anecdotal data about elderly people taking up exercise programs and changing their dietary habits provide reason for more optimism. The critical issue here is the degree to which such changes will sufficiently modify risk factors to justify the disturbance.

In general, moderation seems safest. For example, data from the Alameda County study suggest that not smoking, modest physical activity, moderate weight, and regular meals are associated with lower mortality risks among older populations. As shown in Fig. 5-1, older persons' health habits are generally as good as or better than those of younger people. Although our data are scant, the degree of enthusiasm for active modification will likely vary with the topic addressed.

The best preventive strategies for older persons are those associated with the least risk. The findings from the Treatment on Nonpharmacological Interventions in the Elderly (TONE) study, suggesting that weight loss and sodium restriction could effectively lower blood pressure in older persons, is a good example of such

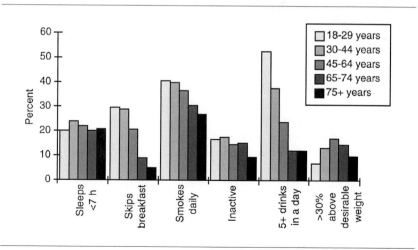

– FIGURE 5-1 – *Personal health habits of people at different ages.* (From U.S. Senate, 1991.)

an approach. Reducing dietary salt intake was shown to lower blood pressure in another study as well. Along the same lines, antioxidant vitamins have been suggested by epidemiological evidence as a means of reducing cardiovascular disease. Several studies have shown protective benefits from using vitamin E to prevent Alzheimer's disease, although the definitive data for either has not yet been seen. A recent review suggests that taking broad vitamin supplements is probably a good idea for most older people (Fletcher and Fairfield, 2002). Hormone replacement therapy (HRT) in women was widely hailed as having multiple benefits including delaying osteoporosis, lowered cholesterol, and prevention of Alzheimer's disease. However, more recent findings suggest that many of these benefits were exaggerated, and that HRT (at least a combination of estrogen and progesterone, the treatment recommended to avoid risks of uterine cancer) may actually increase risks of heart disease, Alzheimer's disease, and stroke, as well as of cancer. The discontinuance of a major trial because of modest but significant risks in several areas makes it unlikely that HRT will play a major role in any preventive program. Its role in treating postmenopausal symptoms is still under evaluation, and will likely become a decision based on risk aversion.

OSTEOPOROSIS

A good example of the conflicted nature of prevention in older persons is the case of osteoporosis. Effective treatments are now available to delay the onset or halt the progression of this disease, which can lead to fractures and disability. Understanding the management of osteoporosis requires thinking systematically about the clinical goals. In this regard, the intellectual exercise is similar to that around hypertension. The real consideration is not necessarily attacking the primary disease but its ultimate effects. In the case of osteoporosis, the adverse outcomes are fractures of various types. However, once attention shifts to the actual outcomes of importance new strategies emerge. For example, if the goal is to prevent hip fractures, wearing hip protectors may be as effective, perhaps more so, than improving bone density, because hip fracture is the combined effect of falling and osteoporosis. Indeed, several studies point to the preventive value of wearing hip protectors, although it is not easy to convince older patients, especially those with cognitive impairment, to wear such devices.

The last decade has seen the emergence of a new class of drugs to treat osteoporosis effectively and with modest side effects, but these drugs are expensive, especially over a lifetime. The first line of defense against this disease is a regimen of calcium, vitamin D, and weight-bearing exercise; but this inexpensive and safe approach may be insufficient or hard to sustain. In these instances, drugs may be indicated (although the use of the big three should be continued).

The prime targets for osteoporosis screening are postmenopausal women, but the disease can also affect men. Screening is done by bone mineral density testing. The World Health Organization standard for osteoporosis is a value of 2.5 standard deviations (SD) (often referred to as a T score) or more below the young adult mean value, but the National Osteoporosis Foundation recommends treating when T scores are ≤2 SD below the young adult mean value.

HRT is effective in delaying the course of osteoporosis, but the effects last only as long as the treatment. Given the new evidence of multiple disease risks associated with HRT, this option has effectively been removed from the osteoporosis treatment repertoire.

The class of bisphosphonates shows great promise in increasing bone mass and reducing fracture rates. The major side effects are gastrointestinal and the drugs must be taken on an empty stomach in an upright position. New weekly dosing regimens promise to reduce the side effects and the cost. The ultimate duration of this therapy is still not established. There is some evidence of a sustained effect for up to a year. A number of bisphosphonate products are emerging each year into this lucrative market, each with claims of improved benefits. In addition, other approaches are being actively explored. Nasally administered calcitonin has been tested, but sufficient advantages over bisphosphonates to justify the cost have not yet been established. An intriguing finding has been that the statins, used to treat high cholesterol, have appeared to show a positive effect on bone mass density. This therapeutic effect has not yet been tested in randomized trials. Table 5-5 compares the effectiveness of the available bisphosphonates and other potential treatments. Both bisphosphonates seem to prevent fractures by increasing bone density. Although parathyroid hormone is the most potent approach, it is not widely used because of the cost and administration problems, as well as potential side effects.

GENERIC APPROACHES

An effort to develop a more comprehensive approach to health promotion in a group of older people met with less success. The first lesson to come out of the project was that older persons have their own agenda about what is important to them and what they believe will benefit them. Even after they reached a compromise agenda that included elements both subjects and health professionals felt were valuable, the changes in functioning were not greater than those for the control group.

One area that has received considerable attention, and perhaps created confusion in the minds of both older persons and their clinicians, is exercise. Overall, there is widespread belief that exercise will benefit the individual. However, exercise is not a unidimensional activity. There are various types, and each is directed at a specific target. Table 5-6 summarizes the major types of exercise and the intended benefits of each type. Different approaches to exercise should be pursued to achieve specific goals. Although its role in osteoporosis prevention

TABLE 5-5 RELATIVE EFFECTIVENESS OF VARIOUS OSTEOPOROSIS TREATMENTS

	MEAN % CHANGE IN BONE MASS DENSITY AT 12–18 MONTHS‡		RATE OF FRACTURES		
	LUMBAR SPINE	FEMORAL NECK	VERTEBRAL	NONSPINE	HIP
Alendronate (10 mg)*	+5	+3	↓	↓	↓
Risedronate (5 mg)*	+3	+2	↓	↓	↓
Raloxifene (60 mg)	+3	+2	↓	—	—
Calcitonin (200 IU)*	+1	—	↓	—	—
Parathyroid hormone (20 mg)	+9	+4	↓	↓	—
Hormone replacement therapy‡	+4	+1	↓	↓(Ind)	↓(Ind)

*FDA-approved agent for treating postmenopausal osteoporosis.
†No longer considered a realistic option.
‡Difference between drug and placebo.
↓Direct evidence from randomized trials.
↓(Ind)Indirect evidence from observational studies.
Source: Information provided by Kristine Ensrud, MD, MPH.

TABLE 5-6   TYPES OF EXERCISE

TYPE	PURPOSE/EXPECTED BENEFIT
Aerobic/anaerobic	Cardiovascular conditioning
Resistance/weights	Strength, tone, muscle mass
Antigravity	Prevent osteoporosis
Balance	Prevent falls
Stretching	Flexibility

remains controversial, exercise is generally recommended as a safe approach, with more possible benefits than risks. Less than a third of older persons report regular exercise, to say nothing of vigorous activity. Although evidence suggests that active aerobic exercise is necessary to reduce risk of cardiovascular accidents, even modest amounts of exercise will improve strength, keep joints more limber, promote a sense of well-being, and improve sleep. Recent work has indicated that even severely compromised nursing home residents can benefit from carefully supervised and graded strength-training exercise. Both the direct benefits (e.g., improved muscle strength and activity tolerance) and indirect effects (e.g., being treated with more esteem) allowed residents to function more autonomously (Fiatarone et al., 1994).

Exercise appears to improve both overall well-being and older persons' sense of self-worth. Likewise, occupational therapy has been shown to produce beneficial results for a group of independently living older adults (Clark et al., 1997). Modest efforts at exercise can yield substantial rewards in terms of improved function and reduced use of long-term care.

Epidemiological data suggest that even among persons in their 70's, cessation of smoking will reduce mortality to levels of nonsmokers in a sufficiently short time to justify actively encouraging quitting. Smoking cessation has rapid benefits for risks of both vascular and lung disease.

There is growing enthusiasm for controlling even modest levels of both diastolic and systolic hypertension among the elderly. The European Working Party on High Blood Pressure in the Elderly showed that treatment was associated with a significant reduction in cardiac mortality, a nonsignificant reduction in cerebrovascular mortality, but no reduction in overall mortality. The results from the Systolic Hypertension in the Elderly Program (SHEP) suggest that lowering isolated systolic hypertension can lead to reduced rates of fatal and nonfatal endpoints for stroke, coronary heart disease, and cardiovascular disease.

It is important to distinguish carefully between the value of uncovering elevated blood pressure and the need to control it over a sustained period. Most older persons with hypertension are aware of it; the challenge is to maintain them in a safe range without producing significant side effects. Hypertension is very common among the elderly. Black females have the highest rates, and among white males the rate approaches 40 percent.

The effects of dietary changes are less certain. Weight loss for obese persons makes sense in terms of reducing cardiovascular load and in the management of adult-onset diabetes and hypertension, but hard data suggest that the benefit may be oversold, certainly for the former. The efficacy of changing diet, especially to reduce the amount of fat consumed, has not yet been clearly established.

Cholesterol and low-density lipoproteins (LDLs) are risk factors for heart disease for general populations, but have not been specifically tested in the elderly. However, elevated high-density lipoproteins have been shown to provide a protective factor for strokes in older people. More than 30 percent of white females have high-risk cholesterol levels (greater than 268 mg/dL). Cholesterol-lowering therapy works in older persons, as well as in the middle-aged, who were generally included in such trials. Recommendations for using lipid-lowering drugs in older patients with a history of cardiac or vascular disease are countered by other claims that cholesterol is not a significant risk factor in older persons. At the same time, only approximately 50 percent of older persons put on lipid-lowering medications remain on the regimen after 5 years. The preponderance of support now seems to favor more aggressive treatment of elevated LDL cholesterol, even in quite elderly persons (Aronow, 2002). However, many older patients do not remain on the statin therapy regimens long enough to benefit from them (Benner et al., 2002).

In areas such as weight, cholesterol, and blood pressure, the clinician must weigh the benefits of intervention against the costs (risks). There is a compelling argument that overzealous activity in the name of prevention may cost more in quality of life than it gains in quality years. Some have suggested that the survivor effect should be taken more seriously. Persons who survive to old age may have demonstrated a biological ability that deserves more respect. At the very least, any determination to change lifestyle at this stage of life should be made by the patient after suitable counseling. Nonetheless, older persons should not be denied the opportunity to actively consider the benefits of primary prevention. The growing body of evidence about at least the art of the possible imposes on clinicians a responsibility to provide them with such information.

One area of behavior with great theoretical promise but little immediate practical application is social support. There is some evidence to suggest that those older persons with strong social support systems, or at least perceived support, are at less risk for adverse events, but it is not yet clear how to build such a support system for those without one naturally. Social support likely plays at least two distinct roles: (1) Having (or perhaps just believing one has) a strong support system may reduce the risk of adverse events (through a yet-to-be-elucidated mechanism that likely involves stress). (2) For persons who are disabled and require assistance, having a real support system may prove the difference between staying in the community and needing to enter an institution. It is difficult to assess the availability of that support system in advance.

The perception, even the promise, of such support does not guarantee that the necessary support will be consistently and conveniently available when it is needed. Even well-intentioned family members may find the task too daunting to be able to maintain it.

PREVENTING DISABILITY

Although discussions of prevention tend to focus on the prevention of disease, the context of geriatrics—with its emphasis on functioning—urges a broader approach. When caring for older patients, equal attention must be paid to seeking means to keep them as active as possible. While there may be little that can be done to prevent the occurrence of a disease in an elderly person, much can be done to minimize the impact of that disease. Impairments cannot be allowed to become disabilities. Recent work in studying disability has raised new questions about the possible differences between transient and persistent disabled states. Studies that followed older people closely showed that many of them move in and out of transient states of disability. Hence, measures of disability over long periods may contain elements of both permanent and transient disability. This distinction is important because efforts to prevent disability may be falsely positive if they reflect transient conditions that would have improved on their own.

A major component of the efforts to avoid this transition are contained in geriatric assessment programs. The general approaches of such programs are reviewed in Chap. 3. It is important to note that these programs have been very varied in their composition. Table 3-1 in Chap. 3 summarizes the major randomized controlled trials using different approaches to assessment.

Work on demonstrated performance, especially when combined with timed measures is promising. This additional component provides a way to achieve more variability and may lead to better prediction. It offers a means to detect more subtle change.

The overarching goal of geriatric practice is the improvement, or at least the preservation, of patients' function. In general, function can be thought of as being determined by three principal forces: (1) the patient's overall physical health; (2) the environment; and (3) the patient's motivation. Much of the discussion in this book deals with ways to maximize the patient's health status by proper diagnosis and treatment. Such steps are necessary but not sufficient for good geriatric care. It is essential to appreciate that a person's environment can play a critical role in affecting his or her functioning. Just imagine for a minute what it would be like to be in a country where you did not speak the language or even understand its symbols. Although your capabilities are intact, you cannot function effectively. By a similar token, even after therapy has achieved its maximal effect, a patient's environment can be crucial.

Environment in this case refers to both the physical and psychological setting. It is fairly easy to imagine the physical barriers to functioning. Narrow doorways, poor lighting, and stairs can all serve as barriers.

Occupational therapists can be especially helpful in assessing the patient's environment to suggest modifications and adaptive equipment. The Appendix contains a simple environmental assessment form useful in uncovering hazards.

The psychological barriers are more subtle, but perhaps more important. They refer to the way patients are treated and, especially, the extent to which they are encouraged to do as much for themselves as they can. We noted earlier that a risk-averse environment can engender excessive dependency; so, too, can the pressure to be productive. As long as time is at a premium, care providers will be motivated to do things for patients, rather than encouraging them to perform those tasks themselves, especially if the latter course takes considerably longer. In the name of efficiency, we may be creating dependency. The efforts to encourage self-sufficiency are precisely what is usually called rehabilitation, even when it occurs in a plain wrapper.

The third element of functional effects is the patient's motivation. Today's older patients place especially high trust in their physicians, whom they view as figures of authority. Thus, one of the most subtle but nonetheless important aspects of this approach to prevention—the prevention of inactivity and despair—is the physician's attitude. For the patient, a gain in function or an ability to deal with a chronic problem is essential. It is surely no mean feat. Such behavior should be encouraged and rewarded. Indifference may be enough to discourage the patient from trying.

Other programs can be mobilized in the patient's behalf. Self-help groups are available in many communities to offer support with chronic illness, including stress management and drugless pain-control techniques. Social activity can play an essential role in maintaining function. Pets have proved to be very effective in improving morale and maintaining function.

Special efforts may be necessary to deal with members of the patient's family. Their concern over potentially dangerous accidents may lead them to become overprotective and thus exaggerate the condition of dependency.

IATROGENESIS

Probably the most important preventable problems faced by older persons today are those associated with treatment. Many iatrogenic problems result from the care that has been provided. In some cases, these problems can be traced to oversights and omissions. In other cases, overzealous care can be blamed. Some of the problem is attributable to lack of expertise in managing older persons, but a substantial portion is caused by the inevitable problems of trying to titrate therapy in an environment that is considerably less resilient to error. The more aggressive the treatment, the greater the chance that it will produce adverse effects. As noted in Chap. 4, the therapeutic window (i.e., the space between a therapeutic dose and a toxic dose) narrows with age. As the response to therapy decreases, the susceptibility to toxic side effects increases. These changes are attributable to many factors, including the ability to metabolize drugs, changes in receptor behavior, and an altered chemical environment produced by other simultaneous drugs.

This narrowing of the therapeutic window is perhaps most easily recognized in the pharmacological treatment of older patients. In the face of reduced capacity for metabolizing and excreting many drugs, the older patient can develop high blood levels on "normal" dosages. Changes in receptors may alter sensitivity to chemicals in either direction.

Many older people are at risk of drug problems. A study of community-dwelling elders found that 20 percent of older people taking medications had inappropriate elements, such as potential drug–disease interactions and excessive duration of use. Another study found that more than 20 percent of older persons were taking drugs that an expert panel had identified as inappropriate for this age group. For example, several studies have shown that thrombolytics may have serious adverse consequences when used in elderly patients with acute myocardial infarctions. Although they are actively recommended for younger victims, their use in older persons must be monitored very closely.

Use of numerous drugs transforms the elderly patient into a living chemistry set. Because of their prevalence and importance, drugs are discussed separately in Chap. 14. In this chapter we focus attention on some of the more subtle ways in which other types of treatment can adversely affect older people. In general, many drugs can be discontinued safely. One caveat, however: in the fear of over-medicating older patients, doctors may be tempted to discontinue drugs that were begun at an earlier time. While such a reevaluation is prudent, the decision to discontinue should be made carefully. One study showed that stopping long-term diuretic medications in elderly patients resulted in an exacerbation of heart failure symptoms and a rise in their blood pressure (Walma et al., 1997).

On a more philosophical plane, one can think about aging as a continuously changing relationship between an organism and its environment. As noted in Chap. 1, aging is typified by a decreased capacity to respond to stress. A person's environment can do much to reduce or create stress. Whereas a mature adult is likely to adapt to or alter the environment, the aged individual is greatly affected by changes of setting. In infancy, a person is readily influenced by his or her environment. One of the signs of maturation is the person's ability to function independently of that environment and ultimately to influence that environment. Indeed, one of the attributes that distinguishes humans from other animals is precisely this capacity to shape the environment. With increased age, the delicate balance shifts again to the point where advanced age often means that the individual is heavily affected by the environment. It is hardly surprising, then, that the elderly patient is vulnerable to the variety of stresses imposed by modern medical care. Table 5-7 lists some of the iatrogenic problems elderly patients may suffer.

SPECIAL RISKS OF HOSPITALS

Hospitals are dangerous places for any patient, as reflected in a report from the Institute of Medicine documenting the prevalence of medical errors (Kohn et al., 2000). Most of us are resilient enough to enter an acute care hospital and suffer the vicissitudes of care with the expectation that we will emerge better (certainly in the long run). The calculation of benefits received for risks undertaken needs to be more carefully thought through with older patients.

Just a little thought reveals the litany of familiar hazards of hospitalization—from the risk of nosocomial infection to getting the wrong drug to the stress of major surgery or the danger of certain diagnostic procedures. One meta-analysis estimated the high rate of adverse drug reactions in hospitalized patients in general at almost 7 percent (Lazarou et al., 1998). All these are imposed on the general hazards of bed rest discussed in Chap. 10, Table 10-2. Table 5-8 offers some examples of potential hazards in the hospital. They include problems of both overtreatment and undertreatment.

Elderly patients are more likely to experience an untoward event during a hospital stay. In part, this is because they present with more physical problems; how-

TABLE 5-7   COMMON IATROGENIC PROBLEMS OF OLDER PERSONS

Overzealous labeling
    Dementia
    Incontinence
Underdiagnosis
Bed rest
Polypharmacy
Enforced dependency
Environmental hazards
Transfer trauma

TABLE 5-8   THE HAZARDS OF HOSPITALIZATION

Diagnostic procedures
    Cardiac catheterization
    Arteriography
Therapeutic procedures
    Intravenous therapy
    Urinary catheters
    Nasogastric tube
    Dialysis
    Transfusion
Drugs
    Medication error
    Drug–drug interaction
    Drug reaction
    Drug side effect
Surgery
    Anesthesia
    Infection
    Metabolic imbalance
    Malnutrition
    Hypovolemia
Bed rest
    Hypovolemia and hypertension
    Calcium metabolism
    Fecal impaction
    Urine incontinence
    Thromboembolism
Nosocomial infection
Falls

ever, they are also more vulnerable. Table 5-9 lists patient characteristics associated with increased risk of hospital iatrogenic complications. Of these, only the first two, source of admission and condition on admission, remained significant when other factors were controlled. Because elderly patients are more likely to come from nursing homes and to be in poor condition on admission, they should be considered at high risk for iatrogenic complications.

In a study of patients hospitalized on a general medical service, the incidence of functional symptoms unrelated to diagnosis was over four times higher among patients age 70 years and older than among younger patients. Younger patients were more likely to be treated for symptoms of confusion, but older patients were more likely to be treated for problems of not eating and incontinence (Gillick, et al., 1982). Table 5-10 provides a simple rapid screening test for identifying older patients at risk of functional decline in the hospital. Delirium can be a serious problem in elderly hospitalized patients (see Chap. 6 for a discussion of this condition).

The elderly patient's vulnerability extends to a more subtle level. Admission to a hospital means entering an unfamiliar world. Moreover, the patient enters the hospital at a time of great stress. The anxiety of unknown consequences exists in addition to the physical stress of the illness.

The hospital presents physical and organizational barriers to which the patient must adapt. Not only the geography but the routines are different. The things we

TABLE 5-9   RISK FACTORS FOR IATROGENIC HOSPITAL EVENTS

Admission from nursing home or other hospital
Physician's assessment of overall condition on admission
Age
Number of drugs
Length of stay

TABLE 5-10   RISK FACTORS FOR FUNCTIONAL DECLINE IN ELDERLY HOSPITALIZED PATIENTS

Age 75+
Missing >15 of the first 21 MMSE items
Dependence in 2+ IADL prior to admission
Pressure sore
Baseline functional dependency
History of low social activity

Abbreviations: IADL, independent activities of daily living; MMSE, Mini-Mental State Examination.

Sources: Adapted from Inouye SK, Charpentier PA: Precipitating factors for delirium in hospitalized elderly persons. *JAMA* 275: 852–857, 1996; and Sager MA, Rudberg MA, Jalaloddin M, et al: Hospital admission risk profile (HARP): identifying older patients at risk for functional decline following acute medical illness and hospitalization. *J Am Geriatr Soc* 44: 251–257, 1996.

rely on to preserve our sense of identity—our clothing, our personal effects—are among the first things taken away. It is hardly surprising, then, that many elderly persons who are able to function in their familiar surroundings become disoriented and often agitated in the hospital. Just as a blind person can move flawlessly in familiar surroundings, an older person may have developed a host of adaptive mechanisms to function in his or her home situation, overcoming problems of memory loss and impaired vision.

Transferred into the sterile, rigid hospital room, such an individual may decompensate. The syndrome of "sundowning," whereby older patients in the hospital become agitated and disoriented as dusk falls, is likely a function of visual or hearing impairments, diminished sensory stimuli, and resultant disorientation.

The older person accustomed to coping with nocturia may wander at night in the dark to where the bathroom at home ought to be and wet the floor. In the crisis of urinary urgency, the patient may be unable to scale the side rails and make it to the bathroom in time. To label an individual who suffers such environmentally exacerbated accidents as incontinent is to inflict double jeopardy.

We fail to appreciate the dangers of bed rest for the elderly people. Bed is actually a very dangerous place for an older person. Besides the risk of falling out of bed, enforced immobility can produce many harms. Complications of bed rest are summarized in Table 5-11 and detailed in Chap. 10.

The hospital breeds dependency. Even with younger patients, hospital personnel are accustomed to performing basic functions for the patient. Use of the

TABLE 5-11   POTENTIAL COMPLICATIONS OF BED REST IN OLDER PERSONS

Pressure sores

Bone resorption

Hypercalcemia

Postural hypotension

Atelectasis and pneumonia

Thrombophlebitis and thromboembolism

Urinary incontinence

Constipation and fecal impaction

Decreased muscle strength

Decreased physical work capacity

Contractures

Depression and anxiety

bathroom is by prescription only. Bathing is often a supervised event. Patients are transported from one location to another. Although most of us as patients may have enjoyed being indulged for a while, we soon begin to rail against the imposed dependency. In older patients who need to be urged, encouraged, and cajoled into doing as much for themselves as possible, such an atmosphere can be especially debilitating.

Encouraging patients to act independently necessitates patience and time; unfortunately, both are scarce in the acute care hospital. It is much faster and easier to do a task for a person who performs slowly and uncertainly than to take the time to encourage that person to do that task independently. Moreover, the result of a professionally performed task is usually neater and more in keeping with hospital standards. Thus, well-meaning staff bowing to the pressures for efficiency may be inclined to do things for elderly patients rather than urging the patients to do as much as possible for themselves. This well intentioned behavior fosters dependency at a time when independent function is crucial.

The hospital is notoriously averse to risk taking. Hospital policies are designed to err on the side of caution. Such behavior can further compromise the independent functioning of older patients. Patients who are not allowed to bathe themselves or who are wheeled rather than walked are likely to become less motivated to use their full capacities. Any fears about their ability are likely to increase.

In light of the multiple adverse consequences that may be associated with hospitalizing older people, we might pause to ask why we have not done more to make hospitals more hospitable for them.

Ironically, we have invested great care in minimizing the trauma of hospitalization for children. Creativity in architecture and programs has gone into making pediatric wards as nonthreatening and homelike as possible. Although children are rarely hospitalized and geriatric patients are frequently hospitalized, no similar investment of creativity has been devoted to making the hospital less stressful for frail elderly patients. We know enough about perceptual and functional problems of aging to recognize that even simple architectural modifications can make a hospital stay easier. Use of primary colors, windows at lower heights, better-designed furniture, use of textures and patterns, and better design of rooms can all help the older patient retain maximum functioning capacity.

Special units for managing geriatric patients are beginning to emerge. Staffed by an interdisciplinary team composed of nurses, social worker, physician, and physical or occupational therapist, these units apply techniques of multidimensional functional evaluation to assess the capacity of the geriatric patient.

Likewise, the reports of geriatric assessment units that took patients who had completed a course of acute care hospitalization and were otherwise destined for a nursing home and dramatically altered both their clinical state and their long-term care course, even reducing mortality rates, suggest that much more can be done for older persons while they are in a hospital. Such geriatric units can uncover treatable conditions, provide rehabilitation to improve functional capacity, and develop a plan of care that will allow elderly patients to remain in the community.

An iatrogenic danger to the elderly patient thus lies in underdiagnosis, especially of mundane but critical conditions involving hearing, vision, and dentition. In addition, even more clinically important problems such as thyroid disease or aortic aneurysms may be overlooked unless a careful examination is performed.

LABELING

Perhaps even more dangerous than the cases of underdiagnosis are those of overdiagnosis. The physician who too readily labels a disoriented patient as senile or demented, or who classifies a urinary accident as incontinence, may be sealing the fate of that patient unnecessarily. These two diagnoses are strongly associated with an increased likelihood of nursing home admission and thus should not be made lightly.

Physicians admitting patients to nursing homes are responsible for assuring both themselves and their patients on several scores:

1. The patient truly needs care in such a setting and cannot reasonably get such care elsewhere.
2. The institution is capable of providing the needed care.
3. The patient is prepared for a transfer to the nursing home.

Too frequently, hospital discharge to the nursing home compounds the trauma. Discharge planning is often begun too late. There is insufficient time to find the best facility for the patient's needs or to allow the patient and the patient's family a sufficient role in making the decision for nursing home placement.

Good discharge planning includes at least five critical steps:

1. Adequate identification of those at risk of needing special arrangements on discharge.
2. Assessment to identify problems and strengths.
3. Determination of the risks and benefits associated with alternative modalities of care.
4. Determination of the most suitable vendor among the modality of care selected.
5. Transmission of adequate information to assure a successful transition.

Patients and their families should play an active role in steps 3 and 4. Ideally, they should make the choice after the information has been provided by professionals. In practice, this is rarely the case.

Adequate information about the risks and benefits of alternative modalities is not presented (it may not be known). No encouragement or assistance is provided to help patients and families determine precisely what outcomes they seek to maximize. Little time is allowed to weigh the complexities of the choice. When it comes to choosing among vendors of a given service, real choices may not exist because of the constraints of payment arrangements, including managed care.

As discussed in Chaps. 15 and 16, the nature of nursing home care is changing. The pressure for earlier discharges from hospitals has created a new demand for what has been termed *subacute care*—in essence, care that was formerly provided in hospitals.

SUMMARY

Many useful steps can be taken to improve and protect the health of elderly patients. The elderly patient represents a different risk:benefit ratio than the younger patient. Actions well tolerated in others may produce serious consequences in the old. Bed is a dangerous place for the older patient; confinement to bed rest should be avoided whenever possible.

The physician must guard against several potential iatrogenic problems with elderly patients. Diagnostic labels implying incurable problems (such as dementia and incontinence) should not be used until a careful search for correctable causes has been undertaken. Special attention should be given to the tendency to create dependency through well-intentioned care. By keeping in mind the need to maintain the patient's functioning, the physician can remain sensitive to the effects of the environment to enhance or impede such activity.

References

Aronow WS: Should hypercholesterolemia in older persons be treated to reduce cardiovascular events? *J Gerontol A Biol Sci Med Sci* 57A:M411–M413, 2002.

Benner JS, Glynn RJ, Mogun H et al: Long-term persistence in use of statin therapy in elderly patients. *JAMA* 288:455–461, 2002.

Clark F, Azen SP, Zemke R, et al: Occupational therapy for independent-living older adults: a randomized controlled trial. *JAMA* 278(16):1321–1326, 1997.

Fiatarone MA, O'Neill EF, Ryan ND, et al: Exercise training and nutritional supplementation for physical frailty in very elderly people. *N Engl J Med* 330(25):1769–1775, 1994.

Fletcher RH, Fairfield KM: Vitamins for chronic disease prevention in adults. *JAMA* 287:3127–3129, 2002.

Gillick MR, Serrell NA, Gillick LS: Adverse consequences of hospitalization in the elderly. *Soc Sci Med* 16:1033–1038, 1982.

Goldberg TH, Chavin SI: Preventive medicine and screening in older adults. *J Am Geriatr Soc* 43:344–354, 1997.

Gorbien M, Bishop J, Beers M, et al: Iatrogenic illness in hospitalized elderly people. *J Am Geriatr Soc* 40:1031–1042, 1992.

Kerlikowske K, Salzmann P, Phillips KA, Cauley JA, Cummings SR: Continuing screening mammography in women aged 70 to 79 years. *JAMA* 282:2156–2163, 1999.

Kohn LT, Corrigan JM, Donaldson MS (eds): *To Err is Human: Building a Safer Health System.* Washington, DC, National Academy Press, 2000.

Lazarou J, Pomeranz BH, Corey PN: Incidence of adverse drug reactions in hospitalized patients: a meta-analysis of prospective studies. *JAMA* 279:1200–1205, 1998.

Scheitel SM, Fleming KC, Chutka DS, et al: Geriatric health maintenance. *Mayo Clin Proc* 71:289–302, 1996.

Srivastava M, Deal C: Medical management and prevention of fragility fractures. *Adv Osteoporotic Fracture Manage* 1(2):34–40, 2001.

US Preventive Services Task Force: *Guide to Clinical Preventive Services: Report of the US Preventive Services Task Force,* 2nd ed. Baltimore, MD, Williams & Wilkins, 1996.

Walma EP, Hoes AW, van Dooren C, et al: Withdrawal of long-term diuretic medication in elderly patients: a double-blind randomised trial. *BMJ* 315:464–468, 1997.

Suggested Readings

Gill TM, Williams CS, Mendes de Leon CF, et al: The role of change in physical performance in determining risk for dependence in activities of daily living among nondisabled community-living elderly persons. *J Clin Epidemiol* 50:765–777, 1997.

Hanlon JT, Schmader KE, Boult C, et al: Use of inappropriate prescription drugs by older people. *J Am Geriatr Soc* 50:26–34, 2002.

Institute of Medicine: *Disability in America: Toward a National Agenda for Prevention.* Washington, DC, National Academy Press, 1991.

Ross KS, Carter HB, Pearson JD, Guess HA: Comparative efficiency of prostate-specific antigen screening strategies for prostate cancer detection. *JAMA* 284:1399–1405, 2000.

Singh MAF: Exercise comes of age: rationale and recommendations for a geriatric exercise prescription. *J Gerontol A Biol Sci Med Sci* 57A:M262–M282, 2002.

Walter LC, Covinsky KE: Cancer screening in elderly patients: a framework for decision making. *JAMA* 285:2750–2756, 2001.

Winawer SJ, Fletcher RH, Miller L: Colorectal screening clinical guidelines and rationale. *Gastroenterology* 112:59–62, 1997.

CHAPTER 6

CONFUSION: DELIRIUM AND DEMENTIA

The appropriate diagnosis and management of geriatric patients exhibiting symptoms and signs of confusion can make a critical difference to their overall health and ability to function independently. Confusion can be acute in onset, or it can be manifest by slowly progressive cognitive impairment. The major causes of confusion in the geriatric population are delirium and dementia. As more people live into the tenth decade of life, the chance that they will develop some form of dementia increases substantially. Community-based studies report a prevalence of dementia as high as 47 percent among those 85 years of age and older. Prevalence rates are, however, highly dependent on the criteria used to define dementia (Erkinjuntti et al., 1997). Between 25 and 50 percent of older patients admitted to acute care medical and surgical services are delirious on admission, or develop delirium during their hospital stay. In nursing homes, 50 to 80 percent of those older than age 65 years have some degree of cognitive impairment.

Misdiagnosis and inappropriate management of syndromes causing confusion in geriatric patients can cause substantial morbidity among the patients, hardship to their families, and millions of dollars in health care expenditure. This chapter provides a practical framework for diagnosing and managing geriatric patients who demonstrate confusion. We focus on the most common causes of confusion in the geriatric population—delirium and dementia—although a variety of other disorders can cause confusion.

DEFINING CONFUSION

Imprecise definition of the abnormalities of cognitive function in older patients labeled as "confused" has led to problems in the diagnosis and management of these patients. *Confusion* has been defined as "a mental state in which reactions to environmental stimuli are inappropriate because the person is bewildered, perplexed, or unable to orientate himself" (Stedman's Medical Dictionary, 2000). This type of definition, although descriptive, is too broad and imprecise to be clinically useful. Terms such as "confused" or "confused at times" are also imprecise. Descriptions such as "impairment of mental function" or "cognitive impairment" coupled with careful documentation of the timing and nature of specific abnormalities provide more precise and clinically useful information. Such documentation is best accomplished by means of a thorough mental status examination.

A thorough mental status examination has several basic components that are essential in diagnosing dementia, delirium, or other syndromes (Table 6-1). In evaluating older patients who appear confused, attention should focus on each of these components in a systematic manner. Recording observations in each area is critical to recognizing and evaluating changes over time. Standardized and validated measures of cognitive function such as the Mini-Mental State Examination (see Appendix), and the Time and Change Test (Inouye et al., 1998a) can be helpful screening tools in these assessments, as well as in subsequent monitoring. Several factors may influence performance and interpretation of standard mental status tests, such as prior educational level, primary language other than English, severely impaired hearing, or poor baseline intellectual function. Thus, scores on one or more of these tests should not be used to replace a more comprehensive examination that includes all the components listed in Table 6-1.

Important information can be gleaned unobtrusively from simply observing and interacting with the patient during the history. Is the patient alert and attentive? Does the patient respond appropriately to questions? How is the patient dressed and groomed? Does the patient repeat himself or herself or give an imprecise medical history, suggesting memory impairment? Orientation, insight, and judgment can sometimes be assessed during the history as well.

TABLE 6-1   KEY ASPECTS OF MENTAL STATUS EXAMINATIONS

State of consciousness

General appearance and behavior

Orientation

Memory (short- and long-term)

Language

Visuospatial functions

Executive control functions (planning and sequencing of tasks)

Other cognitive functions (e.g., calculations, proverb interpretation)

Insight and judgment

Thought content

Mood and affect

Questions relating to specific areas of cognitive functioning should be introduced in a nonthreatening manner, because many patients with early deficits respond defensively. Each of the three basic components of memory should be tested: immediate recall (e.g., repeating digits), recent memory (e.g., recalling three objects after a few minutes), and remote memory (e.g., ability to give details of early life). Language and other cognitive functions should be carefully evaluated. Is the patient's speech clear? Can the patient read (and understand) and write? Does there seem to be a good general fund of knowledge (e.g., current events)? Other cognitive functions that can be tested easily include the ability to perform simple calculations (one that relates to making change while shopping, for example) and to copy diagrams. The ability to interpret proverbs abstractly and to list the names of animals (12 names in 1 minute is normal) are sensitive indicators of cognitive function and are easy to test.

Judgment and insight can usually be assessed during the examination without asking specific questions, though input from family members or other caregivers can be helpful and sometimes necessary. Any abnormal thought content should also be noted during the examination; bizarre ideas, mood-incongruent thoughts, and delusions (especially paranoid delusions) may be prominent in older patients with cognitive impairment and are important both diagnostically and therapeutically. Observations during the examination may also detect abnormalities of executive control. Executive function involves the planning, sequencing, and executing of goal-directed activities. These functions are critical to the ability to perform instrumental activities of daily living. Screening tests for executive dysfunction, including the "EXIT" and a Clock-Drawing Test, have been developed and validated (Roman and Royall, 1999). The Clock-Drawing Test can be especially helpful in clinical practice and is performed by asking the patient to draw a clock face with a specific time. Inability to perform this test may be unsuspected and indicate a need for further evaluation.

Throughout the examination, the patient's mood and affect should be assessed. Depression, apathy, emotional liability, agitation, and aggression are common in older patients with cognitive impairment (Lyketsos et al., 2002), and failure to recognize these abnormalities can lead to improper diagnosis and management. In some patients—such as those who are very intelligent or poorly educated, or have low intelligence, as well as those in whom depression is suspected—more detailed neuropsychological testing by an experienced psychologist is helpful in more precisely defining abnormalities in cognitive function and in differentiating between the many and often interacting underlying causes.

DIFFERENTIAL DIAGNOSIS OF CONFUSION

The causes of confusion in the geriatric population are myriad. The differential diagnosis in an older patient who presents with confusion includes disorders of the brain (e.g., stroke, dementia), a systemic illness presenting atypically (e.g., infection, metabolic disturbance, myocardial infarction, congestive heart failure), sensory impairment (e.g., hearing loss), and adverse effects of a variety of drugs or alcohol.

Similar to many other disorders in geriatric patients, confusion often results from multiple interacting processes rather than a single causative factor. Accurate diagnosis depends on specifically defining abnormalities in mental status and cognitive function and on consistent definitions for clinical syndromes. Disorders causing confusion in the geriatric population can be broadly categorized into three groups:

1. Acute disorders, usually associated with acute illness, drugs, and environmental factors (i.e., delirium).
2. More slowly progressive impairment of cognitive function as seen in most dementia syndromes.
3. Impaired cognitive function associated with affective disorders and psychoses.

Old age alone does not cause impairment of cognitive function of sufficient severity to render an individual dysfunctional. Mild, recent memory loss and slowed thinking and reaction time are common. The prognostic and therapeutic implications of mild cognitive impairment are subjects of intensive research. Older patients are often labeled "senile" because they are unable to answer a question or because they are not given adequate time to respond. Other age-associated disorders such as impaired hearing can also lead to mislabeling an older patient as "confused" or "senile."

Three questions are helpful in making an accurate diagnosis of the underlying cause(s) of confusion:

1. Has the onset of abnormalities been acute (i.e., over a few hours or a few days)?
2. Are there physical factors (i.e., medical illness, sensory deprivation, drugs) that may contribute to the abnormalities?
3. Are psychological factors (i.e., depression and/or psychosis) contributing to or complicating the impairments in cognitive function?

These questions focus on identifying treatable conditions, which, when diagnosed and treated, might result in substantially improved cognitive function.

DELIRIUM

Delirium is an acute or subacute alteration in mental status especially common in the geriatric population. The prevalence of delirium in hospitalized geriatric patients is approximately 15 percent on admission (Francis, 1992), and the incidence in this setting may be up to one-third (Inouye et al., 1996; Schor et al., 1992). In the past, a variety of labels have been used to describe delirious patients (including acute confusional state, acute brain syndrome, metabolic encephalopathy, and toxic psychosis). The *Diagnostic and Statistical Manual of Mental Disorders* (DSM-IV-TR) (American Psychiatric Association, 2000) defines diagnostic criteria for delirium (Table 6-2). The key features of this disorder include the following:

- Disturbance of consciousness
- Change in cognition not better accounted for by dementia
- Symptoms and signs developing over a short period of time (hours to days)
- Fluctuation of the symptoms and signs
- Evidence that the disturbances are caused by the physiological consequences of a medical condition

The disturbances of consciousness and attention, with the suddenness of onset and the fluctuating cognitive status, are the major features that distinguish delirium from other causes of impaired cognitive function. Delirium is characterized by difficulty in sustaining attention to external and internal stimuli, sensory misperceptions (e.g., illusions), and a fragmented or disordered stream of thought. Disturbances of psychomotor activity (such as restlessness, picking at bedclothes, attempting to get out of bed, sluggishness, drowsiness, and generally decreased psychomotor activity) and emotional disturbances (anxiety, fear, irritability, anger, apathy) are very common in delirious patients. Neurological signs (except

TABLE 6-2   DIAGNOSTIC CRITERIA FOR DELIRIUM

1. Disturbance of consciousness (that is, reduced clarity of awareness of the environment) in conjunction with reduced ability to focus, sustain, or shift attention

2. A change in cognition (such as memory deficit, disorientation, or language disturbance) or the development of a perceptual disturbance that is not better accounted for by a preexisting, established, or evolving dementia

3. Development of the disturbance during a brief period (usually hours to days) and a tendency for fluctuation during the course of the day

4. Evidence from the history, physical examination, or laboratory findings that the disturbance is caused by:
   a. A general medical condition
   b. A substance intoxication, side effect, or withdrawal

Source: From the American Psychiatric Association, 2000, with permission.

asterixis) are uncommon in delirium. Many hospitalized patients have delirium on only a single day, but the severity and time course of delirium varies considerably. Many factors predispose geriatric patients to the development of delirium, including impaired sensory functioning and sensory deprivation, sleep deprivation, immobilization, transfer to an unfamiliar environment, and psychosocial stresses such as bereavement.

Among hospitalized geriatric patients, several factors are associated with the development of delirium (Schor et al., 1992; Inouye and Charpentier, 1996), including:

- Age greater than 80 years
- Male sex
- Preexisting dementia
- Fracture
- Symptomatic infection
- Malnutrition
- Addition of three or more medications
- Use of neuroleptics and narcotics
- Use of restraints
- Bladder catheters

Rapid recognition of delirium is critical because it is often related to other reversible conditions and its development may be a poor prognostic sign for adverse outcomes including nursing home placement and death (Inouye et al., 1998b). Inouye and colleagues described a strategy to identify delirium, termed the Confusion Assessment Method (CAM) (Inouye et al., 1990). The diagnosis of delirium by the CAM requires the presence of:

- Acute onset and fluctuating course *and*
- Inattention *and*
- Disorganized thinking *or*
- Altered level of consciousness

It is also important to differentiate delirium from dementia, because the latter is not immediately life-threatening, and inappropriately labeling a delirious patient as demented may delay the diagnosis of serious and treatable conditions. It is not possible to make the diagnosis of dementia when delirium is present in a patient with previously normal or unknown cognitive function. The diagnosis of dementia must await the treatment of all of the potentially reversible causes of delirium, as discussed below. Table 6-3 shows some of the key clinical features that are helpful in differentiating delirium from dementia. *Sundowning* is a term that describes an increase in confusion which commonly occurs in geriatric patients, especially those with preexisting dementia, at night. This condition is probably related to sensory deprivation in unfamiliar surroundings (such as the acute care hospital) and patients who "sundown" may actually meet the criteria for delirium.

TABLE 6-3 KEY FEATURES DIFFERENTIATING DELIRIUM FROM DEMENTIA

FEATURE	DELIRIUM	DEMENTIA
Onset	Acute, often at night	Insidious
Course	Fluctuating, with lucid intervals, during day; worse at night	Generally stable over course of day
Duration	Hours to weeks	Months to years
Awareness	Reduced	Clear
Alertness	Abnormally low or high	Usually normal
Attention	Hypoalert or hyperalert, distractible; fluctuates over course of day	Usually normal
Orientation	Usually impaired for time, tendency to mistake unfamiliar for familiar place and persons	Often impaired
Memory	Immediate and recent impaired	Recent and remote impaired
Thinking	Disorganized	Impoverished
Perception	Illusions and hallucinations (usually visual) relatively common	Usually normal
Speech	Incoherent, hesitant, slow or rapid	Difficulty in finding words
Sleep–wake cycle	Always disrupted	Often fragmented sleep
Physical illness or drug toxicity	Either or both present	Often absent, especially in Alzheimer's disease

Source: From Lipkowski, 1987, with permission.

A complete list of conditions that can cause delirium in the geriatric population would be too long to be useful in a clinical setting. Table 6-4 lists some of the common causes of this disorder. Several of them deserve further attention. Each geriatric patient who becomes acutely "confused" should be evaluated to rule out treatable conditions such as metabolic disorders, infections, and causes for decreased cardiac output (i.e., dehydration, acute blood loss, heart failure). Sometimes this workup is unrevealing. Small cortical strokes, which do not produce focal symptoms or signs, can cause delirium. These events may be difficult or impossible to diagnose with certainty, but there should be a high index of suspicion for this diagnosis in certain subgroups of patients—especially those with a history of hypertension, previous strokes, transient ischemic attacks, or cardiac arrhythmias. If delirium recurs, a source of emboli should be sought and associated conditions (such as hypertension) should be treated optimally. Fecal impaction and urinary retention, common in geriatric patients (especially those in acute care hos-

TABLE 6-4   COMMON CAUSES OF DELIRIUM IN GERIATRIC PATIENTS

Metabolic disorders
    Hypoxia
    Hypercarbia
    Hypo- or hyperglycemia
    Hyponatremia
    Azotemia

Infections

Decreased cardiac output
    Dehydration
    Acute blood loss
    Acute myocardial infarction
    Congestive heart failure

Stroke (small cortical)

Drugs (see Table 6-5)

Intoxication (alcohol, other)

Hypo- or hyperthermia

Acute psychoses

Transfer to unfamiliar surroundings (especially when sensory input is diminished)

Other
    Fecal impaction
    Urinary retention

TABLE 6-5   DRUGS THAT CAN CAUSE OR CONTRIBUTE TO DELIRIUM
AND DEMENTIA*

Analgesics	Cardiovascular
Narcotic	Antiarrhythmics
Nonnarcotic	Digoxin
Nonsteroidal antiinflammatory agents	H_2 receptor antagonists
Anticholinergics/antihistamines	Psychotropic drugs
Anticonvulsants	Antianxiety drugs
Antihypertensives	Antidepressant drugs
Antimicrobials	Antipsychotics
	Sedative/hypnotics
Antiparkinsonism drugs	Skeletal muscle relaxants
	Steroids

* See AHCPR guidelines (Costa et al., 1996) and *Medical Letter*, 2002, for a more
complete list.

pitals), can have dramatic effects on cognitive function and may be causes of acute
confusion. The response to relief from these conditions can be just as impressive.

Drugs are a major cause of acute as well as chronic impairment of cognitive
function in older patients (Medical Letter, 2002). Table 6-5 lists commonly prescribed drugs that can cause or contribute to delirium. Every attempt should be made
to avoid or discontinue any medication that may be worsening cognitive function in
a delirious geriatric patient. Environmental factors, especially rapid changes in location (such as being hospitalized, going on vacation, or entering a nursing home) and
sensory deprivation, can precipitate delirium. This is especially true of those with
early forms of dementia (see below). Measures such as preparing older patients for
changes in location, placing familiar objects in the surroundings, and maximizing
sensory input with lighting, clocks, and calendars may help prevent or manage delirium in some patients. A "Hospital Elder Life Program" has been described that may
help prevent delirium, and cognitive and functional decline among high risk older
patients in acute hospitals (Inouye et al., 2000). This program incorporates several
strategies for identifying potentially reversible causes of delirium and medical
behavioral and environmental interventions for patients who develop delirium.

DEMENTIA

Dementia is a clinical syndrome involving a sustained loss of intellectual
functions and memory of sufficient severity to cause dysfunction in daily living.
Its key features include:

- A gradually progressing course (usually over months to years)
- No disturbance of consciousness

Dementia in the geriatric population can be grouped into two broad categories:

1. Reversible or partially reversible dementias
2. Nonreversible dementias

Reversible Dementias

While it is especially important to rule out treatable and potentially reversible causes of dementia in individual patients, these dementias account for fewer than 20 percent of all causes of dementia in most series (Costa et al., 1996; Clarfield, 1988). Moreover, finding a reversible cause does not guarantee that the dementia will improve after the putative cause has been treated.

Table 6-6 lists causes of reversible dementia. These disorders can be detected by careful history, physical examination, and selected laboratory studies. Drugs known to cause abnormalities in cognitive function (see Table 6-5) should be discontinued whenever feasible. There should be a high index of suspicion regarding excessive alcohol intake in older patients. The incidence of alcohol consumption varies considerably in different populations but is easily missed and can cause dementia as well as delirium, depression, falls, and other medical complications.

One particular disorder, *depressive pseudodementia*, deserves special emphasis. This term has been used to refer to patients who have reversible or partially

TABLE 6-6   CAUSES OF POTENTIALLY REVERSIBLE DEMENTIAS

Neoplasms	Autoimmune disorders
Metabolic disorders	Central nervous system vasculitis, temporal arteritis
Trauma	Disseminated lupus erythematosus
Toxins	Multiple sclerosis
Alcoholism	Drugs (see Table 6-5)
Heavy metals	Nutritional disorders
Organic poisons	Psychiatric disorders
Infections	Depression
	Other disorders (e.g., normal-pressure hydrocephalus)

Sources: From Costa et al., 1996, and Katzman et al., 1988, with permission.

reversible impairments of cognitive function caused by depression. Depression may coexist with dementia in more than one-third of outpatients with dementia, and in an even greater proportion in nursing homes. The interrelationship between depression and dementia is complex. Many patients with early forms of dementia become depressed. Sorting out how much of the cognitive impairment is caused by depression and how much by an organic factor(s) can be difficult. Some clinical characteristics can be helpful in diagnosing depressive pseudodementia, including prominent complaints of memory loss, patchy and inconsistent cognitive deficits on exam, and frequent "don't know" answers. Detailed neuropsychological testing, performed by a psychologist or other health care professional skilled in the use of these tools, can be helpful in many patients. At times, even after a complete assessment, uncertainty still exists regarding the role of depression in producing intellectual deficits. Under these circumstances, a careful trial of antidepressants (in rare instances, electroconvulsive therapy) is justified to facilitate the diagnosis and may help improve overall (but not cognitive) functioning. Older patients who develop reversible cognitive impairment while depressed appear at relatively high risk for developing dementia over the following few years, and their cognitive function should be followed closely over time.

Nonreversible Dementias

Several different classifications have been recommended for the nonreversible dementias. The Agency for Health Care Policy and Research (AHCPR) guideline on Alzheimer's and related dementias (Costa et al., 1996) lists four basic categories, based on the work of Katzman et al. (1988) (Table 6-7):

1. Degenerative diseases of the central nervous system
2. Vascular disorders
3. Trauma
4. Infections

Alzheimer's disease, other degenerative disorders, and vascular dementias account for a vast majority of dementias in the geriatric population, and are the focus of discussion in this chapter.

Alzheimer's and Other Degenerative Diseases   Alzheimer's disease accounts for close to two-thirds of dementias in the geriatric population. Dementia with Lewy bodies (DLB) accounts for up to 25 percent of dementias in some series, and may overlap with Alzheimer's and Parkinson's dementia (Small et al., 1997; McKeith et al., 1996). In addition to the characteristic pathological findings, DLB is characterized by

* Detailed visual hallucinations

TABLE 6-7   CAUSES OF NONREVERSIBLE DEMENTIAS

Degenerative diseases
    Alzheimer's disease
    Dementia associated with Lewy bodies
    Parkinson's disease
    Pick's disease
    Huntington's disease
    Progressive supranuclear palsy
    Others

Vascular dementias
    Occlusive cerebrovascular disease (multiinfarct dementia)
    Binswanger's disease
    Cerebral embolism(s)
    Arteritis
    Anoxia secondary to cardiac arrest, cardiac failure of carbon monoxide
        intoxication

Traumatic dementia
    Craniocerebral injury
    Dementia pugilistica

Infections
    Acquired immunodeficiency syndrome
    Opportunistic infections
    Creutzfeldt-Jakob disease
    Progressive multifocal leukoencephalopathy
    Postencephalitic dementia

Sources: From Costa et al., 1996, and Katzman et al., 1988, with permission.

• Parkinsonian signs
• Alterations of alertness and attention

Table 6-8 lists the diagnostic criteria for Alzheimer's disease (AD). Family history and increasing age are the primary risk factors for AD. Approximately 6 to 8 percent of persons older than age 65 have AD. The prevalence doubles every 5 years, so that nearly 30 percent of the population older than age 85 has AD. By the age of 90, almost 50 percent of persons with a first-degree relative suffering from AD might develop the disease themselves. Rare genetic mutations on chromosomes 1, 14, and 21 cause early onset familial forms of AD, and some forms of late-onset AD are linked to chromosome 12 (Small et al., 1997). The strongest genetic linkage with late-onset AD identified thus far is the apolipoprotein E epsilon-4 (APOE-E4) allele on chromosome 19.

TABLE 6-8   DIAGNOSTIC CRITERIA FOR ALZHEIMER'S DEMENTIA

A. The development of multiple cognitive deficits manifested by both:
  1. Memory impairment (impaired ability to learn new information or to recall previously learned information)
  2. One (or more) of the following cognitive disturbances:
     a. Aphasia (language disturbance)
     b. Apraxia (impaired ability to perform motor activities despite intact motor function)
     c. Agnosia (failure to recognize or identify objects despite intact sensory function)
     d. Disturbance in executive functioning (that is, planning, organizing, sequencing, abstracting)
B. The cognitive deficits cause severe impairment in social or occupational functioning and represent a major decline from a previous level of functioning
C. The course is characterized by gradual onset and continuing cognitive decline
D. The cognitive deficits are not due to any of the following:
  1. Other central nervous system conditions that cause progressive deficits in memory and cognition (e.g., cerebrovascular disease, Parkinson's disease, Huntington's disease, subdural hematoma, normal-pressure hydrocephalus, brain tumor)
  2. Systemic conditions known to cause dementia (for example, hypothyroidism, vitamin deficiencies, hypercalcemia, neurosyphilis, HIV infection)
E. The deficits do not occur exclusively during the course of a delirium
F. The disturbance is not better accounted for by another axis I disorder (for example, major depressive disorder, schizophrenia)

Source: From the American Psychiatric Association, 2000, with permission.

The relative risk of AD associated with one or more copies of this allele in whites is approximately 2.5. However, APOE-E4 does not appear to confer increased risk for AD among African Americans or Hispanics. One study suggests, however, that the cumulative risks of AD to age 90 in the general population, adjusted for education and sex, are four times higher for African Americans and two times higher for Hispanics than for whites (Tang et al., 1998). Because the presence of one or more APOE-E4 alleles is neither sensitive nor specific, there is disagreement on recommending it as a screening test for AD (Small et al., 1997; Mayeux et al., 1998). Until more sensitive and specific tests become available, routine screening, even among high-risk populations, is generally not recommended.

Other possible risk factors for AD include previous head injury, female sex, lower education level, and other yet-to-be-identified susceptibility genes. Possible protective factors include the use of estrogen, antioxidants, and nonsteroidal antiinflammatory drugs. The clinical significance of these possible protective effects, however, remains to be proven.

Vascular Dementias   Vascular dementias, predominately caused by multiple infarcts *(multiinfarct dementia),* account for approximately 15 percent of dementia in the geriatric population. Multiinfarct dementia can occur alone or in combination with other disorders that cause dementia. Autopsy studies suggest that cerebrovascular disease may play an important role in the presence and severity of symptoms of AD (Snowdon et al., 1997). Multiinfarct dementia results when a patient has sustained recurrent cortical or subcortical strokes. Many of these strokes are too small to cause permanent or residual focal neurological deficits or evidence of strokes on computed tomography (CT). Magnetic resonance imaging (MRI) may be more sensitive in detecting small infarcts, but there has been a tendency to overinterpret some of these findings as more MRI scans are being done. Table 6-9 identifies characteristics of patients likely to have multiinfarct dementia and compares the clinical characteristics of primary degenerative and multiinfarct dementias. A key feature of multiinfarct dementia is the stepwise deterioration in cognitive functioning, as illustrated in Fig. 6-1. Another form of vascular form of dementia has been described, termed *senile dementia of the Binswanger type,* which may be impossible to differentiate clinically from multiinfarct dementia. It has become increasingly important to differentiate vascular from other dementias because patients with the former may benefit from more aggressive treatment of hypertension and other cardiovascular risk factors (Forette et al., 2002; Murray et al., 2002), whereas new pharmacological treatments for AD may not help patients with vascular forms of dementias.

EVALUATION

The AHCPR practice guideline (Costa et al., 1996) and a consensus statement of the American Association of Geriatric Psychiatry, the Alzheimer's Association, and the American Geriatrics Society (Small et al., 1997) have updated recommendations for the evaluation of patients suspected of having a dementia syndrome. The first step is to recognize clues that dementia may be present. Table 6-10 lists symptoms that should suggest further evaluation. Patients suspected of having dementia should undergo the following:

- Focused history and physical examination, including assessment for delirium and depression and identification of comorbid conditions (e.g., sensory impairment, physical disability)

TABLE 6-9   ALZHEIMER'S DISEASE VERSUS MULTIINFARCT DEMENTIA: COMPARISON OF CLINICAL CHARACTERISTICS

CHARACTERISTICS	ALZHEIMER'S DISEASE	MULTIINFARCT DEMENTIA
Demographic		
Sex	Women more commonly affected	Men more commonly affected
Age	Generally over age 75 years	Generally over age 60 years
History		
Time course of deficits	Gradually progressive	Stuttering or episodic, with stepwise deterioration
History of hypertension	Less common	Common
History of stroke(s), transient ischemic attack(s), or other focal neurological symptoms	Less common	Common
Examination		
Hypertension	Less common	Common
Focal neurological signs	Uncommon	Common
Signs of atherosclerotic cardiovascular disease	Less common	Common
Emotional lability	Less common	More common

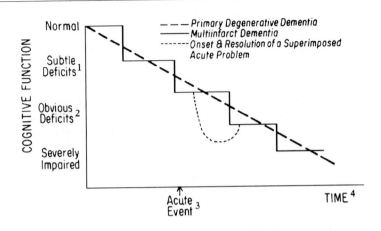

— FIGURE 6-1 —   *Primary degenerative dementia versus multiinfarct dementia: comparison of time courses. [1] Recognized by patient, but only detectable on detailed testing. [2] Deficits recognized by family and friends. [3] See text for explanation. [4] Exact time courses are variable; see text.*

- A functional status assessment (see Chap. 3)
- A mental status examination (see above and Table 6-1)
- Selected laboratory studies to rule out reversible dementia and delirium

Table 6-11 outlines key aspects of the history. Because many physical illnesses and drugs can cause cognitive dysfunction, active medical problems and use of prescription and nonprescription drugs (including alcohol) should be reviewed. The nature and severity of the symptoms should be characterized. What are the deficits? Does the patient admit to them or is the family member describing them? How is the patient reacting to the problems? The responses to these questions can be helpful in differentiating between dementia and depressive pseudodementia. The onset of symptoms and the rate of progression are particularly important. The sudden onset of cognitive impairment (over a few days) should prompt a search for one of the underlying causes of delirium listed in Table 6-4. Irregular, stepwise decrements in cognitive function (as opposed to a more even and gradual loss) favor a diagnosis of multiinfarct dementia (see Table 6-9 and Fig. 6-1). Patients with dementia are often brought for evaluation at a time of sudden worsening of cognitive function (as illustrated by the broken line in Fig. 6-1) and may even meet the criteria for delirium. These sudden changes may be triggered by a number of acute events (a small stroke without focal signs, acute physical illness, drugs, changes in environment, or personal loss such as the death or departure of a relative). Only a careful history (or familiarity with the patient) will

TABLE 6-10 SYMPTOMS THAT MAY INDICATE DEMENTIA

- Learning and retaining new information
  Is repetitious; has trouble remembering recent conversations, events, appointments; frequently misplaces objects.
- Handling complex tasks
  Has trouble following a complex train of thought or performing tasks that require many steps, such as balancing a checkbook or cooking a meal.
- Reasoning ability
  Is unable to respond with a reasonable plan to problems at work or home, such as knowing what to do if the bathroom is flooded; shows uncharacteristic disregard for rules of social conduct.
- Spatial ability and orientation
  Has trouble driving, organizing objects around the house, finding his or her way around familiar places.
- Language
  Has increasing difficulty with finding the words to express what he or she wants to say and with following conversations.
- Behavior
  Appears more passive and less responsive, is more irritable than usual, is more suspicious than usual, misinterprets visual or auditory stimuli.

Source: From Costa et al., 1996, with permission.

help to determine when an acute event has been superimposed on a preexisting dementia. Appropriate management of the acute event will, in many instances, result in improvement in cognitive function (see Fig. 6-1, broken line).

The history should also include specific questions about common problems requiring special attention in patients with dementia. These problems may include wandering, dangerous driving and car crashes, disruptive behavior (e.g., verbal agitation, physical aggression, and nighttime agitation), delusions or hallucinations, insomnia, poor hygiene, malnutrition, and incontinence. They require careful management and most often substantial involvement of family or other caregivers.

A social history is especially important in patients with dementia. Living arrangements and social supports should be assessed. Along with functional status, these factors play a major role in the management of patients with dementia and are of critical importance in determining the necessity for institutionalization. A patient with dementia and weak social supports may require institutionalization at a higher level of function than will a patient with strong social supports. In addition to the lack of availability of a spouse, child, or other relative who can

TABLE 6-11   EVALUATING DEMENTIA: THE HISTORY

Summarize active medical problems and current physical complaints
List drugs (including over-the-counter preparations and alcohol)
Cardiovascular and neurological history
Characterize the symptoms
 Nature of deficits (memory versus other cognitive functions)
 Onset and rate of progression
 Impaired function (e.g., managing money or medications)
 Associated psychological symptoms
  Depression
  Anxiety or agitation
  Paranoid ideation
  Psychotic thought processes (delusions and/or hallucinations)
Ask about special problems
 Wandering (and getting lost)
 Dangerous driving and car crashes
 Disruptive or self-endangering behaviors
 Verbal agitation
 Physical aggression
 Insomnia
 Poor hygiene
 Malnutrition
 Incontinence
Assess the social situation
 Living arrangements
 Social supports
 Availability of relatives and other caregivers
 Employment and health of caregivers

serve as a caregiver, the caregiver's employment and/or poor health can play an important role in determining the need for institutional care.

A general physical examination should focus particularly on cardiovascular and neurological assessment. Hypertension and other cardiovascular findings and focal neurological signs (such as unilateral weakness or sensory deficit, hemianopsia, Babinski reflex) favor a diagnosis of multiinfarct dementia. Pathological reflexes (such as the glabellar sign and grasp, snout, and palmomental reflexes) are nonspecific and occur in many forms of dementia as well as in a small proportion of normal aged persons. These frontal lobe release signs—as well as impaired stereognosis or graphesthesia, gait disorder, and abnormalities on cerebellar testing—are significantly more common in patients with Alzheimer's disease than in age-matched controls. Parkinsonian signs (tremor, bradykinesia, muscle rigidity) should be sought because they may indicate either dementia associated with Lewy bodies or frank Parkinson's disease.

A careful mental status examination (see Table 6-1) and a standardized mental status test should be performed. Although practice guidelines indicate that no single test is clearly superior, the Mini-Mental State Examination and the Time and Change Test are rapid tests that can be used in clinical practice (see Appendix). Neuropsychological testing can be helpful when there is a normal mental status score but also functional and/or behavioral changes (this can occur in patients with high baseline intelligence) or when there is a low score without functional deficits (this can occur in patients with lower educational levels). Neuropsychological testing can also be helpful in differentiating depression and dementia and in pinpointing specific cognitive strengths and weaknesses for patients, families, and health providers.

Selected diagnostic studies are useful in ruling out reversible forms of dementia (Table 6-12). Although CT and MRI scans of the head are expensive, many clinicians and experts order one of these tests for patients with dementia of recent onset in whom no other clinical findings explain the dementia and in those with focal neurological signs or symptoms. Cerebral atrophy on one of these scans

TABLE 6-12   EVALUATING DEMENTIA: RECOMMENDED DIAGNOSTIC
             STUDIES

Blood studies
  Complete blood count
  Glucose
  Urea nitrogen
  Electrolytes
  Calcium and phosphorous
  Liver function tests
  Thyroid stimulating hormone
  Vitamin B_{12} and folate
  Serologic test for syphilis
  Human immunodeficiency virus antibodies (if suspected)
Radiographic studies
  Computed tomography (or magnetic resonance imaging) of the head
Other studies
  Neuropsychological testing (selected patients; see text)

does not establish the diagnosis of Alzheimer's disease; it can occur with normal aging as well as with several specific disease processes. The scan is thus recommended to rule out treatable causes (e.g., subdural hematoma, tumors, normal-pressure hydrocephalus). CT and MRI each have advantages and disadvantages. They are roughly equivalent in the detection of most remediable structural lesions. MRI will demonstrate more lesions than CT in patients with multiinfarct dementia, but will also demonstrate white matter changes of uncertain clinical significance (Small et al., 1997). Position emission tomography (PET) scanning is increasingly available, but remains largely a research tool. PET scanning quantitates glucose metabolism and reveals decreases in specific areas (e.g., frontotemporal) that are highly associated with Alzheimer's disease. PET scan abnormalities can precede the development of clinical deficits by several years in patients at risk for Alzheimer's disease.

MANAGEMENT OF DEMENTIA

General Principles

Although complete cure is not available for the vast majority of dementias, optimal management can provide improvements in the ability of these patients to function, as well as in their overall well-being and that of their families and other caregivers. Table 6-13 outlines key principles for the management of dementia.

If causes of reversible or partially reversible forms of dementia are identified (see Table 6-6), they should be specifically treated. Small strokes (lacunar infarcts), which can cause further deterioration of cognitive function in patients with AD, as well as those with vascular dementia, may be prevented by controlling hypertension; thus hypertension should be aggressively treated in patients with dementia as long as side effects can be avoided. Other specific diseases such as Parkinson's disease should be optimally managed. The treatment of these and other medical conditions is especially challenging because treatment (usually drugs) may have adverse effects on cognitive function.

Pharmacological Treatment of Dementia

There are three basic approaches to the pharmacological treatment of dementia:

1. Agents that enhance cognition and function
2. Drug treatment of coexisting depression

TABLE 6-13   KEY PRINCIPLES IN THE MANAGEMENT OF DEMENTIA

Optimize the patient's function
   Treatment underlying medical conditions (e.g., hypertension, Parkinson's disease)
   Avoid use of drugs with central nervous system side effects (unless required for management of psychological or behavioral disturbances— see Chap. 14)
   Assess the environment and suggest alterations if necessary
   Encourage physical and mental activity
   Avoid situations stressing intellectual capabilities; use memory aids whenever possible
   Prepare the patient for changes in location
   Emphasize good nutrition
Identify and manage complications
   Wandering
   Dangerous driving
   Behavioral disorders
   Depression (see Chap. 7)
   Agitation or aggressiveness
   Psychosis (delusions, hallucinations)
   Malnutrition
   Incontinence (see Chap. 8)
Provide ongoing care
   Reassessment of cognitive and physical function
   Treatment of medical conditions
Provide medical information to patient and family
   Nature of the disease
   Extent of impairment
   Prognosis
Provide social service information to patient and family
   Local Alzheimer's Association
   Community health care resources (day centers, homemakers, home health aides)
   Legal and financial counseling
   Use of advance directives
Provide family counseling for
   Identification and resolution of family conflicts
   Handling anger and guilt
   Decisions on respite or institutional care
   Legal concerns
   Ethical concerns (see Chap. 17)

3. Pharmacological treatment of complications such as paranoia, delusions, psychoses, and agitation (verbal and physical)

Drug treatment of depression is discussed in detail in Chap. 7. Pharmacological treatments including antipsychotics and sedatives are discussed in Chap. 14.

The primary pharmacological approach to the treatment of AD has been the use of cholinesterase inhibitors. Some evidence suggests that these drugs are also effective for DLB and multiinfarct dementia. There are four approved drugs of this class on the market (tacrine, donepezil, rivastigmine, and galantamine). Randomized, placebo-controlled clinical trials suggest that these drugs can have clinically important positive effects on cognitive function, and may improve or prevent decline in overall function and potentially delay nursing home admission. Tacrine is potentially hepatotoxic, and is generally not prescribed for this reason. No studies have compared the other three drugs in this class to each other. Gastrointestinal side effects can be problematic and include nausea, vomiting, and diarrhea. On the other hand, the benefits of these drugs include slight improvements in cognitive function (e.g., generally less than 3 points on a Mini-Mental State Exam), improvements in behavior, and a substantial several month delay in the progression of cognitive impairment and the development of related behavioral symptoms.

Other drugs, including estrogen (in women), vitamin E, ginkgo biloba, and nonsteroidal antiinflammatory agents, are commonly used to prevent dementia. There is, however, no evidence that these drugs are effective in preventing or treating dementia (most evidence suggests they are not). The role of these agents in preventing dementia is under active investigation. Many geropsychiatrists and geroneurologists do prescribe vitamin E in addition to a cholinesterase inhibitor for patients with new onset and early dementia.

Nonpharmacological Management

A variety of supportive measures and other nonpharmacological management techniques are useful in improving the overall function and well-being of patients with dementia and their families (see Table 6-13). These interventions range from specific recommendations for caregivers, such as alterations in the physical environment, the use of memory aids, the avoidance of stressful tasks, and preparation for the patient's move to another living setting with a higher level of care, to more general techniques, such as providing information and counseling services. Many nursing homes have developed "special care units" for dementia patients. With few exceptions, however (Rovner et al., 1996), there is little evidence that such units improve outcomes (Phillips et al., 1997). Assisted-living facilities are now establishing specialized dementia units, with optimally designed environments, trained staff, and intensive activities programming, and without the more hospital-like environment typical of many nursing homes.

The provision of ongoing care is especially important in the management of dementia patients. Reassessment of the patient's cognitive abilities can be helpful in identifying potentially reversible causes for deteriorating function and in making specific recommendations to family and other caregivers. The family is the primary target of strategies to help manage dementia patients in noninstitutional settings. Caring for relatives with dementia is physically, emotionally, and financially stressful. Information on the disease itself and the extent of impairment and on community resources helpful in managing these patients can be of critical importance to family and caregivers. The local chapter of the Alzheimer's Association and the Area Agency on Aging are examples of community resources that can provide education and linkages with appropriate services. Anticipating and teaching family members strategies to cope with common behavioral problems associated with dementia—such as wandering, incontinence, day–night reversal, and nighttime agitation—can be of critical importance. Hazardous driving that can result in car crashes is an especially troublesome problem. Several states now require reporting patients with dementia who maintain drivers' licenses. There remain, however, no validated methods of assessing driving capabilities and safety among individuals with early dementia. Wandering may be especially hazardous for the dementia patient's safety and is associated with falls. Incontinence is common and often very difficult for families to manage (see Chap. 8). Books providing information and suggestions for family management techniques are very useful (see Suggested Readings). Support groups for families of patients with Alzheimer's disease through the Alzheimer's Association are available in most large cities. Family counseling can be helpful in dealing with a variety of issues such as anger, guilt, decisions on institutionalization, handling the patient's assets, and terminal care. Dementia patients and their families should also be encouraged to discuss and document their wishes, using a durable power of attorney for health care or an equivalent mechanism early in the course of the illness (see Chap. 17). Family members should be encouraged to seek respite care periodically to provide time for themselves. Some communities have formal respite care programs available. In the absence of such programs, informal arrangements can often be made to relieve the primary family caregivers for short periods of time at regular intervals. Such relief will help the caregiver to cope with what is generally a very stressful situation. Often a multidisciplinary group of health professionals—made up of a physician, a nurse, a social worker, and, when needed, rehabilitation therapists, a lawyer, and a clergy member—must coordinate efforts to manage these patients and provide support to family and caregivers.

References

American Psychiatric Association: *Diagnostic and Statistical Manual of Mental Disorders,* 4th ed., Text Revision. Washington, DC, APA, 2000.

Clarfield AM: The reversible dementias: do they reverse? *Ann Intern Med* 109:476–186, 1988.

Costa PT Jr, Williams TF, Somerfield M, et al: *Recognition and Initial Assessment of Alzheimer's Disease and Related Dementias.* Clinical Practice Guideline No. 19. Rockville, MD, US Department of Health and Human Services, Public Health Service, Agency for Health Care Policy and Research. AHCPR Publication No. 97–0702. November 1996.

Erkinjuntti T, Ostbye T, Steenhuis R, et al: The effect of different diagnostic criteria on the prevalence of dementia. *N Engl J Med* 337:1667–1674, 1997.

Forette F, Seux M-L, Staessen JA, et al: The prevention of dementia with antihypertensive treatment. *Arch Intern Med* 162:2046–2052, 2002.

Francis J: Delirium in older patients. *J Am Geriatr Soc* 40:829–838, 1992.

Inouye SK, Bogardus ST, Baker DI, Leo-Summers L, Cooney LM: The hospital elder life program: a model of care to prevent cognitive and functional decline in older hospitalized patients. *J Am Geriatr Soc* 48:1697–1706, 2000.

Inouye SK, Charpentier PA: Precipitating factors of delirium in hospitalized elderly persons: predictive model and interrelationship with baseline vulnerability. *JAMA* 275:852–857, 1996.

Inouye SK, Robison JT, Froehlich TE, Richardson ED: The time and change test: a simple screening test for dementia. *J Gerontol A Biol Sci Med Sci* 53A(4):M281–M286, 1998a.

Inouye SK, Rushing JT, Foreman MD, Palmer RM, Pompei P: Does delirium contribute to poor hospital outcomes? *J Gen Intern Med* 13:234–242, 1998b.

Inouye SK, van Dyck CH, Alessi CA, et al: Clarifying confusion: the confusion assessment method: a new method for detection of delirium. *Ann Intern Med* 113:941–948, 1990.

Katzman R, Lasker B, Bernstein N: Advances in the diagnosis of dementia: accuracy of diagnosis and consequences of misdiagnosis of disorders causing dementia, in Terry RD (ed): *Aging and the Brain,* 17–62. New York, Raven Press, 1988.

Lipowski ZJ: Delirium (acute confusional states). *JAMA* 258:1789–1792, 1987.

Lyketsos CG, Lopez O, Jones B, et al: Prevalence of neuropsychiatric symptoms in dementia and mild cognitive impairment. *JAMA* 288(12):1475–1483, 2002.

Mayeux R, Saunders AM, Shea S, et al: Utility of the apolipoprotein E genotype in the diagnosis of Alzheimer's disease. *N Engl J Med* 338:506–511, 1998.

McKeith LG, Galasko D, Kosaka K, et al: Consensus guidelines for the clinical and pathologic diagnosis of dementia with Lewy bodies (DLB): report on the consortium of DLB international workshop. *Neurology* 47:1113–1124, 1996.

Medical Letter: Drugs that may cause psychiatric symptoms. *Med Lett* 44(1134):59–62, 2002.

Murray MD, Lane KA, Gao S, et al: Preservation of cognitive function with antihypertensive medications. *Arch Intern Med* 162:2090–2096, 2002.

Phillips C, Sloane P, Hawes C, et al: Effects of residence in Alzheimer disease special care units on functional outcomes. *JAMA* 278:1340–1344, 1997.

Roman GC, Royall DR: Executive control function: a rational basis for the diagnosis of vascular dementia. *Alzheimer Dis Assoc Disord* 13:S69–S80, 1999.

Rovner BW, Steele CD, Shmuely Y, Folstein MF: A randomized trial of dementia care in nursing homes. *J Am Geriatr Soc* 44:7–13, 1996.

Schor JD, Levkoff SE, Lipsitz LA, et al: Risk factors for delirium in hospitalized elderly. *JAMA* 267:827–831, 1992.

Small GW, Rabins PV, Barry PP, et al: Diagnosis and treatment of Alzheimer disease and related disorders. *JAMA* 278:1363–1371, 1997.

Snowdon DA, Greiner LH, Mortimer JA, et al: Brain infarction and the clinical expression of Alzheimer's disease: the nun study. *JAMA* 277:813–817, 1997.

Stedman's Medical Dictionary, New York, Lippincott Williams & Wilkins, 2000.

Tang MX, Stern Y, Marder K, et al: The ApoE-E4 allele and the risk of Alzheimer disease among African Americans, whites, and Hispanics. *JAMA* 279:751–755, 1998.

Suggested Readings

Cohen-Mansfield J: Nonpharmacologic interventions for inappropriate behaviors in dementia. *Am J Geriatr Psychiatry* 9:361–381, 2001.

Geldmacher DS, Whitehouse PJ: Evaluation of dementia. *N Engl J Med* 335:330–336, 1996.

Gomez-Tortosa E, Ingraham AO, Irizarry MC, Hyman BT: Dementia with Lewy bodies. *J Am Geriatr Soc* 46:1449–1458, 1998.

Mace NL (ed): Dementia care: patient, family and community. Baltimore, MD, Johns Hopkins University Press, 1990.

Martin JB: Molecular basis of the neurodegenerative disorders. *N Engl J Med* 340(25):1970–1980, 1999.

Mayeux R, Sano M: Treatment of Alzheimer's disease. *N Engl J Med* 341(22):1670–1679, 1999.

Silverman DHS, Small GW, Chang CY, et al: Positron emission tomography in evaluation of dementia: regional brain metabolism and long-term outcome. *JAMA* 286(17):2120–2127, 2001.

Williams ME: *The American Geriatrics Society's Complete Guide to Aging and Health.* New York, American Geriatrics Society, 1995.

CHAPTER 7

DIAGNOSIS AND MANAGEMENT OF DEPRESSION

Depression is probably the most common example of the nonspecific and atypical presentation of illness in the geriatric population. The signs and symptoms of depression can be the result of a variety of treatable physical illnesses or the presenting manifestations of a major or minor depressive episode. Frequently, depression and physical illness(es) coexist in older patients. Thus, it is not surprising that treatable depressions are often overlooked in geriatric patients with physical illnesses and that treatable physical illnesses are often not managed optimally in geriatric patients diagnosed as having depression.

Sorting out the complex interrelationships between symptoms and signs of depression caused by physical illnesses and those caused primarily by an affective disorder or related psychiatric diagnosis challenges individuals caring for the geriatric population. Recognition and appropriate management of the onset or recurrence of geriatric depression are critical for improving quality of life and function, as well as for potentially preventing medical morbidity, optimizing health care use, and forestalling premature death. This chapter addresses these issues from the perspective of the nonpsychiatrist, recognizing that the optimal management of most of these patients should involve psychiatrists and psychologists experienced with and interested in the geriatric population.

AGING AND DEPRESSION

Symptoms and signs of depression are common in the geriatric population. The prevalence of major depression among community-dwelling older people is 1 to 2 percent, and an additional 2 percent suffer from dysthymia (a chronic depressive disorder characterized by functional impairment and at least 2 years of depressive symptoms). The prevalence of subsyndromal depression (i.e., symptoms of depression that do not meet standard criteria for major depression) approaches 25 percent (Lebowitz et al., 1997). The prevalence of these conditions is even higher among geriatric patients in acute care hospitals and nursing homes. Major depression is found in up to 22 percent and other depressive syndromes in up to 28 percent of acutely hospitalized older patients (Koenig, 1997). Among institutionalized older persons, major depression is found in close to 15 percent, with another 15 to 20 percent having depressive symptoms; incidence rates of these disorders in nursing homes are in a similar range (Rovner et al., 1991; Parmalee et al., 1992a). Depression is highly associated with mortality in the nursing home population (Rovner et al., 1991; Parmalee et al., 1992b). Suicide is disturbingly common in the geriatric population and its incidence continues to increase. Older white males have the highest rate of suicide—up to six times that in the general population (Lebowitz et al., 1997). Several factors are associated with suicide in the geriatric population (Table 7-1).

Several biological, physical, psychological, and sociological factors predispose older persons to depression (Table 7-2). Aging changes in the central nervous system, such as changes in neurotransmitter concentrations (especially catecholaminergic neurotransmitters), may play a role in the development of geriatric depression. Research is focusing on the central nervous system effects of cytokines, cortisol production, inflammation, and other immune responses, and the role these effects may play in the genesis of depression among medically ill geriatric patients (Lebowitz et al., 1997).

The incidence of several specific diseases associated with symptoms of depression, the prevalence of chronic medical conditions, and the frequency of medication usage increase with age. Each of these factors can predispose older people to depression. Vascular disease in particular may play an important role in geriatric depression. Depressed geriatric patients often have comorbid vascular disorders accompanied by lesions in the basal ganglia and prefrontal areas of the brain. These patients commonly display motor retardation, lack of insight, and impairment of executive functions (Lebowitz et al., 1997).

Other psychosocial factors also predispose older people to depression. Losses are common in the geriatric population. Physical losses can mean a reduction in the ability for self-care, often leading to loss of independence; markedly reduced sensory capacities (especially vision and hearing) can result in isolation and sensory deprivation. Both can play a role in the development of depression. Memory loss and loss of other intellectual functions (dementia) are commonly associated with depression (see Chap. 6). Losses of job, income, and social supports (especially the death of family members and friends) increase with age and can predispose older people to bereavement and frank depression.

SYMPTOMS AND SIGNS OF DEPRESSION

Many common symptoms and signs can represent depression in geriatric patients. Several factors may make these difficult to interpret.

TABLE 7-1   FACTORS ASSOCIATED WITH SUICIDE IN THE GERIATRIC POPULATION

FACTOR	HIGH RISK	LOW RISK
Sex	Male	Female
Religion	Protestant	Catholic or Jewish
Race	White	Nonwhite
Marital status	Widowed or divorced	Married
Occupational background	Blue-collar low-paying job	Professional or white-collar job
Current employment status	Retired or unemployed	Employed full or part time
Living environment	Urban	Rural
	Living alone	Living with spouse or
	Isolated	other relatives
	Recent move	Living in close-knit neighborhood
Physical health	Poor health	Good health
	Terminal illness	
	Pain and suffering	
Mental health	Depression (current or previous)	Happy and well adjusted
	Alcoholism	Positive self-concept
	Low self-esteem	and outlook
	Loneliness	Sense of personal
	Feeling rejected, unloved	control over life
Personal background	Broken home	Intact family of origin
	Dependent personality	Independent, assertive,
	History of poor interpersonal relationships	flexible personality
		History of close
	Family history of mental illness	friendships
		No family history of
	Poor marital history	mental illness
	Poor work record	No previous suicide attempts
		No history of suicide in family
		Good marital history
		Good work record

Source: From Osgood, 1985, with permission.

TABLE 7-2   FACTORS PREDISPOSING OLDER PEOPLE TO DEPRESSION

Biological
    Family history (genetic predisposition)
    Prior episode(s) of depression
    Aging changes in neurotransmission

Physical
    Specific diseases (see Table 7-5)
    Chronic medical conditions (especially with pain or loss of function)
    Exposure to drugs (see Table 7-6)
    Sensory deprivation (loss of vision or hearing)
    Loss of physical function

Psychological
    Unresolved conflicts (e.g., anger, guilt)
    Memory loss and dementia
    Personality disorders

Social
    Losses of family and friends (bereavement)
    Isolation
    Loss of job
    Loss of income

- Aging changes, as well as several common medical conditions, can lead to the physical appearance of depression, even when depression is not present.
- Nonspecific physical symptoms (such as fatigue, weakness, anorexia, diffuse pain) may represent a variety of treatable medical illnesses as well as depression.
- Specific physical symptoms, relating to every major organ system, can represent depression as well as physical illness in geriatric patients.
- Depression can exacerbate symptoms of coexisting physical illnesses.

The physical appearance of older patients suspected of being depressed should be interpreted cautiously. Aging changes such as graying and loss of hair, wrinkled skin, loss of teeth (with altered facial architecture), stooped posture, and slowed gait can present an image of depression. Several medical conditions can further emphasize the physical appearance of depression. Parkinson's disease, which manifests itself by masked facies, bradykinesia, and stooped posture, can be misinterpreted as depression. Patients with presbycusis may appear withdrawn and disinterested simply because they cannot hear enough of normal conversation to participate actively; therefore they withdraw out of frustration. The psychomotor retardation of hypothyroidism may offer the physical appearance of depression. Systemic illnesses—such as disseminated tuberculosis, malignancy, and malnutrition (alone or resulting from a medical condition)—can produce a depressed appearance. Moreover, true depression commonly accompanies many of these medical conditions in geriatric patients (Small et al., 1996; Koenig, 1997).

Symptoms must also be interpreted very cautiously. Many different symptoms can represent depression, physical illness, or a combination of both. Table 7-3 lists several examples of somatic symptoms that may actually represent, or be exacerbated by, depression in older patients. Depression presenting primarily with physical symptoms, which as been termed *masked depression,* is especially common in the geriatric population for several reasons. Many of today's older generation were

TABLE 7-3   EXAMPLES OF PHYSICAL SYMPTOMS THAT CAN REPRESENT DEPRESSION

SYSTEM	SYMPTOM
General	Fatigue
	Weakness
	Anorexia
	Weight loss
	Anxiety
	Insomnia (see Table 7-4)
	"Pain all over"
Cardiopulmonary	Chest pain
	Shortness of breath
	Palpitations
	Dizziness
Gastrointestinal	Abdominal pain
	Constipation
Genitourinary	Frequency
	Urgency
	Incontinence
Musculoskeletal	Diffuse pain
	Back pain
Neurological	Headache
	Memory disturbance
	Dizziness
	Paresthesias

raised in an atmosphere that inhibited the expression of emotion. Finding direct expression of feelings of sadness, guilt, and anger difficult, they may somaticize these emotions and complain of physical symptoms. In addition, many older persons with diminished sensory input from losses of vision, hearing, or touch may overrespond to internal cues (such as their heartbeat and gastrointestinal motility) and focus on these concerns when they are feeling anxious and depressed.

Insomnia is an example of a very common yet nonspecific symptom in the geriatric population. Although it is one of the key symptoms in diagnosing different forms of depression, a variety of factors may underlie this complaint (Table 7-4).

TABLE 7-4   KEY FACTORS IN EVALUATING THE COMPLAINT OF INSOMNIA

Sleep disturbance should be carefully characterized
  Delayed sleep onset
  Frequent awakenings
  Early morning awakenings

Physical symptoms can underlie insomnia (from patient and bed partner)
  Symptoms of physical illnesses
    Pain from musculoskeletal disorders
    Orthopnea, paroxysmal nocturnal dyspnea or cough
    Nocturia
    Gastroesophageal reflux
  Symptoms suggestive of periodic leg movements
  Symptoms suggestive of sleep apnea
    Loud or irregular snoring
    Awakening sweating, anxious, tachycardiac
    Excessive movement
    Morning drowsiness

Aging changes occurring in sleep patterns
  Increased sleep latency
  Decreased time in deeper stages of sleep
  Increased awakenings

Behavioral factors can affect sleep patterns
  Daytime naps
  Earlier bedtime

Medications can affect sleep
  Hypnotic withdrawal
  Alcohol (causes sleep fragmentation)

Persistent complaints of sleep disturbance are, in fact, associated with depression among community-dwelling older people. In addition to depression, insomnia may be caused by other psychiatric disorders as well as several types of medical problems. For example, orthopnea and nocturia caused by congestive heart failure, abdominal discomfort from reflux esophagitis, or anxiety and restlessness from hyperthyroidism can underlie the complaint of insomnia. A careful history should help identify these and other medical conditions that might be contributing to the problem. Insomnia can also be caused by the effects of (or withdrawal from) several types of drugs and alcohol. As more older patients with sleep disturbances have undergone detailed analysis (including continuous observation during sleep and monitoring by polysomnography), other conditions have been detected, including sleep apnea and periodic leg movements. As much as one-third of the geriatric population may have a specific sleep disorder. Obstructive sleep apnea is the most common of these disorders and results not only in complaints of insomnia but also in nighttime hypoxia with associated risks for cardiac arrhythmias and myocardial and cerebral infarction. Specific symptoms, which are often elicited from the bed partner, should prompt consideration for referral to a sleep center, because hypnotics may exacerbate the conditions. Other more specific treatments are available, including continuous positive airway pressure, dental appliances, and uvulopalatopharyngoplasty. Aging itself is associated with changes in sleep patterns, such as daytime naps, early bedtime, increased time until onset of sleep, decreases in the absolute and relative amounts of the deeper stages of sleep, and increased periods of wakefulness, which could contribute to the complaint of insomnia. Thus there is a lengthy differential diagnosis of insomnia in the older patient; the complaint should not be attributed simply to aging or depression and treated with a sedating antidepressant or hypnotic before other potential causes are considered.

DEPRESSION ASSOCIATED WITH MEDICAL CONDITIONS

Symptoms and signs of depression are associated with medical conditions in the geriatric population in several ways.

- Some diseases can result in the physical appearance of depression, even when depression is not present (e.g., Parkinson's disease).
- Many diseases can either directly cause depression or elicit a reaction of depression. The latter is especially true of conditions that cause or produce fear of chronic pain, disability, and dependence.
- Drugs used to treat medical conditions can cause symptoms and signs of depression.
- The environment (factors such as isolation, sensory deprivation, forced dependency) in which medical conditions are treated can predispose to depression.

Depression among older patients with medical illnesses is associated with high levels of functional impairment (Covinsky et al., 1997) and health care costs (Unutzer et al., 1997). A wide variety of physical illnesses can present with or be accompanied by symptoms and signs of depression (Table 7-5). Any medical condition associated with systemic involvement and metabolic disturbances can have profound effects on mental function and affect. The most common among these are fever, dehydration, decreased cardiac output, electrolyte disturbances, and hypoxia. Hyponatremia (whether from disease process or drugs) and hypercalcemia (associated especially with malignancy) may also cause older patients to appear depressed. Systemic diseases, especially malignancies and endocrine disorders, are often associated with symptoms of depression. Depression—accompanied by anorexia, weight loss, and back pain—is commonly present in patients with cancer of the pancreas. Among the endocrine disorders, thyroid and parathyroid conditions are most commonly accompanied by symptoms of depression. Most hypothyroid patients manifest psychomotor retardation, irritability, or depression. Hyperthyroidism may also present as withdrawal and depression in older patients—so-called apathetic thyrotoxicosis. Hyperparathyroidism, with attendant hypercalcemia, can simulate depression and is often manifest by apathy, fatigue, bone pain, and constipation. Other systemic physical conditions—such as infectious diseases, anemia, and nutritional deficiencies—can also have prominent manifestations of depression in the geriatric population.

Because cardiovascular and nervous system diseases are among the most threatening and potentially disabling, they can precipitate symptoms of depression. Myocardial infarction, with attendant fear of shortened life span and restricted lifestyle, commonly precipitates depression. Stroke is often accompanied by depression, but the depression may not always correlate with the extent of physical disability. Patients in whom stroke has produced substantial disability (e.g., hemiparesis, aphasia) can become depressed in response to their loss of function; others whose stroke has produced only minor degrees of physical disability (but in theory may have affected areas of the brain controlling emotion) can also become depressed. Other causes of brain damage, especially in the frontal lobes, such as tumors and subdural hematomas, can also be associated with depression. Older individuals with dementia, both Alzheimer's and multiinfarct dementia, may have prominent symptoms of depression (see Chap. 6). Patients with Parkinson's disease also have a high incidence of clinically diagnosed depression. Depression that develops in response to the chronic pain, loss of function and self-esteem, dependence, and fear of death that accompany physical illness can become severe. Many older individuals who commit suicide have an active physical illness at the time of death.

Symptoms of depression are often caused not only by physical illness but also by the treatment of medical conditions. A variety of psychological responses to hospitalization (including depression) have been observed in older

TABLE 7-5   MEDICAL ILLNESSES ASSOCIATED WITH DEPRESSION

Metabolic disturbances
    Dehydration
    Azotemia, uremia
    Acid–base disturbances
    Hypoxia
    Hypo- and hypernatremia
    Hypo- and hyperglycemia
    Hypo- and hypercalcemia
Endocrine
    Hypo- and hyperthyroidism
    Hyperparathyroidism
    Diabetes mellitus
    Cushing's disease
    Addison's disease
Infections
Cardiovascular
    Congestive heart failure
    Myocardial infarction
Pulmonary
    Chronic obstructive lung disease
    Malignancy
Gastrointestinal
    Malignancy (especially pancreatic)
    Irritable bowel
Genitourinary
    Urinary incontinence
Musculoskeletal
    Degenerative arthritis
    Osteoporosis with vertebral compression or hip fracture
    Polymyalgia rheumatica
    Paget's disease
Neurologic
    Dementia (all types)
    Parkinson's disease
    Stroke
    Tumors
Other
    Anemia (of any cause)
    Vitamin deficiencies
    Hematologic or other systemic malignancy

Source: From Levenson and Hall, 1981, with permission.

patients. Isolation, sensory deprivation, and immobilization, common in hospitalized patients with physical illness, can cause or contribute to depressive symptoms. Iatrogenic complications such as fecal impaction and urinary retention or incontinence can also cause psychological symptoms, including those of depression. Drugs are the most common cause of treatment-induced symptoms and signs of depression. Although a wide variety of pharmacologic agents can produce symptoms of depression (Table 7-6), antihypertensive agents and sedatives are probably the most common drugs that cause symptoms and signs of depression in the geriatric population (Medical Letter, 2002). The mechanisms by which various drugs cause these effects differ and are poorly understood in many instances. Some drugs—such as alcohol, sedatives, antipsychotics, and antihypertensives—have direct effects on the central nervous system. Thus, depressive symptoms, especially new symptoms, should raise a high index of suspicion about the role of drug and/or alcohol abuse. Whenever possible, drugs that can potentially produce these symptoms should be discontinued.

TABLE 7-6   DRUGS THAT CAN CAUSE SYMPTOMS OF DEPRESSION

Antihypertensives	Psychotropic agents
Angiotensin-converting enzyme	Sedatives
inhibitors	Barbiturates
Clonidine	Benzodiazepines
Hydralazine	Meprobamate
Propranolol	Antipsychotics
Reserpine	Chlorpromazine
Analgesics	Haloperidol
Narcotics	Thiothixene
Antiparkinsonism drugs	Hypnotics
Levodopa	Chloral hydrate
Antimicrobials	Benzodiazepines
Sulfonamides	Steroids
Isoniazid	Corticosteroids
Cardiovascular preparations	Estrogens
Digitalis	Others
Diuretics	Antiepileptics
Lidocaine	Alcohol
Hypoglycemic agents	Cancer chemotherapeutic agents
	Cimetidine

Source: After Levenson and Hall, 1981, with permission, and the Medical Letter, 2002.

DIAGNOSING DEPRESSION

In view of the prevalence of symptoms and signs of depression in the geriatric population; aging changes that may complicate the diagnosis; and the interrelationship between depression and its signs and symptoms, medical illnesses, and treatment effects—how is the diagnosis of depression made?

Several general principles are helpful.

- Questions that screen for depressive symptoms, or the use of a depression scale, may be helpful in identifying depressed geriatric patients. However, somatic components of many depression scales are less useful in older patients because of the high prevalence of physical symptoms and medical illnesses.
- Nonspecific or multiple somatic symptoms that are suggestive of depression should not be diagnosed as such until physical illnesses have been excluded.
- Somatic symptoms unexplained by physical findings or diagnostic studies, especially those of relatively sudden onset in an older person who is not usually hypochondriacal, should raise the suspicion of depression.
- Drugs used to treat medical illnesses (see Table 7-6), sedatives, hypnotics, and alcohol abuse should be considered as potential causes for symptoms and signs of depression.
- Standard diagnostic criteria should be the basis for diagnosing various forms of depression in the geriatric population, but several differences may distinguish depression in older, as opposed to younger, patients.
- Major depressive episodes should be differentiated from other diagnoses such as uncomplicated bereavement, bipolar disorder, dysthymic disorder, minor depression, and adjustment disorders with a depressed mood.
- Consultation with experienced geriatric psychiatrists and/or psychologists should be obtained whenever possible to help diagnose and manage depressive disorders.
- Whenever there is uncertainty about the diagnosis, a judicious (but adequate) therapeutic trial of an antidepressant can be very helpful.

Several differences in the presentation of depression can make the diagnosis much more challenging and difficult in older people, as compared to younger people (Table 7-7). The most common clinical problem is differentiating major depressive episodes from other forms of depression. Table 7-8 outlines the criteria for major depression. Table 7-9 lists some of the key features that can aid in distinguishing major depression from other conditions. In addition, as much as 25 percent of community-dwelling and 50 percent of medically ill older patients and nursing home residents suffer from minor or "subsyndromal depression." While the depressive symptoms may not be as

TABLE 7-7   SOME DIFFERENCES IN THE PRESENTATION OF DEPRESSION IN THE OLDER POPULATION, AS COMPARED WITH THE YOUNGER POPULATION

1. Somatic complaints, rather than psychological symptoms, often predominate in the clinical picture.
2. Older patients often deny having a dysphoric mood.
3. Apathy and withdrawal are common.
4. Feelings of guilt are less common.
5. Loss of self-esteem is prominent.
6. Inability to concentrate, with resultant impairment of memory and other cognitive functions, is common (see Chap. 6).

severe as in major depression, they are associated with the development of major depression, physical disability, and heavy use of health services (Lebowitz et al., 1997).

Like the early stages of dementia, depression may go unrecognized unless specific questions are asked. Many older patients who commit suicide have been seen by their physicians within the previous few weeks. At a minimum, all geriatric patients should periodically be asked such a screening question. Specific questions about other common depressive symptoms can also be added to the system review (e.g., sleep disturbance, appetite changes, trouble concentrating, lack of energy, loss of interest). Positive responses should be followed up by further questioning, especially about suicidal ideation. Table 7-10 provides examples of screening questions. A commonly used depression scale is provided in the Appendix.

Because of the overlap of symptoms and signs of depression and physical illness and the close association between many medical conditions and depression, older patients presenting with what appears to be a depression should have physical illnesses carefully excluded.

This can almost always be accomplished by a thorough history, physical examination, and basic laboratory studies (Table 7-11). Other diagnostic studies can provide helpful objective data in patients with persistent somatic symptoms that are difficult to distinguish from psychosomatic complaints (e.g., masked depression). For example, echocardiography and radionuclide cardiac scans can help rule out organic heart disease as a basis for chest pain, fatigue, and dyspnea. Pulmonary function tests can exclude intrinsic lung disease as a cause for chronic shortness of breath. A new complaint of constipation may be related to

TABLE 7-8 SUMMARY CRITERIA FOR MAJOR DEPRESSIVE EPISODE

A. Five (or more) of the following symptoms have been present nearly every day during the same 2-week period and represent a change from previous functioning: at least one is either (1) depressed mood or (2) loss of interest or pleasure. Symptoms that are clearly caused by a general medical condition should not be counted.

(1) Depressed mood most of the day

(2) Markedly diminished interest or pleasure in all, or almost all, activities most of the day

(3) Significant weight loss when not dieting or weight gain, or decrease or increase in appetite

(4) Insomnia or hypersomnia

(5) Psychomotor agitation or retardation

(6) Fatigue or loss of energy

(7) Feelings of worthlessness or excessive or inappropriate guilt (which may be delusional)

(8) Diminished ability to think or concentrate, or indecisiveness

(9) Recurrent thoughts of death (not just fear of dying), recurrent suicidal ideation without a specific plan, or a suicide attempt or a specific plan for committing suicide

The symptoms

B. Do not meet criteria for a mixed episode.

C. Cause clinically significant stress or impairment in social, occupational, or other important areas of functioning.

D. Are not due to the direct physiological effects of a substance or a general medical condition.

E. Are not better accounted for by bereavement, the symptoms persist for longer than 2 months or are characterized by marked functional impairment, morbid preoccupation with worthlessness, suicidal ideation, psychotic symptoms, or psychomotor retardation.

Source: Adapted from American Psychiatric Association, 2000.

TABLE 7-9   MAJOR DEPRESSION VERSUS OTHER FORMS OF DEPRESSION

DIAGNOSTIC CLASSIFICATION	KEY FEATURES DISTINGUISHING FROM MAJOR DEPRESSION
Bipolar disorders	The patient may meet, or have met in the past, criteria for major depression but is having or has had one more manic episode; the latter are characterized by distinct periods of a relatively persistent elevated or irritable mood and other symptoms such as increased activity, restlessness, talkativeness, flight of ideas, inflated self-esteem, and distractibility.
Cyclothymic disorder	There are numerous periods during which symptoms of depression and mania are present but not of sufficient severity or duration to meet the criteria for a major depressive or manic episode; in addition to a loss of interest and pleasure in most activities, the periods of depression are accompanied by other symptoms such as fatigue, insomnia or hypersomnia, social withdrawal, pessimism, and tearfulness.
Dysthymic disorder	Patient usually exhibits a prominently depressed mood, marked loss of interest or pleasure in most activities, and other symptoms of depression; the symptoms are not of sufficient severity or duration to meet the criteria for a major depressive episode, and the periods of depression may be separated by up to a few months of normal mood.
Adjustment disorder with depressed mood	The patient exhibits a depressed mood, tearfulness, hopelessness, or other symptoms in excess of a normal response to an identifiable psychosocial or physical stressor; the response is not an exacerbation of another psychiatric condition, occurs within 3 months of the onset of the stressor, eventually remits after the stressor ceases (or the patient adapts to the stressor), and does not meet the criteria for other forms of depression or uncomplicated bereavement.

TABLE 7-9   MAJOR DEPRESSION VERSUS OTHER FORMS OF DEPRESSION
(*Continued*)

DIAGNOSTIC CLASSIFICATION	KEY FEATURES DISTINGUISHING FROM MAJOR DEPRESSION
Uncomplicated bereavement	This is a depressive syndrome that arises in response to the death of a loved one—its onset is not more than 2 to 3 months after the death, and the symptoms last for variable periods of time; the patient generally regards the depression as a normal response—guilt and thoughts of death refer directly to the loved one; morbid preoccupation with worthlessness, marked or prolonged functional impairment, and marked psychomotor retardation are uncommon and suggest the development of major depression.

depression but may also be caused by hypothyroidism or colonic disease; thus a test for occult blood in the stool, barium enema or colonoscopy, and thyroid function tests can be helpful in the evaluation of this symptom.

MANAGEMENT

General Considerations

Several treatment modalities are available to manage depression in older persons (Table 7-12). Both pharmacological treatment and psychotherapy have some effectiveness in mild to moderate depression in the outpatient geriatric population (McCusker et al., 1998). A randomized controlled trial has documented the effectiveness of a depression treatment program that includes both nonpharmacological and pharmacological treatment coordinated by a care manager with the support of mental health expertise (Unutzer et al., 2002). The choice of treatment(s) for an individual patient depends on many factors, including the primary disorder causing the depression, the severity of symptoms, the availability and

TABLE 7-10   EXAMPLES OF SCREENING QUESTIONS FOR DEPRESSION

For each of the following questions, which description comes closest to the way you have been feeling *during the past month*?

	ALL THE TIME	MOST OF THE TIME	SOME OF THE TIME	A LITTLE OF THE TIME	NONE OF THE TIME
a. How much of the time *during the past month* have you been a very nervous person?	1	2	3	4	5
b. *During the past month,* how much of the time have you felt calm and peaceful?	1	2	3	4	5
c. How much of the time *during the past month* have you felt downhearted and blue?	1	2	3	4	5
d. *During the past month,* how much of the time have you been a happy person?	1	2	3	4	5
e. How often *during the past month* have you felt so down in the dumps that nothing could cheer you up?	1	2	3	4	5
f. *During the past month,* how often did you feel like life isn't worth living anymore?	1	2	3	4	5

Source: Adapted from Stewart et al., 1988, with permission.

TABLE 7-11   DIAGNOSTIC STUDIES HELPFUL IN EVALUATING APPARENTLY
DEPRESSED GERIATRIC PATIENTS WITH SOMATIC SYMPTOMS

BASIC EVALUATION
History
Physical examination
Complete blood count
Erythrocyte sedimentation rate
Serum electrolytes, glucose, and calcium
Renal function tests
Liver function tests
Thyroid function tests

EXAMPLES OF OTHER POTENTIALLY HELPFUL STUDIES	
SYMPTOM OR SIGN	DIAGNOSTIC STUDY
Pain	Appropriate radiologic procedure (e.g., bone film, bone scan, GI series)
Chest pain	ECG, noninvasive cardiovascular studies (e.g., exercise stress test, echocardiography, radionuclide scans)
Shortness of breath	Chest films, pulmonary function tests, pulse oximetry arterial blood gases
Constipation	Test for occult blood in stool, barium enema, thyroid function tests
Focal neurological signs or symptoms	CT or MRI scan, EEG

Abbreviations: CT = computed tomography; ECG = electrocardiography; EEG = electroencephalography; GI = gastrointestinal; MRI = magnetic resonance imaging.

TABLE 7-12   TREATMENT MODALITIES FOR GERIATRIC DEPRESSION

Nonpharmacological
Supportive measures
   Information and encouragement
   Environmental alterations
   Activities (physical and mental)
   Involvement of family and friends
   Ongoing interest and care
Psychotherapy
   Individual
   Group
Electroconvulsive
Pharmacologic
   Antidepressants (see Table 7-13)
   Sedatives for associated anxiety or agitation (see Chap. 14)
   Antipsychotics for associated psychoses (see Chap. 14)

practicality of the various treatment modalities, and underlying conditions that might contraindicate a specific form of treatment (e.g., disorders of vision and hearing that make psychotherapy difficult or severe cardiovascular disease that precludes the use of certain antidepressants).

When a specific active medical condition or drug is suspected as the cause of or contributor to the symptoms and signs of depression, these factors should be attended to before other therapies are initiated unless the depression is severe enough to warrant immediate treatment (e.g., the patient is delusional or suicidal). Treatment of the medical condition should be optimized and all drugs that could be worsening the depression should be discontinued if medically feasible.

Nonpharmacological Management

Supportive measures, such as those listed in Table 7-12, and psychotherapy are often ignored, but they can be very helpful in managing depressed patients; they may also be useful adjuncts to other treatments for patients with more severe depressions. Standard approaches to psychotherapy, such as cognitive–behavioral therapy and interpersonal therapy, are effective in depressed geriatric patients. However, no single approach appears to be more effective than others. Geriatric patients with depressions caused by uncomplicated bereavement, adjustment disorders related to a psychosocial stress (retirement, family conflicts, etc.) or physical conditions (myocardial infarction, stroke, hip fracture, etc.), dysthymic disorder, and minor depression may respond well to supportive measures and psychotherapeutic approaches.

Many depressed patients have hearing impairments, other physical disabilities, or cognitive impairment that can make group and individual psychotherapy difficult. Behavioral treatment may be effective in some dementia patients who are depressed (Teri et al., 1997). Outpatient psychiatric "partial hospitalization" programs are available in many communities and may be especially helpful in managing frail depressed patients who are isolated during the day.

If pharmacological treatment is contraindicated by medical conditions or fails, or if rapid relief from depression is desired (as might be the case in delusional, suicidal, or extremely vegetative patients), electroconvulsive therapy (ECT) should be considered. ECT is relatively safe and can be highly effective in the geriatric population. Certain added precautions are necessary in older patients with hypertension and cardiac arrhythmias (such as close cardiac monitoring and diminished doses of pretreatment atropine), and cardiology consultation is advisable in these situations. Adequate pretreatment muscle relaxation will help avoid musculoskeletal complications, which are of special concern in those patients with osteoporosis. Posttreatment confusion and memory loss is usually mild and improves as the depression subsides.

Pharmacological Treatment

When symptoms and signs of depression are of sufficient severity and duration to meet the criteria for major depression (see Table 7-8), or if the depression is producing marked functional disability or interfering with recovery from other illnesses, drug treatment should be considered.

When pharmacological treatment is initially considered, the patient and family should be educated to understand that an adequate therapeutic trial may take at least 4 to 6 weeks. If this is not discussed, patients may become discouraged by a lack of a rapid response to therapy.

Several types of drugs are available to treat depression in the geriatric population (Table 7-13). While many antidepressants have been studied in these patients, limitations in study designs, outcome measures, patient characteristics, and sample sizes make the clinical utility of several of these agents difficult to assess (Rigler et al., 1998). Experts recommend at least 6 months of therapy beyond recovery for patients with their first onset of depression in late life, and at least 12 months for those with recurrent depression. Some older patients with recurrent depression may need to be treated indefinitely (Lebowitz et al., 1997).

TABLE 7-13   CHARACTERISTICS OF SELECTED ANTIDEPRESSANTS FOR GERIATRIC PATIENTS

DRUG*	RECOMMENDED STARTING DAILY DOSAGE	DAILY DOSAGE RANGE	LEVEL OF SEDATION	ELIMINATION HALF-LIFE †	COMMENTS
Selective serotonin reuptake inhibitors					
Citalopram (Celexa)	10–20 mg	20–30 mg	Very low	Very long	Less inhibition of hepatic cytochrome P450
					May cause somnolence, insomnia, anorexia
Escitalopram (Lexapro)	10 mg	10 mg	Very low	Very long	Side effects as for citalopram
Fluoxetine (Prozac)	5–10 mg	20–60 mg	Very low	Very long	Inhibits hepatic cytochrome P450 ‡
					Must be discontinued 6 weeks before initiating monamine oxidase inhibitor
Paroxetine (Paxil)	10 mg	10–50 mg	Very low	Long	Inhibits hepatic cytochrome P450 ‡
					Has anticholinergic side effects
Sertraline (Zoloft)	25 mg	50–200 mg	Very low	Very long	Less inhibition of cytochrome P450
Serotonin–norepinephrine reuptake blockers					
Venlafaxine (Effexor)	25 mg	75–225 mg	Very low	Intermediate	Reduced clearance with renal or hepatic impairment
					Can cause dose-related hypertension
					Must be tapered over 1–2 weeks when discontinuing

Tricyclic antidepressants

Nortriptyline (Pamelor, others)	10–30 mg	25–150 mg	Mild	Long	Lower but still substantial anticholinergic effects § Blood levels can be monitored
Other agents †					
Bupropion (Wellbutrin)	50–100 mg	150–450 mg	Mild	Intermediate	Divided doses necessary
Mirtazapine (Remeron)	15 mg	15–45 mg	Mild	Long	Reduced clearance with renal impairment May cause or exacerbate hypertension
Nefazodone (Serzone)	100 mg	200–400 mg	Mild	Short	Potent inhibitor of cytochrome P450 ‡ Can increase concentrations of terfenadine, astemizole, and cisapride Has antianxiety effects
Trazodone (Desyrel)	25–50 mg	75–400 mg	Moderate– high	Short	Can cause hypotension May be useful in low doses as a hypnotic

* Other less-commonly used antidepressants are discussed in the text.
† Short = <8 h; intermediate = 8–20 h; long = 20–30 h; very long = > 30 h. Half- lives may vary in older patients and some drugs have active metabolites.
‡ See text for drug interactions.
§ See text for anticholinergic side effects.

The selective serotonin reuptake inhibitors (SSRIs) have replaced tricyclics as the first-line drug treatment for geriatric depression. Studies suggest that these agents are useful in treating depressed older people, but they have not been well studied in frail and medically ill geriatric patients. In one randomized, placebo-controlled trial, paroxetine was beneficial in older patients with dysthymia and more severely impaired patients with minor depression (Williams et al., 2000). All SSRIs are metabolized by the liver and excreted by the kidney. Fluoxetine and its partially active metabolite have especially long half-lives. In addition, fluoxetine and paroxetine are potent inhibitors of the hepatic cytochrome P450 microsomal enzyme system. Toxicity can occur when these drugs are used concurrently with drugs that are metabolized by this system. Elevated levels or toxicity can occur with several drugs used relatively commonly in the geriatric population, including:

- Antiarrhythmics (type 1C)
- Anticonvulsants
- Antipsychotics
- Astemizole
- Benzodiazepines
- Beta blockers
- Calcium-channel blockers
- Carbamazepine
- Cisapride
- Codeine
- Erythromycin
- Oral hypoglycemics
- Terfenadine
- Theophylline
- Tricyclics
- Warfarin

The major side effects of SSRIs include gastrointestinal symptoms (nausea, vomiting, diarrhea), agitation, weight loss, sexual dysfunction, akathisia, and parkinsonian effects. These agents are also associated with the syndrome of inappropriate antidiuretic hormone (SIADH) and may thus cause or contribute to hyponatremia.

Tricyclic antidepressants may be effective, but they have anticholinergic and potential cardiovascular side effects. These include dry mouth, constipation, gastroesophageal reflux, blurred vision, cognitive impairment, tachycardia, and postural hypotension. Tricyclics and SSRIs are associated with falls and hip fracture (Thapa et al., 1998). In one study of older depressed patients with ischemic heart disease, paroxetine was associated with significantly fewer adverse cardiac events (2 percent) than was nortriptyline (18 percent) (Roose et al., 1998). Postural hypotension is a special concern in frail geriatric patients already at risk for falls. Tricyclics, like SSRIs, are associated with SIADH.

Other antidepressants—such as venlafaxine, bupropion, mirtazapine, and nefazodone—are available (see Table 7-13). Experience with these drugs suggest that they may be useful in geriatric depression. Both venlafaxine and mirtazapine should be used carefully in patients with underlying hypertension. Nefazodone may be useful in depressed older patients with prominent anxiety. This drug cannot, however, be used in conjunction with cisapride or the antihistamines terfenadine and astemizole, as it inhibits their metabolism and may thereby lead to life-threatening ventricular arrhythmias.

Methylphenidate (Ritalin) in small doses (10 mg one to three times a day) has been effective and safe in some geriatric patients with retarded depressions and cardiovascular disease. Its effects may diminish over time, and anorexia can be a side effect. Monoamine oxidase inhibitors (such as isocarboxazid, phenelzine, and tranylcypromine) have been used in geriatric patients, but necessitate a relatively strict diet (avoidance of tyramine-rich foods) and can cause prominent hypotension. SSRIs must be discontinued 2 weeks (6 weeks for fluoxetine) before initiating treatment with one of these drugs.

For patients with bipolar disorder, lithium is useful in treating the manic phase of the illness and in preventing recurrent depression. It may also enhance the effects of other antidepressants in treating unipolar depression. Lithium has a very narrow therapeutic:toxic ratio and must be used very carefully in the geriatric population. Its renal clearance is diminished, and blood levels can be influenced by diuretics and angiotensin-converting enzyme (ACE) inhibitors. Blood levels should be monitored once or twice weekly until a stable dosage is achieved and then at least monthly. Dosages of 150 to 300 mg three times a day generally yield adequate blood levels in the elderly (0.3 to 0.6 mEq/L for maintenance). Older patients are particularly susceptible to lithium toxicity, especially tremor and delirium. Hypothyroidism can occur in patients on lithium, and thyroid function tests should be monitored periodically in patients on chronic therapy.

Depressed geriatric patients with psychotic features (paranoid and other types of delusions, hallucinations) may also require antipsychotic drug treatment. These drugs, as well as sedative and hypnotic agents (which are also useful in some depressed older patients with prominent anxiety or psychomotor agitation), are discussed in Chap. 14.

References

American Psychiatric Association: *Diagnostic and Statistical Manual of Mental Disorders,* 4th ed., Text Revision. Washington, DC, American Psychiatric Association, 2000.

Blazer D, Hughes DC, George LK: The epidemiology of depression in an elderly community population. *Gerontologist* 27:281–287, 1987.

Covinsky KE, Fortinsky RH, Palmer RM, et al: Relation between symptoms of depression and health status outcomes in acutely ill hospitalized older persons. *Ann Intern Med* 126:417–425, 1997.

Katon W, Raskind M: Treatment of depression in the medically ill with methylphenidate. *Am J Psychiatry* 137:963–965, 1980.

Koenig HG: Differences in psychosocial and health correlates of major and minor depression in medically ill older adults. *J Am Geriatr Soc* 45:1487–1495, 1997.

Lebowitz BD, Pearson JL, Schneider LS, et al: Diagnosis and treatment of depression late in life. *JAMA* 278:1186–1190, 1997.

Levenson AJ, Hall RCW (eds): *Neuropsychiatric Manifestations of Physical Disease in the Elderly.* New York, Raven Press, 1981.

McCusker J, Cole M, Keller E, et al: Effectiveness of treatments of depression in older ambulatory patients. *Arch Intern Med* 158:705–712, 1998.

Medical Letter: Drugs that may cause psychiatric symptoms. *Med Lett* 44(1134):59–62, 2002.

Osgood NJ: *Suicide in the Elderly.* Rockville, MD, Aspen, 1985.

Parmelee PA, Katz IR, Lawton MP: Incidence of depression in long-term care settings. *J Gerontol* 47:M189–M196, 1992a.

Parmelee PA, Katz IR, Lawton MP: Depression and mortality among institutionalized aged. *J Gerontol* 47:P3–P10, 1992b.

Rigler SK, Studenski S, Duncan PW: Pharmacologic treatment of geriatric depression: key issues in interpreting the evidence. *J Am Geriatr Soc* 46:106–110, 1998.

Roose SP, Laghriss-Thode F, Kennedy JS, et al: Comparison of paroxetine and nortriptyline in depressed patients with ischemic heart disease. *JAMA* 279:287–291, 1998.

Rovner BW, German PS, Brant LJ, et al: Depression and mortality in nursing homes. *JAMA* 265:993–996, 1991.

Small GW, Birkett M, Meyers BS, et al: Impact of physical illness on quality of life and antidepressant response in geriatric major depression. *J Am Geriatr Soc* 44:1220–1225, 1996.

Stewart AL, Hays RD, Ware JE: The MOS short-form general health survey: reliability and validity in a patient population. *Med Care* 26:724–735, 1988.

Teri L, Logsdon RG, Uomoto J, et al: Behavioral treatment of depression in dementia patients: a controlled clinical trial. *J Gerontol Psychol Sci* 52(4):P159–P166, 1997.

Thapa PB, Gideon P, Cost TW, et al: Antidepressants and the risk of falls among nursing home residents. *N Engl J Med* 339:875–882, 1998.

Unutzer J, Patrick DL, Simon G, et al: Depressive symptoms and the cost of health services in HMO patients aged 65 years and older. *JAMA* 277:1618–1623, 1997.

Unutzer J, Katon W, Callahan CM, et al: Collaborative care management of late-life depression in the primary care setting. *JAMA* 288(22):2836–2845, 2002.

Williams JW Jr, Barret J, Oxman T, et al: Treatment of dysthymia and minor depression in primary care. *JAMA* 284(12):1519–1526, 2000.

Suggested Readings

Finkel SI: Efficacy and tolerability of antidepressant therapy in the old-old. *J Clin Psychiatry* 57:23–28, 1996.

Hay DP, Rodriguez MM, Franson KL: Treatment of depression in late life. *Clin Geriatr Med* 14:33–46, 1998.

Kelly KG, Zisselman M: Update on electroconvulsive therapy (ECT) in older adults. *J Am Geriatr Soc* 48:560–566, 2000.

Kennedy GJE: *Suicide and Depression in Late Life: Critical Issues in Treatment, Research, and Public Policy.* New York, Wiley, 1996.

Martin LM, Fleming KC, Evans JM: Recognition and management of anxiety and depression in elderly patients. *Mayo Clin Proc* 70:999–1006, 1995.

CHAPTER 8

INCONTINENCE

Incontinence is a common, disruptive, and potentially disabling condition in the geriatric population. It is defined as the involuntary loss of urine or stool in sufficient amount or frequency to constitute a social and/or health problem. Figure 8-1 illustrates the prevalence of urinary incontinence. Incontinence is a heterogeneous condition, ranging in severity from occasional episodes of dribbling small amounts of urine to continuous urinary incontinence with concomitant fecal incontinence. Incontinent older persons are not always severely demented, bedridden, or in nursing homes. Many, both in institutions and in the community, are ambulatory and have good mental function.

Approximately 33 percent of women age 65 and above and 15 to 20 percent of men older than 65 years have some degree of urinary incontinence. Between 5 and 10 percent of community-dwelling older adults have incontinence more often than weekly and/or use a pad for protection from urinary accidents. The prevalence is as high as 60 to 80 percent in many long-term care institutions. In both community and institutional settings, incontinence is associated with both impaired mobility and poor cognition.

Physical health, psychological well-being, social status, and the costs of health care can all be adversely affected by incontinence (Table 8-1). Urinary incontinence is curable in many geriatric patients, especially those who have adequate mobility and mental functioning.

Even when it is not curable, incontinence can always be managed in a manner that will keep patients comfortable, make life easier for caregivers, and minimize the costs of caring for the condition and its complications. Despite some change in the social perception of incontinence because of television advertisements and public media and educational efforts, many older patients are embarrassed and frustrated by their incontinence and either deny it or do not discuss it with a health professional. It is therefore essential that specific questions about incontinence be included in periodic assessments and that incontinence be noted as a problem when it is detected in institutional settings. Examples of such questions include the following:

"Do you have trouble with your bladder?"
"Do you ever lose urine when you don't want to?"
"Do you ever wear padding to protect yourself in case you lose urine?"

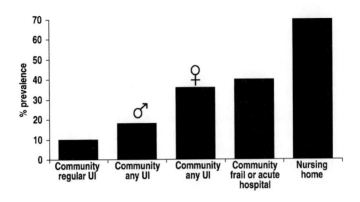

— FIGURE 8-1 —   *Prevalence of urinary incontinence in the geriatric population.*
"Regular UI" is more often than weekly and/or the use of a pad.

TABLE 8-1   POTENTIAL ADVERSE EFFECTS OF URINARY INCONTINENCE

Physical heath
  Skin breakdown
  Recurrent urinary tract infections
  Falls (especially with nighttime incontinence)

Psychological health
  Isolation
  Depression
  Dependency

Social consequences
  Stress on family, friends, and caregivers
  Predisposition to institutionalization

Economic costs
  Supplies (padding, catheters, etc.)
  Laundry
  Labor (nurses, housekeepers)
  Management of complications

This chapter briefly reviews the pathophysiology of geriatric incontinence and provides detailed information on the evaluation and management of this condition. Although most of the chapter focuses on urinary incontinence, much of the pathophysiology also applies to fecal incontinence, which is briefly addressed at the end of the chapter.

NORMAL URINATION

Continence requires effective functioning of the lower urinary tract, adequate cognitive and physical functioning, motivation, and an appropriate environment (Table 8-2). Thus, the pathophysiology of geriatric incontinence can relate to the anatomy and physiology of the lower urinary tract as well as to functional psychological and environmental factors. Several anatomic components participate in normal urination (Fig. 8-2). At the most basic level, urination is governed by reflexes centered in the sacral micturition center. Afferent pathways (via somatic and autonomic nerves) carry information on bladder volume to the spinal cord as the bladder fills. Motor output is adjusted accordingly (Fig. 8-3). Thus, as the

TABLE 8-2   REQUIREMENTS FOR CONTINENCE

Effective lower urinary tract function
  Storage
    Accommodation by bladder of increasing volumes of urine under low
      pressure
      Closed bladder outlet
      Appropriate sensation of bladder fullness
      Absence of involuntary bladder contractions
  Emptying
      Bladder capable of contraction
      Lack of anatomic obstruction to urine flow
      Coordinated lowering of outlet resistance with bladder contractions

Adequate mobility and dexterity to use toilet or toilet substitute and to
  manage clothing

Adequate cognitive function to recognize toileting needs and to find a toilet
  or toilet substitute

Motivation to be continent

Absence of environmental and iatrogenic barriers such as inaccessible toilets
  or toilet substitutes, unavailable caregivers, or drug side effects

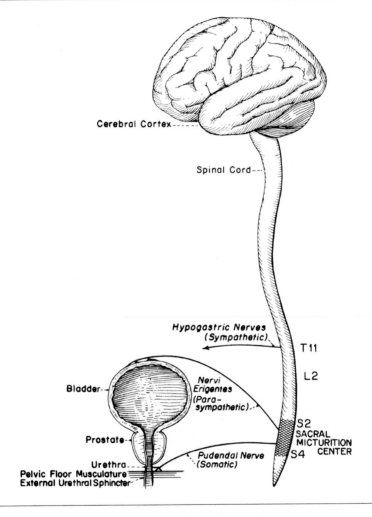

— FIGURE 8-2 — *Structural components of normal micturition.*

bladder fills, sympathetic tone closes the bladder neck, relaxes the dome of the bladder, and inhibits parasympathetic tone; somatic innervation maintains tone in the pelvic floor musculature (including striated muscle around the urethra).

When urination occurs, sympathetic and somatic tones diminish, and parasympathetic cholinergically mediated impulses cause the bladder to contract. All these processes are under the influence of higher centers in the brainstem, cerebral cortex, and cerebellum. This is a simplified description of a very com-

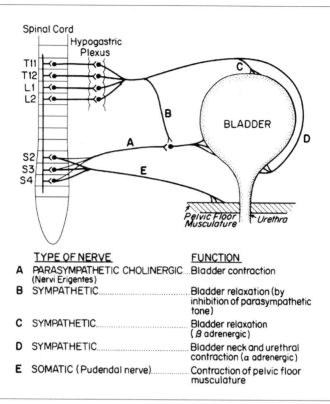

Spinal Cord
Hypogastric
Plexus
T11
T12
L1
L2

B

BLADDER

A

D

S2
S3
S4

E

Pelvic Floor
Musculature

Urethra

TYPE OF NERVE	FUNCTION
A PARASYMPATHETIC CHOLINERGIC (Nervi Erigentes)	Bladder contraction
B SYMPATHETIC	Bladder relaxation (by inhibition of parasympathetic tone)
C SYMPATHETIC	Bladder relaxation (β adrenergic)
D SYMPATHETIC	Bladder neck and urethral contraction (α adrenergic)
E SOMATIC (Pudendal nerve)	Contraction of pelvic floor musculature

— FIGURE 8-3 — *Peripheral nerves involved in micturition.*

plex process, and the neurophysiology of urination remains incompletely understood. It appears, however, that the cerebral cortex exerts a predominantly inhibitory influence and the brainstem facilitates urination. Thus, loss of the central cortical inhibiting influences over the sacral micturition center from diseases such as dementia, stroke, and parkinsonism can produce incontinence in elderly patients. Disorders of the brainstem and suprasacral spinal cord can interfere with the coordination of bladder contractions and lowering of urethral resistance, and interruptions of the sacral innervation can cause impaired bladder contraction and problems with continence.

Normal urination is a dynamic process, requiring the coordination of several physiological processes. Figure 8-4 depicts a simplified schematic diagram of the pressure-volume relationships in the lower urinary tract, similar to measurements made in urodynamic studies. Under normal circumstances, as the bladder fills, bladder pressure remains low (e.g., <115 cm H_2O). The first urge to void is variable but generally occurs between 150 and 300 mL, and normal

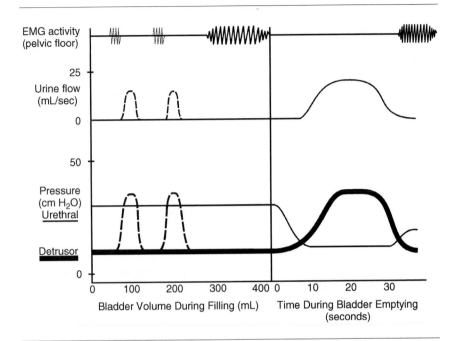

— FIGURE 8-4 — *Schematic of the dynamic function of the lower urinary tract during bladder filling (left) and emptying (right). As the bladder fills, true detrusor pressure (thick line at bottom) remains low (less than 5 to 10 cm H_2O) and does not exceed urethral resistance pressure (thin line at bottom). As the bladder fills to capacity (generally 300 to 600 mL), pelvic floor and sphincter activity increase as measured by electromyography (EMG, top). Involuntary detrusor contractions (illustrated by dashed lines) occur commonly among incontinent geriatric patients (see text). They may be accompanied by increased EMG activity in attempts to prevent leakage (dashed lines at top). If detrusor pressure exceeds urethral pressure during an involuntary contraction, as shown, urine will flow. During bladder emptying, detrusor pressure rises, urethral pressure falls, and EMG activity ceases in order for normal urine flow to occur.*

bladder capacity is 300 to 600 mL. When normal urination is initiated, true detrusor pressure (bladder pressure minus intraabdominal pressure) increases, urethral resistance decreases, and urine flow occurs when detrusor pressure exceeds urethral resistance. If at any time during bladder filling total intravesicular pressure (which includes intraabdominal pressure) exceeds outlet resistance, urinary leakage will occur. This will happen if, for example, intraabdominal pressure rises *without* a rise in true detrusor pressure when someone with low outlet or urethral sphincter weakness coughs or sneezes. This would be defined as *genuine stress incontinence* in urodynamic terminology. Alternatively, the bladder can contract involuntarily and cause urinary leakage. This would be defined as *detrusor motor instability* or *detrusor hyperreflexia* in patients with neurological disorders.

CAUSES AND TYPES OF INCONTINENCE

Basic Causes

There are four basic categories of causes for geriatric urinary incontinence (Fig. 8-5). Determining the cause(s) is essential to proper management.

It is very important to distinguish between urological and neurological disorders that cause incontinence and other problems (such as diminished mobility and/or mental function, inaccessible toilets, and psychological problems), which can cause or contribute to the condition. As is the case for a number of other common geriatric problems discussed in this text, multiple disorders often interact to cause urinary incontinence, as depicted in Fig. 8-5.

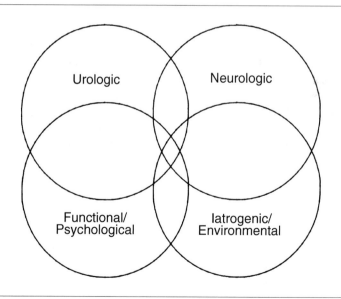

— FIGURE 8-5 — *Basic underlying causes of geriatric urinary incontinence.*

Aging alone does *not* cause urinary incontinence. Several age-related changes can, however, contribute to its development.

In general, with age, bladder capacity declines, residual urine increases, and involuntary bladder contractions become more common (see Fig. 8-4). These contractions are found in up to 80 percent of older incontinent patients, as well as in 5 to 10 percent of older women and in 33 percent or more of older men with no or minimal urinary symptoms. Combined with impaired mobility, these contractions account for a substantial proportion of incontinence in frail geriatric patients.

Aging is associated with a decline in bladder outlet and urethral resistance pressure in women. This decline, which is related to diminished estrogen influence and laxity of pelvic structures associated with prior childbirths, surgeries, and deconditioned muscles, predisposes to the development of stress incontinence (Fig. 8-6). Decreased estrogen can also cause atrophic vaginitis and urethritis, which can, in turn, cause symptoms of dysuria and urgency and predispose to the development of urinary infection and urge incontinence. In men, prostatic enlargement is associated with decreased urine flow rates and detrusor motor instability and can lead to urge and/or overflow types of incontinence (see below). Aging is also associated with abnormalities of arginine vasopressin (AVP) levels. Lack of the normal diurnal rhythm of AVP secretion may contribute to nocturnal polyuria, and predispose many older people to nighttime incontinence.

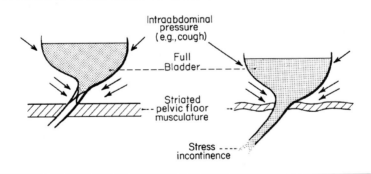

— FIGURE 8-6 — *Simplified schematic depicting age-associated changes in pelvic floor muscle, bladder, and urethra-vesicle position, predisposing to stress incontinence. Normally (left), the bladder and outlet remain anatomically inside the intraabdominal cavity, and rises in pressure contribute to bladder outlet closure. Age-associated changes (e.g., estrogen deficiency, surgeries, childbirth) can weaken the structures maintaining bladder position (right); in this situation, increases in intraabdominal pressure can cause urine loss (stress incontinence).*

Reversible Factors Causing or Contributing to Incontinence

Numerous potentially reversible conditions and medications may cause or contribute to geriatric incontinence (Tables 8-3 and 8-4).

The term *acute incontinence* refers to those situations in which the incontinence is of sudden onset, usually related to an acute illness or an iatrogenic problem, and subsides once the illness or medication problem has been resolved. *Persistent incontinence* refers to incontinence that is unrelated to an acute illness and persists over time.

TABLE 8-3   REVERSIBLE CONDITIONS THAT CAUSE OR CONTRIBUTE TO GERIATRIC URINARY INCONTINENCE

CONDITION	MANAGEMENT
Conditions affecting the lower urinary tract	
Urinary tract infection (symptomatic with frequency, urgency,dysuria, etc.)	Antimicrobial therapy.
Atrophic vaginitis/urethritis	Oral or topical estrogen.
Postprostatectomy	Behavioral intervention. Avoid further surgical therapy until it is clear condition will not resolve.
Stool impaction	Disimpaction; appropriate use of stool softeners, bulk-forming agents, and laxatives if necessary; implement high fiber intake, adequate mobility, and fluid intake.
Drug side effect (see Table 8-4)	Discontinue or change therapy if clinically appropriate. Dosage reduction or modification (e.g., flexible scheduling of rapid-acting diuretics) may also help.
Increased urine production	
Metabolic (hyperglycemia, hypercalcemia)	Better control of diabetes mellitus. Therapy for hypercalcemia depends on underlying cause.
Excess fluid intake	Reduction in intake of diuretic fluids (e.g., caffeinated beverages).

TABLE 8-3   REVERSIBLE CONDITIONS THAT CAUSE OR CONTRIBUTE
TO GERIATRIC URINARY INCONTINENCE (*Continued*)

CONDITION	MANAGEMENT
Volume overload	Support stockings.
Venous insufficiency with edema	Leg elevation.
	Sodium restriction.
	Diuretic therapy.
Congestive heart failure	Medical therapy.
Impaired ability or willingness to reach a toilet	
Delirium	Diagnosis and treatment of underlying cause(s) of acute confusional state.
Chronic illness, injury, or restraint that interferes with mobility	Regular toileting. Use of toilet substitutes. Environmental alterations (e.g., bedside commode, urinal).
Psychological	Remove restraints if possible. Appropriate pharmacologic and/or nonpharmacologic treatment.

Source: From Fantl, Newman, et al., 1996a, with permission.

Potentially reversible conditions can play a role in *both* acute and persistent incontinence. A search for these factors should be undertaken in all incontinent geriatric patients.

The causes of acute and reversible forms of urinary incontinence can be remembered by the acronym DRIP (Table 8-5).

Many older persons, because of urinary frequency and urgency, especially when they are limited in mobility, carefully arrange their schedules (and may even limit social activities) in order to be close to a toilet. Thus, an acute illness (e.g., pneumonia, cardiac decompensation, stroke, lower extremity or vertebral fracture) can precipitate incontinence by disrupting this delicate balance.

Hospitalization, with its attendant environmental barriers (such as bed rails, poorly lit rooms), and the immobility that often accompanies acute illnesses can contribute to acute incontinence. Acute incontinence in these situations is likely to resolve with resolution of the underlying acute illness. Unless an indwelling or external catheter is necessary to record urine output accurately, this type of incontinence should be managed by environmental manipulations, scheduled toilet-

TABLE 8-4   MEDICATIONS THAT CAN AFFECT CONTINENCE

TYPE OF MEDICATION	POTENTIAL EFFECTS ON CONTINENCE
Diuretics	Polyuria, frequency, urgency
Anticholinergics	Urinary retention, overflow incontinence, stool impaction

Psychotropics
  Tricyclic
    Antidepressants
	Anticholinergic actions, sedation

Antipsychotics	Anticholinergic actions, sedation, immobility
Sedative-hypnotics	Sedation, delirium, immobility, muscle relaxation
Narcotic analgesics	Urinary retention, fecal impaction, sedation, delirium
α-Adrenergic blockers	Urethral relaxation
α-adrenergic agonists	Urinary retention
Angiotensin-converting enzyme inhibitors	Cough precipitating stress incontinence
β-Adrenergic agonists	Urinary retention
Calcium-channel blockers	Urinary retention
Alcohol	Polyuria, frequency, urgency, sedation, delirium, immobility
Caffeine	Polyuria, bladder irritation

TABLE 8-5   ACRONYM FOR POTENTIALLY REVERSIBLE CONDITIONS*

D	Delirium
R	Restricted mobility, retention
I	Infection, inflammation, impaction
P	Polyuria, pharmaceuticals

* See Tables 8-3 and 8-4.

ings, the appropriate use of toilet substitutes (e.g., urinals, bedside commodes) and pads, and careful attention to skin care. In a substantial proportion of patients, incontinence may persist for several weeks after hospitalization and should be evaluated as for persistent incontinence (see below).

Fecal impaction is a common problem in both acutely and chronically ill geriatric patients. Large impactions may cause mechanical obstruction of the bladder outlet in women and may stimulate involuntary bladder contractions induced by sensory input related to rectal distention. Whatever the underlying mechanism, relief of fecal impaction can lead to improvement and sometimes resolution of the urinary incontinence.

Urinary retention with overflow incontinence should be considered in any patient who suddenly develops urinary incontinence. Immobility, anticholinergic and narcotic drugs, and fecal impaction can all precipitate overflow incontinence in geriatric patients. In addition, this condition may be a manifestation of an underlying process causing spinal cord compression and presenting acutely.

Any acute inflammatory condition in the lower urinary tract that causes frequency and urgency can precipitate incontinence. Treatment of an acute cystitis, vaginitis, or urethritis can restore continence.

Conditions that cause polyuria, including hyperglycemia and hypercalcemia, as well as diuretics (especially the rapid-acting loop diuretics), can precipitate acute incontinence. Some older people drink excessive amounts of fluids, and others ingest a large amount of caffeine without understanding the prominent effects it can have on the bladder. Patients with volume-expanded states, such as congestive heart failure and lower extremity venous insufficiency, may have polyuria at night, which can contribute to nocturia and nocturnal incontinence.

As in the case of many other conditions discussed throughout this text, a wide variety of medications can play a role in the development of incontinence in elderly patients via several different mechanisms (see Table 8-4). Whether the incontinence is acute or persistent, the potential role of these medications in causing or contributing to the patients' incontinence should be considered. Whenever feasible, stopping the medication, switching to an alternative, or modifying the dosage schedule can be an important component (and possibly the only one necessary) of the treatment for incontinence.

▨ Persistent Incontinence

Persistent forms of incontinence can be classified clinically into four basic types. As depicted in Fig. 8-7, these types can overlap. Thus, an individual patient may have more than one type simultaneously. While this classification does not include all the neurophysiological abnormalities associated with incontinence, it is helpful in approaching the clinical assessment and treatment of incontinence in the geriatric population.

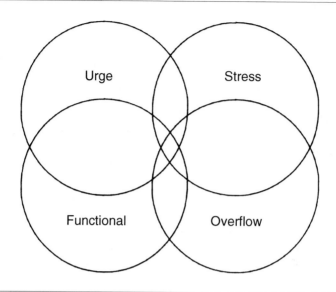

— FIGURE 8-7 — *Basic types of persistent geriatric urinary incontinence.*

Three of these types—stress, urge, and overflow—result from one or a combination of two basic abnormalities in lower genitourinary tract function: (1) Failure to store urine, caused by a hyperactive or poorly compliant bladder or by diminished outflow resistance (2) Failure to empty bladder, caused by a poorly contractile bladder or by increased outflow resistance. Table 8-6 shows the clinical definitions and common causes of persistent urinary incontinence. *Stress incontinence* is common in older women, especially in ambulatory clinic settings. It may be infrequent and involve very small amounts of urine and need no specific treatment in women who are not bothered by it. On the other hand, it may be so severe and bothersome that it necessitates surgical correction. It is most often associated with weakened supporting tissues and consequent hypermobility of the bladder outlet and urethra caused by lack of estrogen and/or previous vaginal deliveries or surgery (see Fig. 8-6). Obesity and chronic coughing can exacerbate this condition. Women who have had previous vaginal repair and/or surgical bladder neck suspension may develop a weak urethra (intrinsic sphincter deficiency [ISD]). These women generally present with severe incontinence and symptoms of constant wetting with any activity.

This condition should be suspected during office evaluation if a woman loses urine involuntarily with coughing in the supine position during a pelvic examination when her bladder is relatively empty. In general, women with ISD are less responsive to nonsurgical treatment but may benefit from periurethral injections

TABLE 8-6 BASIC TYPES AND CAUSES OF PERSISTENT URINARY
INCONTINENCE

TYPES	DEFINITION	COMMON CAUSES
Stress	Involuntary loss of urine (usually small amounts) with increases in intraabdominal pressure (e.g., cough, laugh, exercise)	Weakness of pelvic floor musculature and urethral hypermobility Bladder outlet or urethral sphincter weakness
Urge	Leakage of urine (variable but often larger volumes) because of inability to delay voiding after sensation of bladder fullness is perceived	Detrusor overactivity, isolated or associated with one or more of the following: Local genitourinary condition such as tumors, stones, diverticuli, or outflow obstruction Central nervous system disorders such as stroke, dementia, parkinsonism, spinal cord injury
Overflow	Leakage of urine (usually small amounts) resulting from mechanical forces on an overdistended bladder or from other effects of urinary retention on bladder and sphincter function	Anatomic obstruction by prostate, stricture, cystocele Acontractile bladder associated with diabetes mellitus or spinal cord injury Neurogenic (detrusor-sphincter dyssynergy), associated with multiple sclerosis and other suprasacral spinal cord lesions
Functional	Urinary accidents associated with inability to toilet because of impairment of cognitive and/or physical functioning, psychological unwillingness, or environmental barriers	Severe dementia and other neurological disorders Psychological factors such as depression and hostility

or a surgical sling procedure (see below). Stress incontinence is unusual in men but can occur after transurethral surgery and/or radiation therapy for lower urinary tract malignancy when the anatomic sphincters are damaged.

Urge incontinence can be caused by a variety of lower genitourinary and neurological disorders (see Table 8-6). Patients with urge incontinence typically present with irritative symptoms of an overactive bladder, including frequency (voiding more than every 2 hours), urgency, and nocturia (two or more voids during usual sleeping hours). Urge incontinence is most often, but not always, associated with detrusor motor instability or detrusor hyperreflexia (see Fig. 8-4). Some patients have a poorly compliant bladder without involuntary contractions (e.g., radiation or interstitial cystitis, both relatively unusual conditions).

Other patients have symptoms of an overactive bladder but do not exhibit detrusor motor instability on urodynamic testing. Some patients with neurological disorders have detrusor hyperreflexia on urodynamic testing but do not have urgency and are incontinent without any warning symptoms ("unconscious incontinence"). The above-described patients are generally treated as if they had urge incontinence if they empty their bladders and do not have other correctable genitourinary pathology. A subgroup of older incontinent patients with detrusor motor instability also have impaired bladder contractility—emptying less than one-third of their bladder volume with involuntary contractions on urodynamic testing (Resnick and Yalla, 1987; Elbadawi et al., 1993). This condition has been termed *detrusor hyperactivity with impaired contractility* (DHIC). Patients with DHIC may present with symptoms that are not typical of urge incontinence and may strain to complete voiding. These patients may be difficult to manage because of their urinary retention.

Urinary retention with *overflow incontinence* can result from anatomic or neurogenic outflow obstruction, a hypotonic or acontractile bladder, or both. The most common causes include prostatic enlargement, diabetic neuropathic bladder, and urethral stricture. Low spinal cord injury and anatomic obstruction in females (caused by pelvic prolapse and urethral distortion) are less common causes of overflow incontinence. Several types of drugs can also contribute to this type of persistent incontinence (see Table 8-4). Some patients with suprasacral spinal cord lesions (e.g., multiple sclerosis) develop detrusor-sphincter dyssynergy and consequent urinary retention, which must be treated in a similar manner as overflow incontinence; in some instances a sphincterotomy is necessary. The symptoms of overflow incontinence are nonspecific and urinary retention is easily missed on physical examination. Thus, a postvoid residual determination must be performed to exclude this condition.

The term *functional incontinence* refers to incontinence associated with the inability or lack of motivation to reach a toilet on time. Factors that contribute to functional incontinence (such as inaccessible toilets and psychological disorders) can also exacerbate other types of persistent incontinence. Patients with incontinence that appears to be predominantly related to functional factors may also have abnormalities of the lower genitourinary tract. In some patients, it can be very difficult to determine whether the functional factors or the genitourinary factors predominate without a trial of specific types of treatment. However, no matter what specific treatments are prescribed, patients with functional incontinence require systematic toileting assistance as a component of their management plan.

These basic types of incontinence may occur in combination, as depicted by the overlap in Fig. 8-7. Older women commonly have a combination of stress and urge incontinence (generally referred to as *mixed incontinence*). Frail geriatric patients often have urge incontinence with detrusor instability as well as functional disabilities that contribute to their incontinence.

EVALUATION

Basic Evaluation

The first step in evaluating incontinent patients is to identify the incontinence by direct observation or the screening questions discussed earlier. In patients with the sudden onset of incontinence (especially when associated with an acute medical condition and hospitalization), the reversible factors that can cause acute incontinence (see Tables 8-3, 8-4, and 8-5) can be ruled out by a brief history, physical examination, postvoid residual determination, and basic laboratory studies (urinalysis, culture, serum glucose or calcium). Table 8-7 shows the basic components of the evaluation of persistent urinary incontinence. Practice guidelines suggest that the basic evaluation should include a focused history, targeted physical examination, urinalysis, and postvoiding residual (PVR) determination (Fantl, Newman, et al., 1996; American Medical Directors Association, 1996). The history should focus on the characteristics of the incontinence, current medical problems and medications, the most bothersome symptom(s), and the impact of the incontinence on the patient and caregivers (Table 8-8). Bladder records or voiding diaries such as those shown in Fig. 8-8 (for outpatients) and Fig. 8-9 (for institutionalized patients) can be helpful in initially characterizing symptoms as well as in following the response to treatment.

Physical examination should focus on abdominal, rectal, and genital examinations and an evaluation of lumbosacral innervation (Table 8-9). During the history and physical examination, special attention should be given to factors such as mobility, mental status, medications, and accessibility of toilets that may either be causing the incontinence or interacting with urological and neurological disorders to worsen the condition. The pelvic examination in women should include careful inspections of the labia and vagina for signs of inflammation suggestive of atrophic vaginitis and for pelvic prolapse. Most older women have some

TABLE 8-7   COMPONENTS OF THE DIAGNOSTIC EVALUATION OF
            PERSISTENT URINARY INCONTINENCE

All patients
    History, including bladder record
    Physical examination
    Urinalysis
    Postvoid residual determination
Selected patients*
    Laboratory studies
        Urine culture
        Urine cytology
        Blood glucose, calcium
        Renal function tests
        Renal ultrasonography
    Gynecologic evaluation
    Urological evaluation
    Cystourethroscopy
    Urodynamic tests
        Simple
            Observation of voiding
            Cough test for stress incontinence
            Simple (single channel) cystometry
        Complex
            Urine flowmetry
            Multichannel cystometrogram
            Pressure-flow study
            Leak-point pressure
            Urethral pressure profilometry
            Sphincter electromyography
            Videourodynamics

* See text and Table 8-9.

degree of pelvic prolapse (e.g., grade 1 or 2 cystocele as depicted in Fig. 8-10).
Not all incontinent older women with these degrees of prolapse need gynecological evaluation (see below).

   A clean urine sample should be collected for urinalysis. For men who are
frequently incontinent, making a "clean-catch" specimen difficult to obtain, a
clean specimen can be obtained using a condom catheter after cleaning the
penis (Ouslander et al., 1987). For women, a clean specimen can be obtained

TABLE 8-8   KEY ASPECTS OF AN INCONTINENT PATIENT'S HISTORY

Active medical conditions, especially neurologic disorders, diabetes
  mellitus, congestive heart failure, venous insufficiency

Medications (see Table 8-4)

Fluid intake pattern
  Type and amount of fluid (especially before bedtime)

Past genitourinary history, especially childbirth, surgery, dilatations, urinary
  retention, recurrent urinary tract infections

Symptoms of incontinence
  Onset and duration
  Type—stress vs. urge vs. mixed vs. other
  Frequency, timing, and amount of incontinence episodes and of continent
    voids (see Figs. 8-8 and 8-9)

Other lower urinary tract symptoms
  Irritative—dysuria, frequency, urgency, nocturia
  Voiding difficulty—hesitancy, slow or interrupted stream, straining,
    incomplete emptying
  Other—hematuria, suprapubic discomfort

Other symptoms
  Neurological (indicative of stroke, dementia, parkinsonism, normal
    pressure hydrocephalus, spinal cord compression, multiple sclerosis)
  Psychological (depression)
  Bowel (constipation, stool incontinence)
  Symptoms suggestive of volume-expanded state (e.g., lower extremity
    edema, shortness of breath while horizontal or with exertion)

Environmental factors
  Location and structure of bathroom
  Availability of toilet substitutes

Perceptions of incontinence
  Patient's concerns or ideas about underlying cause(s)
  Most bothersome symptoms(s)
  Interference with daily life
  Severity (e.g., is it enough of a problem for you to consider surgery?)

BLADDER RECORD

Day: _____

Date: _____ / _____ .
month   day

INSTRUCTIONS:

1) In the 1st column make a mark every time during the 2-hour period you urinate into the toilet

2) Use the 2nd column to record the amount you urinate (if you are measuring amounts)

3) In the 3rd or 4th column, make a mark every time you accidentally leak urine

Time Interval	Urinated in Toilet	Amount	Leaking Accident	or	Large Accident	Reason for Accident *
6-8 am						
8-10 am						
2-4 pm						
4-6 pm						
6-8 pm						
8-10 pm						
10-12 pm						
Overnight						

Number of pads used today: _____

* For example, if you coughed and have a leaking accident, write "cough".
If you had a large accident after a strong urge to urinate, write "urge".

— FIGURE 8-8 — *Example of a bladder record for ambulatory care settings.*

by cleaning the urethral and perineal area and having the patient void into a disinfected bedpan (Ouslander et al., 1995d). Persistent microscopic hematuria (>5 red blood cells per high-power field) in the absence of infection is an indication for further evaluation to exclude a tumor or other urinary tract pathology.

Because the prevalence of "asymptomatic bacteriuria" roughly parallels the prevalence of incontinence, incontinent geriatric patients commonly have significant bacteriuria. In the initial evaluation of incontinent noninstitutionalized patients, especially those in whom the incontinence is new or worsening, otherwise asymptomatic bacteriuria should be treated before further evaluation is undertaken. In the nursing home population, we do not recommend eradicating

INCONTINENCE MONITORING RECORD

INSTRUCTIONS: EACH TIME THE PATIENT IS CHECKED:
1) Mark *one* of the circles in the BLADDER section at the hour closest to the time the patient is checked.
2) Make an X in the BOWEL section if the patient has had an incontinent or normal bowel movement.

| 🌢 = Incontinent, small amount | ∅ = Dry | X = Incontinent BOWEL |
| ● = Incontinent, large amount | ⩟ = Voided correctly | X = Normal BOWEL |

PATIENT NAME _____ ROOM # _____ DATE _____

| | BLADDER | | | BOWEL | | | |
	INCONTINENT OF URINE	DRY	VOIDED CORRECTLY	INCONTINENT X	NORMAL X	INITIALS	COMMENTS
12 am	● ●	○	△ cc ___				
1	● ●	○	△ cc ___				
2	● ●	○	△ cc ___				
3	● ●	○	△ cc ___				
4	● ●	○	△ cc ___				
5	● ●	○	△ cc ___				
6	● ●	○	△ cc ___				
7	● ●	○	△ cc ___				
8	● ●	○	△ cc ___				
9	● ●	○	△ cc ___				
10	● ●	○	△ cc ___				
11	● ●	○	△ cc ___				
12 pm	● ●	○	△ cc ___				
1	● ●	○	△ cc ___				
2	● ●	○	△ cc ___				
3	● ●	○	△ cc ___				
4	● ●	○	△ cc ___				
5	● ●	○	△ cc ___				
6	● ●	○	△ cc ___				
7	● ●	○	△ cc ___				
8	● ●	○	△ cc ___				
9	● ●	○	△ cc ___				
10	● ●	○	△ cc ___				
11	● ●	○	△ cc ___				
TOTALS:							

— FIGURE 8-9 — *Example of a record to monitor bladder and bowel functions in institutional settings. This type of record is especially useful for implementing and following the results of various training procedures and other treatment protocols. (From Ouslander et al., 1986a, with permission.)*

TABLE 8-9   KEY ASPECTS OF AN INCONTINENT PATIENT'S PHYSICAL
EXAMINATION

Mobility and dexterity
   Functional status compatible with ability to self-toilet
   Gait disturbance (parkinsonism, normal-pressure hydrocephalus)

Mental status
   Cognitive function compatible with ability to self-toilet
   Motivation
   Mood and effect

Neurological
   Focal signs (especially in lower extremities)
   Signs of parkinsonism
   Sacral arc reflexes

Abdominal
   Bladder distension
   Suprapubic tenderness
   Lower abdominal mass

Rectal
   Perianal sensation
   Sphincter tone (resting and active)
   Impaction
   Masses
   Size and contour of prostate

Pelvic
   Perineal skin condition
   Perineal sensation
   Atrophic vaginitis (friability, inflammation, bleeding)
   Pelvic prolapse (i.e., cystocele, rectocele; see Fig. 8-10)
   Pelvic mass
   Other anatomic abnormality

Other
   Lower extremity edema or signs of congestive heart failure (if nocturia is
   a prominent complaint)

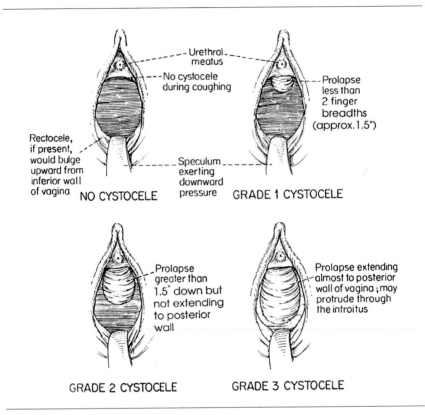

Urethral meatus
No cystocele during coughing
Rectocele, if present, would bulge upward from inferior wall of vagina
NO CYSTOCELE
Speculum exerting downward pressure

Prolapse less than 2 finger breadths (approx. 1.5")
GRADE 1 CYSTOCELE

Prolapse greater than 1.5" down but not extending to posterior wall
GRADE 2 CYSTOCELE

Prolapse extending almost to posterior wall of vagina; may protrude through the introitus
GRADE 3 CYSTOCELE

— FIGURE 8-10 — *Example of a grading system for cystoceles.* (From Ouslander et al., 1989a, with permission.)

bacteriuria unless symptoms of a urinary tract infection are present, because eradicating bacteriuria does not affect the severity of chronic, stable incontinence (Ouslander et al., 1995a). However, the new onset of incontinence, worsening incontinence, unexplained fever, and declines in mental and/or functional status may be the manifestations of a urinary tract infection in this population.

A PVR determination should be done either by catheterization or ultrasonogram to detect urinary retention, which cannot always be detected by physical examination. A portable ultrasonographic device that calculates residual urine is available (Diagnostic Ultrasound, Redmond, WA).

Patients with residual volumes of more than 200 mL should be considered for further evaluation. The need for further evaluation in patients with lesser degrees of retention should be determined on an individual basis, considering the patients' symptoms and the degree to which they complain of straining or are observed to strain with voiding.

Further Evaluation

The need for further evaluation and the specific diagnostic procedures listed in Table 8-7 should be determined on an individual basis. Clinical practice guidelines state that not all incontinent geriatric patients require further evaluation. Patients who have unexplained polyuria should have their blood glucose and calcium levels determined. Patients with significant urinary retention should have renal function tests and be considered for renal ultrasound and urodynamic testing to determine whether obstruction, impaired bladder contractility, or both are present. Persistent microscopic hematuria in the absence of infection is an indication for urine cytology and urological evaluation, including cystoscopy. Even in the absence of hematuria, patients with the recent and sudden onset of irritative urinary symptoms who have risk factors for bladder cancer (heavy smoking, industrial exposure to aniline dyes) should be considered for these evaluations. Women with marked pelvic prolapse (see Fig. 8-10) should be referred for gynecological evaluation.

Complex urodynamic testing is essential to determine the cause(s) of urinary retention and for any older patient for whom surgical intervention is being considered. Simple urodynamic tests, which can be performed without expensive equipment (including observation for straining during voiding, a cough test for stress incontinence with a comfortably full bladder, and simple cystometry) may be helpful in determining the cause(s) of incontinence in settings in which access to complex urodynamic testing is limited.

Table 8-10 summarizes criteria for referral for further evaluation, and Fig. 8-11 summarizes the overall approach to the evaluation of geriatric urinary incontinence.

MANAGEMENT

General Principles

Several therapeutic modalities can be used in managing incontinent geriatric patients (Table 8-11). Treatment can be especially helpful if specific diagnoses are made and attention is paid to all factors that may be contributing to the incontinence in a given patient. Even when cure is not possible, the comfort and satisfaction of both patients and caregivers can almost always be enhanced.

Special attention should be given to the management of acute incontinence, which is most common among older patients in acute care hospitals. Acute incontinence may be transient if managed appropriately; on the other hand, inappropriate management may lead to a permanent problem. The most common approach to incontinent geriatric patients in acute care hospitals is indwelling catheterization.

TABLE 8-10   CRITERIA FOR CONSIDERING REFERRAL OF INCONTINENT
PATIENTS FOR UROLOGICAL, GYNECOLOGICAL, OR
URODYNAMIC EVALUATION

CRITERIA	DEFINITION	RATIONALE
History		
Recent history of lower urinary tract or pelvic surgery or irradiation	Surgery or irradiation involving the pelvic area or lower urinary tract within the past 6 months.	A structural abnormality relating to the recent procedure should be sought.
Recurrent symptomatic urinary tract infections	Two or more symptomatic episodes in a 12-month period.	A structural abnormality or or pathological condition in the urinary tract predisposing to infection should be excluded.
Risk factors for bladder cancer	Recent or sudden onset of irritative symptoms, history of heavy smoking, or exposure to aniline dyes.	Urine for cytology and cystoscopy to exclude bladder cancer should be considered.
Physical examination		
Marked pelvic prolapse	A prominent cystocele that descends the entire height of the vaginal vault with coughing during speculum examination.	Anatomic abnormality may underlie the pathophysiology of the incontinence, and selected patients may benefit from surgical repair.
Marked prostatic enlargement and/ or suspicion of cancer	Gross enlargement of the prostate on digital exam; prominent induration or asymmetry of the lobes.	An evaluation to exclude prostate cancer may be appropriate and have therapeutic implications.
Postvoid residual		
Difficulty passing a 14-Fr straight catheter	Impossible catheter passage, or passage requiring considerable force, or a larger, more rigid catheter.	Anatomic blockage of the urethra or bladder neck may be present.

TABLE 8-10   CRITERIA FOR CONSIDERING REFERRAL OF INCONTINENT
PATIENTS FOR UROLOGICAL, GYNECOLOGICAL, OR
URODYNAMIC EVALUATION (*Continued*)

CRITERIA	DEFINITION	RATIONALE
Postvoid residual volume >200	Volume of urine remaining in the bladder within a few minutes after the patient voids spontaneously in as normal a fashion as possible.	Anatomic or neurogenic obstruction or poor bladder contractility may be present.
Urinalysis Hematuria	Greater than 5 red blood cells per high-power field on repeated microscopic exams in the absence of infection.	A pathological condition in the urinary tract should be excluded.
Therapeutic trial Failure to respond	Persistent symptoms that are bothersome to the patient after adequate trials of behavioral and/or drug therapy.	Urodynamic evaluation may help guide specific therapy

In some instances, this is justified by the necessity for accurate measurement of urine output during the acute phase of an illness. In many instances, however, it is unnecessary and poses a substantial and unwarranted risk of catheter-induced infection. Although it may be more difficult and time-consuming, making toilets and toilet substitutes accessible and combining this with some form of scheduled toileting is probably a more appropriate approach in patients who do not require indwelling catheterization. Newer launderable or disposable and highly absorbent bed pads and undergarments may also be helpful in managing these patients. These products may be more costly than catheters but probably result in less morbidity (and, therefore, overall cost) in the long run. All of the potential reversible factors that can cause or contribute

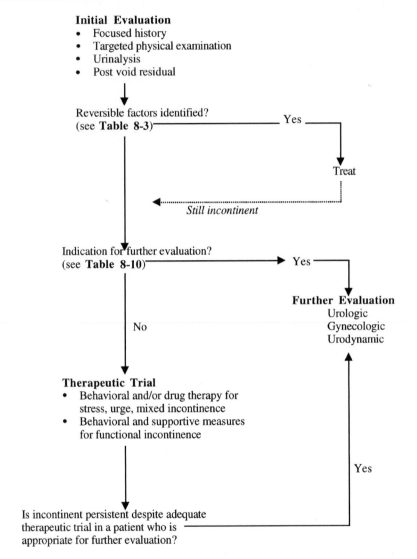

— FIGURE 8-11 —   *Algorithm protocol for evaluating incontinence.*

TABLE 8-11   TREATMENT OPTIONS FOR GERIATRIC URINARY
             INCONTINENCE

Nonspecific supportive measures
    Education
    Modifications of fluid and medication intake
    Use of toilet substitutes
    Environmental manipulations
    Garments and pads

Behavioral interventions (see Table 8-13)
    Patient-dependent
        Pelvic muscle exercises
        Bladder training
        Bladder retraining (see Table 8-14)
    Caregiver-dependent
        Scheduled toileting
        Habit training
        Prompted voiding (see Table 8-15)

Drugs (see Table 8-16)
    Bladder relaxants
    α-Agonists
    α-Antagonists
    Estrogen

Periurethral injections
Surgery
    Bladder neck suspension or sling
    Removal of obstruction or pathological lesion

Mechanical devices
    Urethral plugs, clamps
    Artificial sphincters

Catheters
    External
    Intermittent
    Indwelling

to incontinence (see Tables 8-3, 8-4, and 8-5) should be attended to in order to maximize the potential for regaining continence.

Supportive measures are critical in managing all forms of incontinence and should be used in conjunction with other, more specific treatment modalities. A positive attitude, education, environmental manipulations, the appropriate use of toilet substitutes, avoidance of iatrogenic contributions to incontinence, modifications of diuretic and fluid intake patterns, and good skin care are all important.

Specially designed incontinence undergarments and pads can be very helpful in many patients but must be used appropriately. They are now being marketed on television and are readily available in stores. Although they can be effective, several caveats should be noted:

1. Garments and pads are a nonspecific treatment. They should not be used as the first response to incontinence or before some type of diagnostic evaluation is done.
2. Many patients are curable if treated with specific therapies, and some have potentially serious factors underlying their incontinence that must be diagnosed and treated.
3. Pants and pads can interfere with attempts at behavioral intervention and thereby foster dependency.
4. Many disposable products are relatively expensive and are not covered by Medicare or other insurance.

To a large extent the optimal treatment of persistent incontinence depends on identifying the type(s). Table 8-12 outlines the primary treatments for the basic types of persistent incontinence in the geriatric population. Each treatment modality is briefly discussed below. Behavioral interventions have been well studied in the geriatric population. These interventions are recommended by guidelines as an initial approach to therapy in many patients because they are generally noninvasive and nonspecific (i.e., patients with stress and/or urge incontinence respond equally well) (Fantl et al., 1991; Ouslander et al., 1995a).

Behavioral Interventions

Many types of behavioral interventions have been described for the management of urinary incontinence. The term *bladder training* has been used to encompass a wide variety of techniques. It is, however, important to distinguish between procedures that are patient dependent (i.e., necessitate adequate function, learning capability, and motivation of the patient), in which the goal is to restore a normal pattern of voiding and continence, and procedures that are caregiver dependent that can be used for functionally disabled patients, in which the goal is to keep the patient and environment dry. Table 8-13 summarizes behavioral interventions. All the patient-dependent procedures generally involve the patient's

TABLE 8-12 PRIMARY TREATMENTS FOR DIFFERENT TYPES OF
GERIATRIC URINARY INCONTINENCE

Type of incontinence	Primary treatments
Stress	Pelvic muscle (Kegel) exercises Other behavioral interventions (see Table 8-13) α-Adrenergic agonists Estrogen Periurethral injections Surgical bladder neck suspension or sling
Urge	Bladder relaxants Estrogen (if atrophic vaginitis present) Bladder training (including pelvic muscle exercises)
Overflow	Surgical removal of obstruction Bladder retraining (see Table 8-14) Intermittent catheterization Indwelling catheterization
Functional	Behavioral interventions (caregiver dependent; see Tables 8-13 and 8-15) Environmental manipulations Incontinence undergarments and pads

continuous self-monitoring, using a record such as the one depicted in Fig. 8-8; the caregiver-dependent procedures usually involve a record such as the one shown in Fig. 8-9.

Pelvic muscle (Kegel) exercises are an essential component of patient-dependent behavioral interventions. These exercises consist of repetitive contractions and relaxations of the pelvic floor muscles.

The exercises may be taught by having the patient interrupt voiding to get a sense of the muscles being used or by having women squeeze the examiner's fingers during a vaginal examination (without doing a Valsalva maneuver, which is the opposite of the intended effect). A randomized trial has documented that many young-old women (mean age in the mid to upper sixties) can be taught these exercises during an office exam and derive significant reductions in incontinence (Burgio et al., 2002).

Many women, however, especially those older than age 75, require biofeedback to help them identify the muscles and practice the exercises. One exercise

TABLE 8-13   EXAMPLES OF BEHAVIORAL INTERVENTIONS FOR URINARY INCONTINENCE

PROCEDURE	DEFINITION	TYPES OF INCONTINENCE	COMMENTS
Patient dependent			
Pelvic muscle (Kegel) exercises	Repetitive contraction and relaxation of pelvic floor muscles	Stress and urge	Requires adequate function and motivation. Biofeedback often helpful in teaching the exercise
Bladder training	Use of education, bladder records, pelvic muscle, and other behavioral techniques	Stress and urge	Requires trained therapist, adequate cognitive and physical functioning, and motivation.
Bladder retraining	Progressive lengthening or shortening of intervoiding interval, with intermittent catheterization used in patients recovering from overdistention injuries with persistent retention (see Table 8-14)	Acute (e.g., postcatheterization with urge or overflow, poststroke)	Goal is to restore normal pattern of voiding and continence. Requires adequate cognitive and physical function and motivation.

Caregiver dependent			
Scheduled toileting	Routine toileting at regular intervals (scheduled toileting)	Urge and functional	Goal is to prevent wetting episodes. Can be used in patients with impaired cognitive or physical functioning. Requires staff or caregiver availability and motivation.
Habit training	Variable toileting schedule based on patient's voiding patterns	Urge and functional	Goal is to prevent wetting episodes. Can be used in patients with impaired cognitive or physical functioning. Requires staff or caregiver availability and motivation.
Prompted voiding	Offer opportunity to toilet every 2 h during the day; toilet only on request; social reinforcement; routine offering of fluids (see Table 8-15)	Urge, stress, mixed, functional	Same as above. 25-40% of nursing home residents respond well during the day and can be identified during a 3-day trial (see text and Table 8-15)

is a 10-second squeeze and a 10-second relaxation. Most older women will have to build endurance gradually to this level. Once learned, the exercises should be practiced many times throughout the day (up to 40 exercises per day) and, importantly, should be used in everyday life during situations (e.g., coughing, standing up, hearing running water) that might precipitate incontinence. Vaginal cones (weights) may be useful adjuncts to pelvic muscle exercises in some patients. Electrical stimulation may also be used to help identify and train pelvic muscles. This technique (using a different frequency of stimulation) may also be useful in suppressing the involuntary bladder contractions associated with urge incontinence. Many older patients are reluctant to purchase the devices for a therapeutic trial.

Biofeedback generally involves the use of vaginal (or rectal) pressure or electromyography (EMG) and abdominal muscle EMG recordings to train patients to contract pelvic floor muscles and relax the abdomen. Studies show that these techniques can be very effective for managing both stress and urge incontinence in the geriatric population Numerous software packages are now available to assist with biofeedback training.

Other forms of patient-dependent interventions include bladder training and bladder retraining. Bladder training involves education, pelvic muscle exercises (with or without biofeedback), strategies to manage urgency, and the regular use of bladder records (see Fig. 8-8). Bladder training is highly effective in selected community-dwelling patients, especially.

Table 8-14 provides an example of a bladder retraining protocol. This protocol is applicable to patients who have had indwelling catheterization for monitoring of urinary output during a period of acute illness or for treatment of urinary retention with overflow incontinence. Such catheters should always be removed as soon as possible, and this type of bladder retraining protocol should enable most indwelling catheters to be removed from patients in acute care hospitals as well as some in long-term care settings. A patient who continues to have difficulty voiding after 1 to 2 weeks of bladder retraining should be examined for other potentially reversible causes of voiding difficulties, such as those mentioned in the preceding discussion of acute incontinence. When difficulties persist, a urological referral should be considered in order to rule out correctable lower genitourinary pathology.

The goal of caregiver-dependent interventions is to prevent incontinence episodes rather than to restore normal patterns of voiding and complete continence. Such procedures are effective in reducing incontinence in selected nursing home residents (Ouslander et al., 1995b). In its simplest form, scheduled toileting involves toileting the patient at regular intervals, usually every 2 h during the day and every 4 h during the evening and night. Habit training involves a schedule of toiletings or prompted voidings that is modified according to the patient's pattern of continent voids and incontinence episodes as demonstrated by a monitoring record such as that shown in Fig. 8-9. Adjunctive techniques to prompt

TABLE 8-14 EXAMPLE OF A BLADDER RETRAINING PROTOCOL

Objective: To restore a normal pattern of voiding and continence after the removal of an indwelling catheter

1. Remove the indwelling catheter (clamping the catheter before removal is not necessary).
2. Treat urinary tract infection if present.
3. Initiate a toileting schedule. Begin by toileting the patient:
   a. Upon awakening
   b. Every 2 h during the day and evening
   c. Before getting into bed
   d. Every 4 h at night
4. Monitor the patient's voiding and continence pattern with a record that allows for the recording of:
   a. Frequency, timing, and amount of continent voids
   b. Frequency, timing, and amount of incontinence episodes
   c. Fluid intake pattern
   d. Postvoid catheter volume
5. If the patient is having difficulty voiding (complete urinary retention or very low urine outputs, e.g., <240 mL in an 8-h period while fluid intake is adequate):
   a. Perform in-and-out catheterization, recording volume obtained, every 6 to 8 h until residual values are <200 mL
   b. Instruct the patient on techniques to trigger voiding (e.g., running water, stroking inner thigh, suprapubic tapping) and to help completely empty bladder (e.g., bending forward, suprapubic pressure, double voiding)
   c. If the patient continues to have high residual volumes after 1–2 weeks, consider urodynamic evaluation
6. If the patient is voiding frequently (i.e., more often than every 2 h):
   a. Perform postvoid residual determination to ensure the patient is completely emptying the bladder
   b. Encourage the patient to delay voiding as long as possible and instruct him or her to use techniques to help completely empty bladder
   c. If the patient continues to have frequency and nocturia with or without urgency and incontinence:
      1. Rule out other reversible causes (e.g., urinary tract infection medication effects, hyperglycemia, and congestive heart failure)
      2. Consider urodynamic evaluation to rule out bladder instability (unstable bladder, detrusor hyperreflexia)

voiding (e.g., running tap water, stroking the inner thigh, or suprapubic tapping) and to facilitate complete emptying of the bladder (e.g., bending forward after completion of voiding) may be helpful in some patients. Prompted voiding has been the best-studied of these procedures. Table 8-15 provides an example of a prompted voiding protocol. Up to 40% of incontinent nursing home residents may become essentially dry during the day with a consistent prompted voiding program (Ouslander et al., 1995b). The success of these interventions is largely dependent on the knowledge and motivation of the caregivers who are implementing them, rather than on the physical functional and mental status of the incontinent patient. Targeting of prompted voiding to selected patients after a 3-day trial (see Table 8-15) may enhance its cost-effectiveness. Quality assurance methods, based on principles of industrial statistical quality control, have been shown to be helpful in maintaining the effectiveness of prompted voiding in nursing homes (Schnelle et al., 1995). However, unless adequate staffing, training, and administrative support for the program persist, the effectiveness of prompted voiding will not be maintained.

▊ Drug Treatment

Table 8-16 lists the drugs used to treat various types of incontinence.

The efficacy of drug treatment has not been as well studied in the geriatric population as it has in younger populations. However, for many patients, especially those with urge or stress incontinence, drug treatment may be very effective. Drug treatment can be prescribed in conjunction with various behavioral interventions. There are few data on the relative efficacy of drug versus behavioral versus combination treatment (Burgio et al., 1998). Treatment decisions should be individualized and will depend in large part on the characteristics and preferences of the patient and the preference of the health care professional.

For urge incontinence, drugs with anticholinergic and relaxant effects on the bladder smooth muscle are used. All of them can have bothersome systemic anticholinergic side effects, especially dry mouth, and they can precipitate urinary retention in some patients.

Men with some degree of outflow obstruction, diabetics, and patients with impaired bladder contractility are at the highest risk for developing urinary retention and should be followed carefully when these drugs are prescribed. Patients with Alzheimer's disease must be followed for the development of drug-induced delirium, which is, however, unusual. The newest bladder relaxant, tolterodine, appears to have an efficacy similar to that of other anticholinergics (Appell, 1997). Tolterodine and oxybutynin are both available in long-acting preparations. Tolterodine has proven efficacy in the geriatric population (Malone-Lee et al., 2001). Some functionally impaired patients may respond to these drugs when they are prescribed in conjunction with prompted voiding (Ouslander et al.,

TABLE 8-15   EXAMPLE OF A PROMPTED VOIDING PROTOCOL FOR A
NURSING HOME

Assessment period (3–5 days)
1. Contact resident every hour from 7 a.m. to 7 p.m. for 2–3 days, then
   every 2 h for 2–3 days
2. Focus attention on voiding by asking them whether he or she is wet or dry
3. Check residents for wetness, record on bladder record, and give feedback
   on whether response was correct or incorrect
4. Whether wet or dry, ask residents if they would like to use the toilet or
   urinal. If they say yes:
   • Offer assistance
   • Record results on bladder record
   • Give positive reinforcement by spending extra time talking with them
   If they say no:
   • Repeat the question once or twice
   • Inform them that you will be back in 1 h and request that they try to
     delay voiding until then
   • If there has been no attempt to void in the last 2–3 h, repeat the request
     to use the toilet at least twice more before leaving
5. Offer fluids

Targeting
1. Prompted voiding is more effective in some residents than others
2. The best candidates are residents who show the following characteristics
   during the assessment period:
   • Void in the toilet, commode, or urinal (as opposed to being incontinent
     in a pad or garment) more than two-thirds of the time
   • Wet on ≤20% of checks
   • Show substantial reduction in incontinence frequency on 2-h prompts
3. Residents who do not show any of these characteristics may be candidates for either:
   • Further evaluation to determine the specific type of incontinence if they
     attempt to toilet but remain frequently wet
   • Palliative management by containment devices and a checking-and-
     changing protocol if they do not cooperate with prompting

Prompted voiding (ongoing protocol)
1. Contact the resident every 2 h from 7 a.m. to 7 p.m.
2. Use same procedures as for the assessment period
3. For nighttime management, use either modified prompted voiding
   schedule or containment device, depending on resident's sleep pattern
4. If a resident who has been responding well has an increase in
   incontinence frequency despite adequate staff implementation of the
   protocol, the resident should be evaluated for reversible factors

TABLE 8-16   DRUGS USED TO TREAT URINARY INCONTINENCE

DRUGS	DOSAGES	MECHANISMS OF ACTION	TYPE OF INCONTINENCE	POTENTIAL ADVERSE EFFECTS
Anticholinergic and antispasmodic agents				
Hyoscamine (Levsin, others)	0.125 mg tid	Increase bladder capacity Diminish involuntary bladder contractions	Urge or mixed with urge predominant	Dry mouth, blurry vision, elevated intraocular pressure, delirium, constipation
Imipramine (Tofranil)*	25–50 mg tid			
Oxybutynin				
Short-acting	2.5–5.0 mg tid			
Long-acting (Ditropan XL)	5–30 mg qd			
Transdermal (Oxytrol)	3.9 mg patch every 4 days			
Tolterodine (Detrol LA)	4 mg qd		Stress	
α-Adrenergic agonists				
Pseudoephedrine (Sudafed)	30–60 mg tid			Headache, tachycardia, elevation of blood pressure
Topical estrogens				
Topical estradiol cream	0.5–1.0 g/ application	Strengthen periurethral tissues Increase periurethral blood flow	Urge associated with atrophic vaginitis Stress	Local irritation

	Dosage	Action	Indication	Side Effects
Vaginal estradiol ring (Estring)	One ring every 3 months			
Cholinergic agonists				
Bethanechol (Urecholine) †	10–30 mg tid	Stimulate bladder contraction	Overflow incontinence with atonic bladder	Bradycardia, hypotension, bronchoconstriction, gastric acid secretion
Alpha-adrenergic antagonists				
Doxazosin (Cardura)	1–4 mg qhs	Relax smooth muscle of urethra and prostatic capsule	Urge incontinence and related irritative symptoms associated with benign prostatic enlargement	Postural hypotension
Tamsulosin (Flowmax)	0.4–0.8 mg/d			
Terazosin (Hytrin)	1–5 mg qhs			

* Imipramine may also cause postural hypotension and cardiac conduction disturbances.
† Most effective if used after acute bladder overdistention in conjunction with bladder retraining (see Table 8-14).

1995c). The *goal* of treatment in these patients may not be to cure the incontinence but to reduce its severity and prevent discomfort and complications.

For stress incontinence, drug treatment involves a combination of an alpha agonist and estrogen. Drug treatment is appropriate for motivated patients who have mild to moderate degrees of stress incontinence, do not have a major anatomic abnormality (e.g., grade 3 cystocele or intrinsic sphincter deficiency), and do not have any contraindications to these drugs. These patients may also respond to concomitant behavioral interventions, as described above. For stress incontinence, estrogen alone is not as effective as it is in combination with an alpha agonist (Fantl, Bump, et al., 1996). Estrogen is also used for the treatment of irritative voiding symptoms and urge incontinence in women with atrophic vaginitis and urethritis. Oral estrogen is probably not as effective as topical estrogen for these symptoms. Vaginal estrogen can be prescribed 5 nights per week for 1 to 2 months initially and then reduced to a maintenance dose of one to three times per week. A vaginal ring that slowly releases estradiol is also available.

Drug treatment for chronic overflow incontinence using a cholinergic agonist or an α-adrenergic antagonist is rarely efficacious.

Bethanechol may be helpful when given for a brief period subcutaneously in patients with persistent bladder contractility problems after an overdistension injury, but it is seldom effective when given over the long term orally. α-adrenergic blockers may be helpful in relieving symptoms associated with outflow obstruction in some patients but are probably not efficacious for long-term treatment of overflow incontinence. These drugs are, however, effective in treating irritative voiding symptoms associated with urge incontinence in men with benign prostatic enlargement (Lepor et al., 1996).

Surgery

Surgery should be considered for older women with stress incontinence that continues to be bothersome after attempts at nonsurgical treatment and in women with a significant degree of pelvic prolapse or ISD. As with many other surgical procedures, patient selection and the experience of the surgeon are critical to success. All women being considered for surgical therapy should have a thorough evaluation, including urodynamic tests, before undergoing the procedure.

Women with mixed stress incontinence and detrusor motor instability may also benefit from surgery, especially if the clinical history and urodynamic findings suggest that stress incontinence is the predominant problem. Many modified techniques of bladder neck suspension can be done with minimal risk and are highly successful in achieving continence over about a 5-year period. Urinary retention can occur after surgery, but it is usually transient and can be managed by a brief period of suprapubic catheterization. Periurethral injection of collagen and other materials is now available and may offer patients with ISD an alternative to surgery. Surgical intervention for patients with ISD involves a perivaginal sling procedure rather than bladder neck suspension.

Surgery may be indicated in men in whom incontinence is associated with anatomically and/or urodynamically documented outflow obstruction. Men who have experienced an episode of complete urinary retention are likely to have another episode within a short period of time and should have a prostatic resection, as should men with incontinence associated with a sufficient amount of residual urine to be causing recurrent symptomatic infections or hydronephrosis. The decision about surgery in men who do not meet these criteria must be an individual one, weighing carefully the degree to which the symptoms bother the patient, the potential benefits of surgery (obstructive symptoms often respond better than irritative symptoms), and the risks of surgery, which may be minimal with newer prostate resection techniques. A small number of older patients, especially men who have stress incontinence related to sphincter damage due to previous transurethral surgery, may benefit from the surgical implantation of an artificial urinary sphincter.

Catheters and Catheter Care

Three basic types of catheters and catheterization procedures are used for the management of urinary incontinence: external catheters, intermittent straight catheterization, and chronic indwelling catheterization.

External catheters generally consist of some type of condom connected to a drainage system. Improvements in design and observance of proper procedure and skin care when applying the catheter will decrease the risk of skin irritation as well as the frequency with which the catheter falls off. Patients with external catheters are at increased risk of developing symptomatic infection. External catheters should be used only to manage intractable incontinence in male patients who do not have urinary retention and who are extremely physically dependent. As with incontinence undergarments and padding, these devices should not be used as a matter of convenience, since they may foster dependency.

Intermittent catheterization can help in the management of patients with urinary retention and overflow incontinence because of an acontractile bladder or DHIC. The procedure can be carried out by either the patient or a caregiver and involves straight catheterization two to four times daily, depending on catheter urine volumes and patient tolerance. In general, bladder volume should be kept to less than 400 mL. In the home setting, the catheter should be kept clean (but not necessarily sterile).

Intermittent catheterization may be useful for certain patients in acute care hospitals and nursing homes, for example following removal of an indwelling catheter in a bladder retraining protocol (see Table 8-14). Nursing home residents, however, may be difficult to catheterize, and the anatomic abnormalities commonly found in older patients' lower urinary tracts may increase the risk of infection as a consequence of repeated straight catheterizations. In addition, using this technique in an institutional setting (which may have an abundance of organisms that are relatively resistant to many commonly used antimicrobial agents) may yield an unacceptable risk of nosocomial infections, and using sterile catheter trays for these procedures would be very expensive; thus, it may be extremely difficult to implement such a program in a typical nursing home setting.

Chronic indwelling catheterization is overused in some settings and increases the incidence of a number of complications, including chronic bacteriuria, bladder stones, periurethral abscesses, and even bladder cancer. Nursing home residents, especially men, managed by this technique are at relatively high risk of developing symptomatic infections. Given these risks, it seems appropriate to recommend that the use of chronic indwelling catheters be limited to certain specific situations (Table 8-17). When indwelling catheterization is used, certain principles of catheter care should be observed in order to attempt to minimize complications (Table 8-18).

FECAL INCONTINENCE

Fecal incontinence is less common than urinary incontinence. Its occurrence is relatively unusual in older patients who are continent with regard to urine; however, a large proportion (30 to 50 percent) of geriatric patients with frequent urinary incontinence also have episodes of fecal incontinence. This coexistence suggests common pathophysiological mechanisms.

TABLE 8-17   INDICATIONS FOR CHRONIC INDWELLING CATHETER USE

Urinary retention that
  Is causing persistent overflow incontinence, symptomatic infections, or
    renal dysfunction
  Cannot be corrected surgically or medically
  Cannot be managed practically with intermittent catheterization

Skin wounds, pressure sores, or irritations that are being contaminated by
  incontinent urine

Care of terminally ill or severely impaired patients for whom bed and clothing
  changes are uncomfortable or disruptive

Preference of patient when toileting or changing cause excessive discomfort

TABLE 8-18   KEY PRINCIPLES OF CHRONIC INDWELLING CATHETER CARE

1. Maintain sterile, closed gravity-drainage system.
2. Avoid breaking the closed system.
3. Use clean techniques in emptying and changing the drainage system; wash hands between patients in institutionalized setting.
4. Secure the catheter to the upper thigh or lower abdomen to avoid perineal contamination and urethral irritation due to movement of the catheter.
5. Avoid frequent and vigorous cleaning of the catheter entry site; washing with soapy water once per day is sufficient.
6. Do not routinely irrigate.
7. If bypassing occurs in the absence of obstruction, consider the possibility of a bladder spasm, which can be treated with a bladder relaxant.
8. If catheter obstruction occurs frequently, increase the patient's fluid intake and acidify the urine with dilute acetic acid irrigations.
9. Do not routinely use prophylactic or suppressive urinary antiseptics or antimicrobials.
10. Do not do surveillance cultures to guide management of individual patients because all chronically catheterized patients have bacteriuria (which is often polymicrobial) and the organisms change frequently.
11. Do not treat infection unless the patient develops symptoms; symptoms may be nonspecific and other possible sources of infection should be carefully excluded before attributing symptoms to the urinary tract.
12. If a patient develops frequent symptomatic urinary tract infections, a genitourinary evaluation should be considered to rule out pathology such as stones, periurethral or prostatic abscesses, and chronic pyelonephritis.

Defecation, like urination, is a physiological process that involves smooth and striated muscles, central and peripheral innervation, coordination of reflex responses, mental awareness, and physical ability to get to a toilet. Disruption of any of these factors can lead to fecal incontinence. The most common causes of fecal incontinence are problems with constipation and laxative use, neurological disorders, and colorectal disorders (Table 8-19). Constipation is extremely common in the geriatric population and, when chronic, can lead to fecal impaction and incontinence. The hard stool (or scybalum) of fecal impaction irritates the rectum and results in the production of mucus and fluid. This fluid leaks around the mass of impacted stool and precipitates incontinence. Constipation is difficult to define; technically it indicates less than three bowel movements per week, although many patients use the term to describe difficult passage of hard stools or a feeling of incomplete evacuation. Poor

TABLE 8-19   CAUSES OF FECAL INCONTINENCE

Fecal impaction

Laxative overuse or abuse

Neurological disorders
    Dementia
    Stroke
    Spinal cord disease/injury

Colorectal disorders
    Diarrheal illness
    Diabetic autonomic neuropathy
    Rectal sphincter damage

dietary and toilet habits, immobility, and chronic laxative abuse are the most common causes of constipation in geriatric patients (Table 8-20).

Appropriate management of constipation will prevent fecal impaction and resultant fecal incontinence. The first step in managing constipation is the identification of all possible contributory factors. If the constipation is a new complaint and represents a recent change in bowel habit, then colonic disease, endocrine or metabolic disorders, depression, or drug side effects should be considered (see Table 8-19).

Proper diet, including adequate fluid intake and bulk, is important in preventing constipation. Crude fiber in amounts of 4 to 6 g (equivalent to 3 or 4 tablespoons of bran) a day is generally recommended. Improving mobility, body positioning during toileting, and the timing and setting of toileting are all important in managing constipation.

Defecation should optimally take place in a private, unrushed atmosphere and should take advantage of the gastrocolic reflex, which occurs a few minutes after eating. These factors are often overlooked, especially in nursing home settings.

A variety of drugs can be used to treat constipation (Table 8-21). These drugs are often overused; in fact, their overuse may cause an atonic colon and contribute to chronic constipation ("cathartic colon").

Laxative drugs can also contribute to fecal incontinence. Rational use of these drugs necessitates knowing the nature of the constipation and quality of the stool. For example, stool softeners will not help a patient with a large mass of already soft stool in the rectum. These patients would benefit from a glycerin or irritant suppositories.

The use of osmotic and irritant laxatives should be limited to no more than three or four times a week.

Fecal incontinence from neurological disorders is sometimes amenable to biofeedback therapy, although most severely demented patients are unable to

TABLE 8-20   CAUSES OF CONSTIPATION

Diet low in bulk and fluid

Poor toilet habits

Immobility

Laxative abuse

Colorectal disorders
   Colonic tumor, stricture, volvulus
   Painful anal and rectal conditions (hemorrhoids, fissures)

Depression

Drugs
   Anticholinergic
   Narcotic

Diabetic autonomic neuropathy

Endocrine or metabolic
   Hypothyroidism
   Hypercalcemia
   Hypokalemia

cooperate. For those patients with end-stage dementia who fail to respond to a regular toileting program and suppositories, a program of alternating constipating agents (if necessary) and laxatives on a routine schedule (such as giving laxatives or enemas three times a week) is often effective in controlling defecation.

Experience suggests that these measures should permit management of even severely demented patients. As a last resort, specially designed incontinence undergarments are sometimes helpful in managing fecal incontinence and preventing complications. Frequent changing is essential, because fecal material, especially in the presence of incontinent urine, can cause skin irritation and predispose to pressure ulcers.

References

American Medical Directors Association: *Urinary Incontinence: Clinical Practice Guideline.* Columbia, MD, AMDA, 1996.

Appell RA: Clinical efficacy and safety of tolterodine in the treatment of overactive bladder: a pooled analysis. *Urology* 50(Suppl 6A):90–96, 1997.

Burgio KL, Locher JL, Goode PS, et al: Behavioral vs. drug treatment for urge urinary incontinence in older women. *JAMA* 280(23):1995–2000, 1998.

TABLE 8-21   DRUGS USED TO TREAT CONSTIPATION

TYPE	EXAMPLES	MECHANISM OF ACTION
Stool softeners and lubricants	Dioctyl sodium succinate Mineral oil	Soften and lubricate fecal mass
Bulk-forming agents	Bran Psyllium mucilloid	Increase fecal bulk and retain fluid in bowel lumen
Osmotic cathartics	Milk of magnesia Magnesium sulfate/ citrate Lactulose Sorbitol	Poorly absorbed and retain fluid in bowel lumen; increase net secretions of fluid in small intestine
Stimulants and irritants	Cascara Senna Bisacodyl Phyenolphthalein	Alter intestinal mucosal permeability; stimulate muscle activity and fluid secretions
Enemas	Tap water Saline Sodium phosphate Oil	Induce reflex evacuations
Suppositories	Glycerin Bisacodyl	Cause mucosal irritation

Burgio KL, Goode PS, Locher JL, et al: Behavioral training with and without biofeedback in the treatment of urge incontinence in older women. *JAMA* 288(18):2293–2299, 2002.

Elbadawi A, Yalla SV, Resnick N: Structural basis of geriatric voiding dysfunction: I. Methods of a prospective ultrastructural/urodynamic study and an overview of the findings. *J Urol* 150:1650–1656, 1993.

Fantl JA, Wyman FJ, McClish DK, et al: Efficacy of bladder training in older women with urinary incontinence. *JAMA* 265:609–613, 1991.

Fantl JA, Newman DK, Colling J, et al: *Urinary Incontinence in Adults: Acute and Chronic Management. Clinical Practice Guideline No. 2, 1996, Update* (AHCPR Publication No. 96-0682). Rockville, MD, US Department of Health and Human Services, Public Health Service, Agency for Health Care Policy and Research, 1996a.

Fantl JA, Bump RC, Robinson D, et al: Efficacy of estrogen supplementation in the treatment of urinary incontinence: the Continence Program for Women Research Group. *Obstet Gynecol* 88:745–749, 1996b.

Lepor H, Williford WO, Barry MJ, et al: The efficacy of terazosin, finasteride, or both in benign prostatic hyperplasia. Veterans Affairs Cooperative Studies Benign Prostatic Hyperplasia Study Group. *N Engl J Med* 335:533–539, 1996.

Malone-Lee JG, Walsh JB, Maugourd MF, et al: Tolterodine: a safe and effective treatment for older patients with overactive bladder. *J Am Geriatr Soc* 49:700–705, 2001.

Ouslander JG, Uman GC, Urman HN: Development and testing of an incontinence monitoring record. *J Am Geriatr Soc* 34:83–90, 1986a.

Ouslander JG, Greengold BA, Silverblatt FJ, et al: An accurate method to obtain urine for culture in men with external catheters. *Arch Intern Med* 147:286–288, 1987.

Ouslander JG, Leach GE, Staskin DR: Simplified tests of lower urinary tract function in the evaluation of geriatric urinary incontinence. *J Am Geriatr Soc* 37:706–714, 1989a.

Ouslander JG, Schapira M, Schnelle J, et al: Does eradicating bacteriuria affect the severity of chronic urinary incontinence among nursing home residents? *Ann Intern Med* 122:749–754, 1995a.

Ouslander JG, Schnelle JF, Uman G, et al: Predictors of successful prompted voiding among incontinent nursing home residents. *JAMA* 273:1366–1370, 1995b.

Ouslander JG, Schnelle JF, Uman G, et al: Does oxybutynin add to the effectiveness of prompted voiding for urinary incontinence among nursing home residents? a placebo-controlled trial. *J Am Geriatr Soc* 43:610–617, 1995c.

Ouslander JG, Schapira M, Schnelle JF: Urine specimen collection from incontinent female nursing home residents. *J Am Geriatr Soc* 43:279–281, 1995d.

Resnick NM, Yalla SV: Detrusor hyperactivity with impaired contractile function: an unrecognized but common cause of incontinence in elderly patients. *JAMA* 257:3076–3081, 1987.

Schnelle JF, McNees P, Crook V, et al: The use of a computer-based model to implement an incontinence management program. *Gerontologist* 35:656–665, 1995.

Suggested Readings

Abrams P, Cardozo L, Khoury S, Wein A (eds): *Incontinence. 2nd International Consultation on Incontinence.* Plymouth, United Kingdom, Plybridge Distributors, 2001.

Barry MJ: A 73-year-old man with symptomatic benign prostatic hyperplasia. *JAMA* 287(24):2178–2184, 1997.

Brown JS, Vittinghoff E, Wyman JF, et al: Urinary incontinence: does it increase risk for falls and fractures? *J Am Geriatr Soc* 48:721–725, 2000.

Ouslander JG (ed): Aging and the lower urinary tract. *Am J Med Sci* 314(4):214–218, 1997.

Ouslander JG, Maloney C, Grasela TH, et al: Implementation of a nursing home urinary incontinence management program with and without tolterodine. *J Am Med Dir Assoc* 2:207–214, 2001.

Ouslander JG, Schnelle JF: Incontinence in the nursing home. *Ann Intern Med* 122:438–449, 1995.

Resnick NM, Ouslander JG (eds): NIH consensus conference on urinary incontinence in adults. *J Am Geriatr Soc* 38:263–386, 1990.

Romero Y, Evans JM, Fleming KC, Phillip SF: Constipation and fecal incontinence in the elderly population. *Mayo Clin Proc* 71:81–92, 1996.

Skelly J, Flint AJ: Urinary incontinence associated with dementia. *J Am Geriatr Soc* 42:286–294, 1995.

Yoshimura N, Chancellor MB: Current and future pharmacological treatment for overactive bladder. *J Urol* 168:1897–1913, 2002.

CHAPTER 9

INSTABILITY AND FALLS

Falls are among the major causes of morbidity in the geriatric population. Falling is not only a problem in its own right; it is often a marker for frailty, and falls may be predictors of death as well as indirect causes (usually through fractures). Close to one-third of those aged 65 years and older living at home suffer a fall each year, and about 1 in 40 of those will be hospitalized. Only about half of the elderly patients hospitalized as the result of a fall will be alive a year later. Among geriatric nursing homes residents, as many as half suffer a fall each year; 10 to 25 percent have serious consequences. Accidents are the fifth leading cause of death in persons older than age 65, and falls account for two-thirds of these accidental deaths. Of deaths from falls in the United States, more than 70 percent occur in the 11 percent of the population older than age 65. However, it may be difficult to separate the effects of the accident from the underlying frailty that led to it. Fear of falling can adversely affect older persons' functional status. Repeated falls and consequent injuries can be important factors in the decision to institutionalize an elderly person.

Table 9-1 lists potential complications of falls. Fractures of the hip, femur, humerus, wrist, and ribs, and painful soft-tissue injuries are the most frequent physical complications. Many of these injuries will result in hospitalization, with the attendant risks of immobilization and iatrogenic illnesses (see Chaps. 5 and 10). Fractures of the hip and lower extremities often lead to prolonged disability because of impaired mobility. A less-common, but important, injury is subdural hematoma. Neurological symptoms and signs that develop days to weeks after a fall should prompt consideration of this treatable problem.

Even when the fall does not result in serious injury, substantial disability may result from fear of falling, loss of self-confidence, and restricted ambulation (either self-imposed or imposed by caregivers).

Falls and their attendant complications should be preventable, but it is easier to identify risk factors for falling than to prevent its occurrence. A growing body of studies suggests that at least some types of falls can be prevented. Moreover, it is possible to prevent the untoward consequences of falls (i.e., fractures) by changing the way old people fall. The potential for prevention together with the use of falling as an indicator of underlying frailty combine to make an

TABLE 9-1   COMPLICATIONS OF FALLS IN ELDERLY PATIENTS

Injuries
   Painful soft-tissue injuries
   Fractures
      Hip
      Femur
      Humerus
      Wrist
      Ribs
   Subdural hematoma

Hospitalization
   Complications of immobilization (see Chap. 10)
   Risk of iatrogenic illnesses (see Chap. 5)

Disability
   Impaired mobility because of physical injury
   Impaired mobility from fear, loss of self-confidence, and restriction of
      ambulation

Risk of institutionalization

Death

understanding of the causes of falls and a practical approach to the evaluation and management of patients with instability and falls important components of geriatric care. Similar to many other conditions described throughout this text, the factors that can contribute to or cause falls are multiple, and very often more than one of these factors plays an important role (Fig. 9-1).

Falling may be a useful indicator of frailty in general. Persons with a history of falling have higher levels of subsequent health care use and poor functional status. Fallers who were thoroughly assessed showed a benefit in functional outcomes over those who were not, even when the cause of the fall could not be determined or treated.

AGING AND INSTABILITY

Several age-related factors contribute to instability and falls (Table 9-2). Most "accidental" falls are caused by one or a combination of these factors interacting with environmental hazards.

Aging changes in postural control and gait probably play a major role in many falls among older persons. Increasing age is associated with diminished proprio-

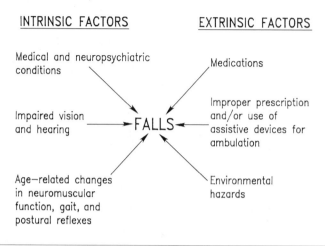

INTRINSIC FACTORS   EXTRINSIC FACTORS

Medical and neuropsychiatric conditions

Medications

Impaired vision and hearing → FALLS ←

Improper prescription and/or use of assistive devices for ambulation

Age–related changes in neuromuscular function, gait, and postural reflexes

Environmental hazards

— FIGURE 9-1 — *Multifactorial causes and potential contributors to falls in older persons.*

ceptive input, slower righting reflexes, diminished strength of muscles important in maintaining posture, and increased postural sway. All these changes can contribute to falling—especially the ability to avoid a fall after encountering an environmental hazard or an unexpected trip. Changes in gait also occur with increasing age. Although these changes may not be sufficiently prominent to be labeled truly pathological, they can increase susceptibility to falls. In general, elderly people do not pick their feet up as high, thus increasing the tendency to trip. Elderly men develop wide-based, short-stepped gaits; elderly women often walk with a narrow-based, waddling gait. Orthostatic hypotension (defined as a drop in systolic blood pressure of 20 mm Hg or more when moving from a lying to a standing position) occurs in approximately 20 percent of older persons. Although not all elderly individuals with orthostatic hypotension are symptomatic, this impaired physiological response could play a role in causing instability and precipitating falls in a substantial proportion of patients. Older people have been shown to experience a postprandial fall in blood pressure as well.

Several pathological conditions that increase in prevalence with increasing age can contribute to instability and falling. Degenerative joint disease (especially of the neck, the lumbosacral spine, and the lower extremities) can cause pain, unstable joints, muscle weakness, and neurological disturbances. Healed fractures of the hip and femur can cause an abnormal and less steady gait. Residual muscle weakness or sensory deficits from a recent or remote stroke can cause instability.

Muscle weakness as a result of disuse and deconditioning (caused by pain and/or lack of exercise) can contribute to an unsteady gait and impair the ability

TABLE 9-2   AGE-RELATED FACTORS CONTRIBUTING TO INSTABILITY
AND FALLS

Changes in postural control
  Decreased proprioception
  Slower righting reflexes
  Decreased muscle tone
  Increased postural sway
  Orthostatic hypotension

Changes in gait
  Feet not picked up as high
  Men: develop flexed posture and wide-based, short-stepped gait
  Women: develop narrow-based, waddling gait

Increased prevalence of pathologic conditions relative to stability
  Degenerative joint disease
  Fractures of hip and femur
  Stroke with residual deficits
  Muscle weakness from disuse and deconditioning
  Peripheral neuropathy
  Diseases or deformities of the feet
  Impaired vision
  Impaired hearing
  Forgetfulness and dementia
  Other specific disease processes (e.g., cardiovascular disease,
    parkinsonism—see Table 9-3)

Increased prevalence of conditions causing nocturia (e.g., congestive heart
  failure, venous insufficiency)

Increased prevalence of dementia

to right oneself after a loss of balance. Diminished sensory input, such as in diabetic and other peripheral neuropathies, visual disturbances, and impaired hearing diminish cues from the environment that normally contribute to stability and
thus predispose one to falls. Impaired cognitive function may result in the creation of, or wandering into, unsafe environments and may lead to falls. Podiatric
problems (bunions, calluses, nail disease, joint deformities, etc.) that cause pain,
deformities, and alterations in gait are common, correctable causes of instability.
Other specific disease processes common in older people (such as Parkinson's
disease and cardiovascular disorders) can cause instability and falls and are discussed further below.

Inability to get up after a fall can be an indication of a poor prognosis. In one study almost half those who fell at least once reported being unable to get up. These older persons had poorer functional outcomes.

CAUSES OF FALLS IN OLDER PERSONS

Table 9-3 outlines the multiple and often interacting causes of falls among older persons. More than half of all falls are related to medically diagnosed conditions, emphasizing the importance of a careful medical assessment for patients who fall (see below). Several studies have examined risk factors for falls among older persons and have found a variety of these factors—including cognitive impairment, disabilities of the lower extremities, gait and balance abnormalities, nocturia, and the number and nature of medications being taken—as important risk factors. Frequently overlooked, environmental factors can increase susceptibility to falls and other accidents. Homes of elderly people are often full of environmental hazards (Table 9-4). Unstable furniture, rickety stairs with inadequate railings, throw rugs and frayed carpets, and poor lighting should be specifically looked for on home visits. Several factors are associated with falls among older nursing home residents (Table 9-5). Awareness of these factors can help prevent morbidity and mortality in these settings. Although attention to the environment makes sense, the role of environmental hazards may be overemphasized (Gill et al., 2000).

Several factors can hinder precise identification of the specific causes for falls. These factors include lack of witnesses, inability of the elderly person to recall the circumstances surrounding the event, the transient nature of several causes [e.g., arrhythmia, transient ischemic attack (TIA), postural hypotension], and the fact that the majority of elderly people who fall do not seek medical attention. Somewhat more detailed information is available on the circumstances surrounding falls in nursing homes (see Table 9-5), but these individuals represent a relatively low proportion and a highly select group among the total senior population.

Close to half of all falls can be classified as accidental. Usually an accidental trip or a slip can be precipitated by an environmental hazard, often in conjunction with factors listed in Table 9-2. Addressing the environmental hazards begins with a careful assessment of the patient's environment. Some older persons have developed a strong attachment to their cluttered surroundings and may need active encouragement to make the necessary changes, but many may simply take such environmental risks for granted until they are specifically identified.

Syncope, "drop attacks," and "dizziness" are commonly cited causes of falls in elderly persons. Indeed, dizziness has been nominated as a possible geriatric syndrome, worthy of fuller exploration (Tinetti et al., 2000). If there is a clear history of loss of consciousness, a cause for true syncope should be sought. Although the complete differential diagnosis of syncope is beyond the scope of

TABLE 9-3   CAUSES OF FALLS

Accidents
    True accidents (trips, slips, etc.)
    Interactions between environmental hazards and factors increasing
      susceptibility (see Table 9-2)
Syncope (sudden loss of consciousness)
Drop attacks (sudden leg weaknesses without loss of consciousness)
Dizziness and/or vertigo
    Vestibular disease
    Central nervous system disease
Orthostatic hypotension
    Hypovolemia or low cardiac output
    Autonomic dysfunction
    Impaired venous return
    Prolonged bed rest
    Drug-induced hypotension
    Postprandial hypotension
Drug-related causes
    Diuretics
    Antihypertensives
    Tricyclic antidepressants
    Sedatives
    Antipsychotics
    Hypoglycemics
    Alcohol
Specific disease processes
    Acute illness of any kind ("premonitory fall")
    Cardiovascular
      Arrhythmias
      Valvular heart disease (aortic stenosis)
      Carotid sinus syncope
    Neurological causes
      Transient ischemic attack (TIA)
      Stroke (acute)
      Seizure disorder
      Parkinson's disease
      Cervical or lumbar spondylosis (with spinal cord or nerve root com-
      pression)
      Cerebellar disease
      Normal-pressure hydrocephalus (gait disorder)
      Central nervous system lesions (e.g., tumor, subdural hematoma)
Idiopathic (no specific cause identifiable)

TABLE 9-4   COMMON ENVIRONMENTAL HAZARDS

Old, unstable, and low-lying furniture

Beds and toilets of inappropriate height

Unavailability of grab bars

Uneven stairs and inadequate railing

Throw rugs, frayed carpets, cords, wires

Slippery floors and bathtubs

Inadequate lighting, glare

Cracked and uneven sidewalks

TABLE 9-5   FACTORS ASSOCIATED WITH FALLS AMONG OLDER
NURSING HOME RESIDENTS

Recent admission

Dementia

Hip weakness

Certain activities (toileting, getting out of bed)

Psychotropic drugs causing daytime sedation

Cardiovascular medications (vasodilators, diuretics)

Polypharmacy

Low staff–patient ratio

Unsupervised activities

Unsafe furniture

Slippery floors

this chapter, some of the more common causes of syncope in older people include vasovagal responses, cardiovascular disorders (such as brady- and tachyarrhythmias and aortic stenosis), acute neurological events (such as TIA, stroke, and seizure), pulmonary embolus, and metabolic disturbances (e.g., hypoxia, hypoglycemia). Cardiovascular causes for syncope are more common in the elderly than in younger populations. A precise cause for syncope may remain unidentified in 40 to 60 percent of elderly patients.

Drop attacks, described as sudden leg weakness causing a fall without loss of consciousness, are probably overdiagnosed in elderly people who fall. They are often attributed to vertebrobasilar insufficiency, frequently precipitated by a change in head position. Only a small proportion of older people who fall have truly had a drop attack. The underlying pathophysiology is poorly understood, and care should be taken to rule out other causes.

Dizziness and unsteadiness are extremely common complaints among elderly people who fall (as well as those who do not). A feeling of light-headedness can be associated with several different disorders, but is a nonspecific symptom and should be interpreted with caution. Patients complaining of light-headedness should be carefully evaluated for postural hypotension and intravascular volume depletion.

Vertigo (a sensation of rotational movement), on the other hand, is a more specific symptom and is probably an uncommon precipitant of falls in the elderly. It is most commonly associated with disorders of the inner ear, such as acute labyrinthitis, Ménière's disease, and benign positional vertigo. Vertebrobasilar ischemia and infarction and cerebellar infarction can also cause vertigo. Patients with vertigo caused by organic disorders often have nystagmus, which can be observed by having the patient quickly lie down and turning the patient's head to the side in one motion. Many older patients with symptoms of dizziness and unsteadiness are anxious, depressed, and chronically afraid of falling, and the evaluation of their symptoms is quite difficult. Some patients, especially those with symptoms suggestive of vertigo, will benefit from a thorough otological examination including auditory testing, which may help clarify the symptoms and differentiate inner-ear from central nervous system (CNS) involvement.

Orthostatic hypotension is best detected by taking the blood pressure and pulse in supine position, after 1 minute in the sitting position, and after 1 and 3 minutes in the standing position. A drop of more than 20 mm Hg in systolic blood pressure is generally considered to represent significant orthostatic hypotension. In many instances, this condition is asymptomatic; however, several conditions can cause orthostatic hypotension or worsen it to a severity sufficient to precipitate a fall.

These conditions include low cardiac output from heart failure or hypovolemia, autonomic dysfunction (which can result from diabetes or Parkinson's disease), impaired venous return (e.g., venous insufficiency), prolonged bed rest with deconditioning of muscles and reflexes, and several different drugs. Simply eating a full meal can precipitate a reduction in blood pressure in an older person that may be worsened and precipitate a fall when the person stands up. The association of orthostatic hypotension with elevated blood pressure but not with the use of antihypertensive medication suggests that treatment of hypertension may improve this condition.

Drugs that should be suspected of playing a role in falls include diuretics (hypovolemia), antihypertensives (hypotension), tricyclic antidepressants (postural hypotension), sedatives (excessive sedation), antipsychotics (sedation, muscle rigidity, postural hypotension), hypoglycemics (acute hypoglycemia), and alcohol (intoxication). Combinations of these drug types may greatly increase the risk of a fall. Psychotropic drugs are commonly prescribed and appear to substantially increase the risk of falls and hip fractures, especially in patients prescribed tricyclic antidepressants.

Many disease processes, especially of the cardiovascular and neurological systems, can be associated with falls. Cardiac arrhythmias are common in ambulatory elderly persons and may be difficult to associate directly with a fall or syncope. In general, cardiac monitoring should document a temporal association between a specific arrhythmia and symptoms (or a fall) before the arrhythmia is diagnosed (and treated) as the cause of falls.

Syncope can be a symptom of aortic stenosis and is an indication of the need to evaluate a patient suspected of having significant aortic stenosis for valve replacement. Aortic stenosis is difficult to diagnose by physical examination alone, and all patients suspected of having this condition should have an echocardiogram.

Some elderly individuals have sensitive carotid baroreceptors and are susceptible to syncope resulting from reflex increase in vagal tone (caused by cough, straining at stool, micturition, etc.), which leads to bradycardia and hypotension. Carotid sinus sensitivity can be detected by bedside maneuvers (see below).

Cerebrovascular disease is often implicated as a cause or contributing factor for falls in older patients. Although cerebral blood flow and cerebrovascular autoregulation may be diminished, these aging changes alone are not enough to cause unsteadiness or falls. They may, however, render the elderly person more susceptible to stresses such as diminished cardiac output, which will more easily precipitate symptoms. Acute strokes (caused by thrombosis, hemorrhage, or embolus) can cause and may initially manifest themselves in falls. TIAs of both the anterior and posterior circulations frequently last only minutes and are often poorly described. Thus, care must be taken in making these diagnoses. Anterior circulation TIAs may cause unilateral weakness and thus precipitate a fall. Vertebrobasilar (posterior circulation) TIAs may cause vertigo, but a history of transient vertigo alone is not a sufficient basis for the diagnosis of a TIA. The diagnosis of posterior circulation TIA necessitates that one or more other symptoms (visual field cuts, dysarthria, ataxia, or limb weakness—which can be bilateral) be associated with vertigo. Vertebrobasilar insufficiency, as mentioned above, is often cited as a cause of drop attacks; in addition, mechanical compression of the vertebral arteries by osteophytes of the cervical spine when the head is turned has also been proposed as a cause of unsteadiness and falling. Both of these conditions are poorly documented, are probably overdiagnosed, and should not be used as causes of a fall simply because nothing else can be found.

Other diseases of the brain and central nervous system can also cause falls. Parkinson's disease and normal-pressure hydrocephalus can cause disturbances of gait, which lead to instability and falls. Cerebellar disorders, intracranial tumors, and subdural hematomas can cause unsteadiness, with a tendency to fall. A slowly progressive gait disability with a tendency to fall, especially in the presence of spasticity or hyperactive reflexes in the lower extremities, should prompt consideration of cervical spondylosis and spinal cord compression. It is especially important to consider these diagnoses because treatment may improve the condition before permanent disability ensues.

Despite this long list, the precise causes of many falls will remain unknown—even after a thorough evaluation. The ultimate test of the etiology for falls is its reversibility. As noted earlier, we are better at finding putative causes than in correcting them.

EVIDENCE ON FALLS PREVENTION

The intense effort to identify risk factors for falls has been matched more recently with interventive efforts. A recent meta-analysis concluded that there was evidence that interventions could prevent the rate of falls, but the cost-effectiveness of falls prevention still remains unclear (RAND, 2002). Table 9-6 summarizes some of the findings from these studies. In general, they suggest that it is possible to reduce the rate of falling, but not the rate of injurious falls. Despite this mixed message, there is growing enthusiasm for undertaking preventive efforts. Moreover, good clinical sense still dictates active efforts to identify remediable risk factors. A randomized trial showed that targeted intervention to reduce the rate of falls did lower the overall rate (as compared with a control group) but there was no significant difference in the rate of serious falls. A meta-analysis of the several studies conducted under the auspices of the Frailty and Injuries: Cooperative Studies of Intervention Techniques (FICSIT) trials showed only modest results. In only two cases did an intervention lead to a significant reduction in falls; exercise and balance were associated with fewer falls, but not with falls with injuries. Tai Chi training was shown to increase the time to a fall but not to a serious fall compared with an educational control group. When a specific fall prevention program was compared with a more general chronic disease prevention program, the falls program achieved lower rates of falls and serious falls at the end of the first year, but by year 2, the differences disappeared. A New Zealand study showed that elderly patients could be taught at home to perform exercises that reduced the rate of falls. A fact to remember when interpreting the effect of exercise in falls prevention is that exercise needs to be sustained, probably for at least 6 months. The dropout rate for many of these exercise programs is quite high (approximately one-third to one-half of participants), suggesting that at least part of the problem in demonstrating an effect may lie in maintaining the intervention.

A successful multifactorial approach to reducing falls among nursing home patients employed training in environmental and personal safety, wheelchair use,

TABLE 9-6 SUMMARY OF FALLS INTERVENTION STUDIES

INTERVENTION	FINDINGS	REFERENCE
Exercise and cognitive-behavioral therapy	No difference in time to first fall	Reinsch et al., 1992
Combination of medication adjustment, behavioral instructions, exercise program	At 1 year RR for falls 0.69; no significant effect on injurious falls	Tinetti et al., 1994
Removing safety hazards, behavior program, strength, range of motion, and proprioception exercises	At 2 years RR for falling 0.85; no significant effect on injurious falls	Hornbrook et al., 1994
Nurse home assessment with and without specific attention to falls risks	Both intervention groups have lower rates of falls and injurious falls after 1 year, but not at 2 years	Wagner et al., 1994
Various exercise programs	RR for falls among general exercise group 0.90, including balance 0.83; no significant effect on injurious falls	FICSIT (Province et al., 1995)
Tai Chi	Relative hazard for falling 0.51	Wolf et al., 1996
Strength and endurance training	Relative hazard for falls 0.53	Buchner et al., 1997
Weight-bearing exercise	Number of falls over 2 years not significant but difference in rate for months 12–18 was significant	McMurdo et al., 1997
Home-based physical therapy exercise program	Hazard ratio for first fall was not significant, but for fall with injury it was 0.61	Campbell et al., 1997
Medical and occupational therapy assessment and referrals	RR for falls at 12 mo 0.39, for recurrent falls 0.33; RR for hospital admission 0.61	PROFET (Close et al., 1999)

TABLE 9-6   SUMMARY OF FALLS INTERVENTION STUDIES (*Continued*)

INTERVENTION	FINDINGS	REFERENCE
Home-based strength and balance exercise program	RR for falls at 2 years 0.69; RR for moderate/severe injury 0.63	Campbell et al., 1999
Home visit by occupational therapist for environmental assessment and modification	Decrease in number of persons falling; among prior fallers, RR of fall was 0.64	Cumming et al., 1999
Falls prevention strategies in nursing homes	Only two-thirds completed 6-mo intervention; no difference in fall rates	McMurdo et al., 2000
Additive model: education, exercise, home safety advice, clinical assessment	Compared to education group, significant reduction in slips and trips, but not falls	Steinberg et al., 2000
Home hazard assessment, information on hazard reduction, installation of safety devices	No significant difference in rate of falls in the home	Stevens et al., 2001
Nurse-delivered home exercise program	Significant decrease in numbers of falls and serious injurious falls	Robertson et al., 2001
Multiple strategies in residential care facilities (education, environmental modifications, reviewing drug regimens, etc.)	Adjusted OR for falls 0.49; adjusted incidence rate for falls 0.60	Jensen et al., 2002

Abbreviations: OR = odds ratio; RR = relative risk.

psychotropic drug management, and transferring and ambulation. Although not immediately connected to reducing fall risks, a study directed at frail nursing home patients showed that moderate exercise improved gait and stair-climbing ability. A multifactorial intervention study among residential care facility residents, which combined staff education with environmental modifications, attention to drug regimens, and exercise programs, reduced the rate of falls significantly. If the falls per se cannot be prevented, the risk of fractures can be reduced by having those at high risk wear external hip protectors (Kannus et al., 2000; Parker, 2001).

Studies of instructional environments suggest that carpeted floors are associated with fewer falls than vinyl floors (Healey, 1994). Likewise, the use of bed alarms is associated with a reduction in the fall rate among hospitalized patients (Tideiksaar et al., 1993). Although many people think of physical restraints as a means of preventing falls, the evidence points in the opposite direction.

EVALUATING THE ELDERLY PATIENT WHO FALLS

Older patients who report a fall (or recurrent falls) that is not clearly the result of an accidental trip or slip should be carefully evaluated, even if the falls have not resulted in serious physical injury. A jointly developed set of recommendations for assessing people who fall has been issued by the American Geriatrics Society, The British Geriatrics Society, and the American Academy of Orthopaedic Surgeons (American Geriatrics Society et al., 2001). Table 9-7 lists the hallmarks of these recommendations. An example of an assessment from for older patients who fall is included in the Appendix. A thorough fall evaluation consists of a detailed history, physical examination, gait and balance assessment, and, in certain instances, selected laboratory studies.

TABLE 9-7   RECOMMENDATIONS FOR FALLS ASSESSMENT

1. All older people should be asked about falls in the prior year.

2. Those with a single prior fall should have a "get-up-and-go test" or its equivalent (rising from a chair without using their arms and walking at a reasonable rate). Those who pass and have no history of falling need nothing further.

3. Those with two or more falls should be given a full falls assessment.

4. Fall assessment consists of:
   • History of fall circumstances, medications, acute or chronic medical problems, and mobility levels
   • Examination of vision, gait and balance, and lower extremity joint function
   • Basic neurological examination (mental status, muscle strength, lower extremity peripheral nerves, proprioception, reflexes, tests of cortical, extrapyramidal, and cerebellar function
   • Basic cardiovascular assessment (heart rate and rhythm, postural pulse and blood pressure, and possibly carotid sinus stimulation test)

Source: American Geriatrics Society, et al., 2001.

The history should focus on the general medical history and medications, the patient's thoughts about what caused the fall, the circumstances surrounding it, any premonitory or associated symptoms (such as palpitations caused by a transient arrhythmia or focal neurological symptoms caused by a TIA), and whether there was loss of consciousness (Table 9-8). A history of loss of consciousness after the fall (which is often difficult to document) is important information and should raise the suspicion of a cardiac event (transient arrhythmia or heart block) or a seizure (especially if there has been incontinence). Falls are often unwitnessed, and elderly patients may not recall any details of the circumstances surrounding the event. Detailed questioning can sometimes lead to identification of environmental factors that may have played a role in the fall and to symptoms that may lead to a specific diagnosis. Many elderly patients will not be able to give details about an unwitnessed fall and will simply report, "I just fell down, I don't

TABLE 9-8   EVALUATING THE ELDERLY PATIENT WHO FALLS: KEY
POINTS IN THE HISTORY

General medical history

History of previous falls

Medications (especially antihypertensive and psychotropic agents)

Patient's thoughts on the cause of the fall
    Was patient aware of impending fall?
    Was it totally unexpected?
    Did patient trip or slip?

Circumstances surrounding the fall
    Location and time of day
    Witnesses
    Relationship to changes in posture, turning of head, cough, urination

Premonitory or associated symptoms
    Light-headedness, dizziness, vertigo
    Palpitations, chest pain, shortness of breath
    Sudden focal neurologic symptoms (weakness, sensory disturbance,
      dysarthria, ataxia, confusion, asphasia)
    Aura
    Incontinence of urine or stool

Loss of consciousness
    What is remembered immediately after the fall?
    Could the patient get up and, if so, how long did it take?
    Can loss of consciousness be verified by a witness?

know what happened." The skin, extremities, and painful soft-tissue areas should be assessed to detect any injury that may have resulted from a fall.

Several other aspects of the physical examination can be helpful in determining the cause(s) (Table 9-9). Because a fall can herald the onset of a variety of acute illnesses ("premonitory" falls), careful attention should be given to vital signs. Fever, tachypnea, tachycardia, and hypotension should prompt a search for an acute illness (such as pneumonia or sepsis, myocardial infarction, pulmonary embolus, or gastrointestinal bleeding). Postural blood pressure and pulse determinations taken supine, sitting, and standing (after 1 and 3 minutes) are critical in the diagnosis and management of falls in older patients. As noted earlier, postural hypotension occurs in a substantial number of healthy, asymptomatic elderly persons as well as in those who are deconditioned from immobility or have venous insufficiency. This finding can also be a sign of dehydration, acute blood loss (occult gastrointestinal bleeding), or a drug side effect. Visual acuity should be assessed for any possible contribution to instability and falls. The cardiovascular examination should focus on the presence of arrhythmias (many of which are easily missed during a brief examination) and signs of aortic stenosis. Because both of these conditions are potentially serious and treatable, yet difficult to diagnose by physical examination, the patient should be referred for continuous monitoring and echocardiography if they are suspected. If the history suggests carotid sinus sensitivity, the carotid can be gently massaged for 5 seconds to observe whether this precipitates a profound bradycardia (50 percent reduction in heart rate) or a long pause (2 seconds). The extremities should be examined for evidence of deformities, limits to range of motion, or active inflammation that might underlie instability and cause a fall.

Special attention should be given to the feet because deformities, painful lesions (calluses, bunions, ulcers), and poorly fitted, inappropriate, or worn-out shoes are common and can contribute to instability and falls.

Neurological examination is also an important aspect of this physical assessment. Mental status should be assessed (see Chap. 6), with a careful search for focal neurological signs. Evidence of muscle weakness, rigidity, or spasticity should be noted, and signs of peripheral neuropathy (especially posterior column signs such as loss of position or vibratory sensation) should be ruled out. Abnormalities in cerebellar function (especially heel-to-shin testing) and signs of Parkinson's disease (such as resting tremor, muscle rigidity, and bradykinesia) should be sought.

Gait and balance assessments are a critical component of the examination and are probably more useful in identifying remediable problems than is the standard neuromuscular exam. Although sophisticated techniques have been developed to assess gait and balance, careful observation of a series of maneuvers is the most practical and useful assessment technique. The "get-up-and-go" test and other practical performance-based balance and gait assessments have been developed. Tables 9-10 and 9-11 provide examples of these types of assessment. Abnormalities on these assessments may be helpful in identifying patients who

TABLE 9-9   EVALUATING THE ELDERLY PATIENT WHO FALLS: KEY
ASPECTS OF THE PHYSICAL EXAMINATION

Vital signs
   Fever, hypothermia
   Respiratory rate
   Pulse and blood pressure (lying, sitting, standing)

Skin
   Turgor
   Pallor
   Trauma

Eyes
   Visual acuity

Cardiovascular
   Arrhythmias
   Carotid bruits
   Signs of aortic stenosis
   Carotid sinus sensitivity

Extremities
   Degenerative joint disease
   Range of motion
   Deformities
   Fractures
   Podiatric problems (calluses; bunions; ulcerations; poorly fitted,
     inappropriate, or worn-out shoes)

Neurological
   Mental status
   Focal signs
   Muscles (weakness, rigidity, spasticity)
   Peripheral innervation (especially position sense)
   Cerebellar (especially heel-to-shin testing)
   Resting tremor, bradykinesia, other involuntary movements
   Observing the patient stand up and walk (the "get-up-and-go" test)

are likely to fall again and potentially remediable problems that might prevent future falls.

There is no specific laboratory workup for an elderly patient who falls. Laboratory studies should be ordered based on information gleaned from the history and physical examination. If the cause of the fall is obvious (such as a slip or a trip) and no suspicious symptoms or signs are detected, laboratory studies are unwarranted. If the history or physical examination (especially vital signs) suggests an acute illness, appropriate laboratory studies (such as complete blood count, electrolytes, blood urea nitrogen, chest films, electrocardiogram) should be ordered. If a transient arrhythmia or heart block is suspected, ambulatory electrocardiographic monitoring should be done. Although the sensitivity and specificity of this procedure for determining the cause of falls in the elderly is unknown, and many elderly people have asymptomatic ectopy, cardiac abnormalities detected on continuous monitoring that are clearly related to symptoms should be treated.

Because it is difficult to diagnose aortic stenosis on physical examination, echocardiography should be considered in all patients with suggestive histories and a systolic heart murmur or those who have a delay in the carotid upstroke. If the history suggests anterior circulation TIA, noninvasive vascular studies should be considered to rule out treatable vascular lesions. Computed tomography (CT) scans and electroencephalograms should be reserved for those patients in whom there is a high suspicion of an intracranial lesion or seizure disorder.

MANAGEMENT

Table 9-12 outlines the basic principles of managing elderly patients with instability problems and a history of falls. Assessment and treatment of physical injury should not be overlooked because it may be helpful in preventing recurrent falls.

When specific conditions are identified by history, physical examination, and laboratory studies, they should be treated in order to minimize the risk of subsequent falls, morbidity, and mortality. Table 9-13 lists examples of treatments for some of the more common conditions. This table is meant only as a general outline; most of these topics are discussed in detail in general textbooks of medicine.

Physical therapy and patient education are important aspects of the management of these elderly patients. Gait training, muscle strengthening, the use of assistive devices, and adaptive behaviors (such as rising slowly, using rails or furniture for balance, and techniques of getting up after a fall) are all helpful in preventing subsequent morbidity from instability and falls.

Environmental manipulations can be critical in preventing further falls. The environments of the elderly are often unsafe (see Table 9-4), and appropriate interventions can often be instituted to improve safety (see Table 9-13). Physical restraints (vests, belts, mittens, geri-chairs, etc.) are commonly used in institutional settings for those felt to be at high risk of falling. Nursing home regulations

TABLE 9-10 EXAMPLE OF A PERFORMANCE- BASED ASSESSMENT OF GAIT

	OBSERVATION	
COMPONENTS	NORMAL	ABNORMAL
Initiation of gait (patient asked to begin walking down hallway at a normal pace using any assistive device they normally walk with)	Begins walking immediately without observable hesitation; initiation of gait is single, smooth motion	Hesitates; multiple attempts; initiation of gait not a smooth motion
Step height (begin observing after first few steps: observe one foot, then the other; observe from side)	Swing foot completely clears floor but by no more than 1–2 in.	Swing foot is not completely raised off floor (may hear scraping) or is raised too high (1–<2 in.)
Step length (observe distance between toe of stance foot and heel of swing foot; observe from side; do not judge first few or last few steps; observe one side at a time)	At least the length of individual's foot between the stance toe and swing heel (step length usually longer but foot length provides basis for observation)	Step length less than described under "normal"
Step symmetry (observe the middle part of the path, not the first or last steps; observe distance between heel of each swing foot and toe of each stance foot)	Step length same or nearly same on both sides for most step cycles	Step length varies between sides, or patient advances with same foot every step

Step continuity	Begins raising heel of one foot (toe off) as heel of other foot touches the floor (heel strike); no breaks or stops in stride; step lengths equal over most cycles	Places entire foot (heel and toe) on floor before beginning to raise other foot; or stops completely between steps; or step length varies over cycles
Path deviation [observe from behind; observe one foot over several strides; observe in relation to line on floor (e. g., tiles) if possible; difficult to assess if patient uses a walker]	Foot follows close to straight line as patient advances	Foot deviates from side to side or toward one direction
Trunk stability (observe from behind; side-to-side motion of trunk may be a normal gait pattern; need to differentiate this from instability)	Trunk does not sway; knees or back are not flexed; arms are not abducted in effort to maintain stability	Any of preceding features present
Walk stance (observe from behind)	Feet should almost touch as one passes other	Feet apart with stepping
Turning while walking	No staggering; turning continuous with walking; steps are continuous while walking; steps are continuous while turning	Staggers; stops before initiating turn; or steps are discontinuous

Source: From Tinetti, 1986, with permission.

TABLE 9-11 EXAMPLE OF A PERFORMANCE BASED-ASSESSMENT OF BALANCE

Maneuver	Normal	Adaptive	Abnormal
Sitting balance	Steady, stable	Holds onto chair to keep upright	Leans, slides down in chair
Arising from chair	Able to arise in a single movement without using arms	Uses arms (on chair or walking aid) to pull or push up and/or moves forward in chair before attempting to rise	Multiple attempts required or unable without human assistance
Immediate standing balance (first 3–5 s)	Steady without holding onto walking aid or other object for support	Steady, but uses walking aid or support grabbing objects for support	Any sign of unsteadiness (e.g., other object for staggering, more than minimal trunk sway)
Standing balance	Steady, able to stand with feet together without holding onto an object for support	Steady, but cannot put feet together	
Balance with eyes closed (with feet as close together as possible)	Steady without holding onto any object with feet together	Steady with feet apart	Any sign of unsteadiness or needs to hold onto an object
Turning balance (360°)	No grabbing or staggering; no need to hold onto any objects; steps are continuous (turn is a flowing movement)	Steps are discontinuous (patient puts one foot completely on floor before raising other foot)	Any sign of unsteadiness or holds onto an object
Nudge on sternum (patient standing with feet as close together as possible; examiner pushes with light, even pressure over sternum three times; reflects ability to withstand displacement)	Steady, able to withstand pressure	Needs to move feet, but able to maintain balance	Begins to fall, or examiner has to help maintain balance

Neck turning (patient asked to turn head side to side and look up while standing with feet as close together as possible)	Able to turn head at least halfway side to side and able to bend head back to look at ceiling; no staggering, grabbing, or symptoms of light-headedness, unsteadiness, or pain	Decreased ability to turn side to side to extend neck, but no staggering, grabbing, or symptoms of light-headedness, unsteadiness, or pain	Any sign of unsteadiness or symptoms when turning head or extending neck
One-leg standing balance	Able to stand on one leg for 5 s without holding onto object for support		Unable
Back extension (ask patient to lean back as far as possible, without holding onto object if possible)	Good extension without holding object or staggering	Tries to extend, but range of motion is decreased or needs to hold object to attempt extension	Will not attempt, no extension seen, or staggers
Reaching up (have patient attempt to remove an object from a shelf high enough to necessitate stretching or standing on toes)	Able to take down object without needing to hold onto other object for support and without becoming unsteady	Able to get object but needs to steady self by holding onto something for support	Unable or unsteady
Bending down (patient is asked to pick up small objects, such as pen, from the floor)	Able to bend down and pick up the object and able to get up easily in single attempt without needing to pull self up with arms	Able to get object and get upright in single attempt but needs to pull self up with arms or hold onto something for support	Unable to bend down or unable to get upright after bending down or takes multiple attempts to upright self
Sitting down	Able to sit down in one smooth movement	Needs to use arms to guide self into chair or not a smooth movement	Falls into chair, misjudges distances (lands off center)

TABLE 9-12   PRINCIPLES OF MANAGEMENT FOR ELDERLY PATIENTS
WITH COMPLAINTS OF INSTABILITY AND/OR FALLS

Assess and treat physical injury

Treat underlying conditions (Table 9–13)

Provide physical therapy and education
  Gait retraining
  Muscle strengthening
  Aids to ambulation
  Properly fitted shoes
  Adaptive behaviors

Alter the environment
  Safe and proper-size furniture
  Elimination of obstacles (loose rugs, etc.)
  Proper lighting
  Rails (stairs, bathroom)

TABLE 9-13   EXAMPLES OF TREATMENT FOR UNDERLYING CAUSES OF FALLS

CONDITION AND CAUSE	POTENTIAL TREATMENT
CARDIOVASCULAR	
Tachyarrhythmias	Antiarrhythmics*
Bradyarrhythmias	Pacemaker*
Aortic stenosis	Valve surgery (for syncope)
Postural hypotension	
Drug-related	Elimination of drugs(s)
With venous insufficiency	Support stockings
	Leg elevation
	Adaptive behaviors
Autonomic dysfunction or	Support stockings
idiopathic	Mineralocorticoids
	ProAmatine (Midodrine hydrochloride)
	Adaptive behaviors

TABLE 9-13   EXAMPLES OF TREATMENT FOR UNDERLYING CAUSES OF FALLS (*Continued*)

CONDITION AND CAUSE	POTENTIAL TREATMENT
NEUROLOGICAL	
Anterior circulation transient ischemic attack (TIA)	Aspirin and/or surgery †
Posterior circulation TIA	Aspirin
Cervical spondylosis (with spinal cord compression)	Physical therapy
	Neck brace
	Surgery
Parkinson's disease	Antiparkinsonian drugs
Visual impairment	Ophthalmological evaluation and specific treatment
Seizure disorder	Anticonvulsants
Normal-pressure hydrocephalus	Surgery (shunt) †
Dementia	Supervised activities
	Hazard-free environment
Benign positional vertigo	Habituation exercises
	Antivertiginous medication
OTHERS	
Foot disorders	Podiatric evaluation and treatment
Gait disorders (miscellaneous)	Properly fitted shoes
	Physical therapy
Drug overuse (e.g., sedatives, alcohol, other psychotropic drugs, antihypertensives)	Elimination of drug(s)

* These treatments may be indicated only if the cardiac disturbance is clearly related to symptoms.
† Risk:benefit ratio must be carefully assessed.

in the Omnibus Budget Reconciliation Act of 1987, and the increasing recognition that physical restraints probably do not decrease and may in fact increase falls and injuries (Tinetti et al., 1992; Neufeld et al., 1999), have led to the reduced and more appropriate use of these devices in many institutional settings.

The same multiorganization group noted earlier has also offered a series of recommendations on interventions. Table 9-14 summarizes these recommendations. Here, too, the scientific strength of the recommendations is limited.

TABLE 9-14   RECOMMENDED FALL INTERVENTIONS TO PREVENT FALLS

1. Among community-dwelling older persons
   - Gait training and advice on appropriate assistive devices
   - Review and modify medication, especially psychotropics
   - Exercise programs that include balance
   - Treat postural hypertension
   - Modify environmental hazards
   - Treat cardiovascular disorders, including arrhythmias
2. In long-term care and assisted-living settings
   - Staff education programs
   - Gait training and advice on appropriate assistive devices
   - Review and modify medication, especially psychotropics

Source: American Geriatrics Society et al., 2001

References

American Geriatrics Society, British Geriatrics Society, American Academy of Orthopaedic Surgeons Panel on Falls Prevention: Guideline for the prevention of falls in older persons. *J Am Geriatr Soc* 49:664–672, 2001.

Buchner DM, Cress ME, deLateur BJ, et al. The effect of strength and endurance training on gait, balance, fall risk and health services use in community-living older adults. *J Gerontol A Biol Sci Med Sci* 52A:M218–M224, 1997.

Campbell AJ, Robertson MC, Gardener MM, et al: Randomised controlled trial of a general practice programme of home-based exercise to prevent falls in elderly women. *BMJ* 315:1065–1069, 1997.

Campbell AJ, Robertson MC, Gardner MM, et al: Falls prevention over 2 years: a randomised controlled trial in women 80 years and older. *Age Ageing* 28:513–518, 1999.

Close J, Ellis M, Hooper R, et al: Prevention of Falls in the Elderly Trial (PROFET): a randomized controlled trial. *Lancet* 353:93–97, 1999.

Cumming RG, Thomas M, Szonyi G, et al: Home visits by an occupational therapist for assessment and modification of environmental hazards: a randomized trial of falls prevention. *J Am Geriatr Soc* 47:1397–1402, 1999.

Fiatarone MA, O'Neill EF, Ryan ND, et al: Exercise training and nutritional supplementation for physical frailty in very elderly people. *N Engl J Med* 330:1769–1775, 1994.

Gill TM, Williams CS, Tinetti ME: Environmental hazards and the risk of nonsyncopal falls in the homes of community-living older persons. *Med Care* 38:1174–1183, 2000.

Healey F: Does flooring type affect risk of injury in older patients? *Nursing Times* 90:40–41, 1994.

Hornbrook MC, Stevens VJ, Wingfield DJ, et al: Preventing falls among community-dwelling older persons: results from a randomized trial. *Gerontologist* 34:16–23, 1994.

Jensen J, Lundin-Olsson L, Nyberg L, Gustafson Y. Fall and injury prevention in older people living in residential care facilities: a cluster randomized trial. *Ann Intern Med* 136:733–741, 2002.

Kannus P, Parkkari J, Niemi S, et al: Prevention of hip fracture in elderly people with use of a hip protector. *N Engl J Med* 343:1506–1513, 2000.

Lauritzen JB , Petersen MM, Lund B: Effect of external hip protectors on hip fractures. *Lancet* 341:11–13, 1993.

Mathias SN, Nayak USL, Isaacs B: Balance in elderly patients: the "get up and go" test. *Arch Phys Med Rehabil* 67:387–389, 1986.

McMurdo MET, Mole PA, Paterson CR: Controlled trial of weight-bearing exercise in older women in relation to bone density and falls. *BMJ* 314:569, 1997.

McMurdo ME, Millar AM, Daly F: A randomized controlled trial of fall prevention strategies in old peoples' homes. *Gerontology* 46(2):83–87, 2000.

Neufeld RR, Libow LS, Foley WJ, Dunbar JM, Cohen C, Breuer B: Restraint reduction reduces serious injuries among nursing home residents. *J Am Geriatr Soc* 47:1202–1207, 1999.

Parker MJ, Gillespie LD, Gillespie WJ: Hip protectors for preventing hip fractures in the elderly (Cochrane Review): Oxford (update software.com): The Cochrane Library, 2001, Issue 2, 2001.

Province MA, Hadley EC, Hornbrook MC, et al: The effects of exercise on falls in elderly patients: a preplanned meta-analysis of the FICSIT trials. *JAMA* 273:1341–1347, 1995.

RAND: Falls prevention interventions in the Medicare population. Contract No. 500–98–0281. Prepared for the Centers for Medicare and Medicaid Services. Santa Monica, CA, RAND, 2002.

Ray WA, Taylor JA, Meador KG, et al: A randomized trial of a consultation service to reduce falls in nursing homes. *JAMA* 278:557–562, 1997.

Reinsch S, MacRae P, Lachenbruch PA, Tobis JS: Attempts to prevent falls and injury: a prospective community study. *Gerontologist* 32:450–456, 1992.

Robertson MC, Devlin N, Gardner MM, Campbell AJ: Effectiveness and economic evaluation of a nurse delivered home exercise programme to prevent falls. 1: randomized controlled trial. *BMJ* 322:697–701, 2001.

Rubenstein LZ, Robbins AS, Josephson KR, et al: The value of assessing falls in an elderly population. *Ann Intern Med* 113:308–316, 1990.

Steinberg M, Cartwright C, Peel N, Willimas G: A sustainable programme to prevent falls and near falls in community-dwelling older people: results of a randomized trial. *J Epidemiol Community Health* 54:227–232, 2000.

Stevens M, Holman CDJ, Bennett N, de Klerk N: Preventing falls in older people: outcome evaluation of a randomized controlled trial. *J Am Geriatr Soc* 49:1448–1455, 2001.

Tideiksaar R, CF Feiner, Maby J: Falls prevention: the efficacy of a bed alarm system in an acute-care setting. *Mt Sinai J Med* 60:522–527, 1993.

Tinetti ME: Performance-oriented assessment of mobility problems in elderly patients. *J Am Geriatr Soc* 34:119–126, 1986.

Tinetti M, Baker D, McAvay G, et al: A multifactorial intervention to reduce the risk of falling among elderly people living in the community. *N Engl J Med* 331:821–827, 1994.

Tinetti ME, Liu W, Ginter SF: Mechanical restraint use and fall-related injuries among residents of skilled nursing facilities. *Ann Intern Med* 116:369–374, 1992.

Tinetti ME, Williams CS, Gill TM: Dizziness among older adults: a possible geriatric syndrome. *Ann Intern Med* 132:337–344, 2000.

Wagner EH, LaCroix AZ, Grothaus L, et al: Preventing disability and falls in older adults: a population-based randomized trial. *Am J Public Health* 84:1800–1806, 1994.

Wolf SL, Barnhart HX, Kutner NG, et al: Reducing frailty and falls in older persons: an investigation of Tai Chi and computerized balance training. *J Am Geriatr Soc* 44:489–497, 1996.

Wolfson L, Whipple R, Amerman P, et al: Gait assessment in the elderly: a gait abnormality rating scale and its relation to falls. *J Gerontol Med Sci* 45:M12–M19, 1990.

Suggested Readings

Agostini JV, Baker DI, Bogardus STJ: Prevention of falls in hospitalized and institutionalized older people: *Making Health Care Safer: A Critical Analysis of Patient Safety Practices.* Rockville, MD, Agency for Healthcare Research and Quality, 2001.

Alexander N: Gait disorders in older adults. *J Am Geriatr Soc* 44:434–451, 1996.

Connell B: Role of the environment in falls prevention. *Clin Geriatr Med* 12:859–880, 1996.

Gillespie LD, Gillespie WJ, Robertson MC, et al: Interventions for preventing falls in elderly people. *Cochrane Database of Syst Rev* 3:CD000340, 2001.

King MB, Tinetti ME: Falls in community-dwelling older persons. *J Am Geriatr Soc* 43:1146–1154, 1995.

Luukinen H, Koski K, Konkanen R: Incidence of injury-causing falls among older adults by place of residence: a population-based study. *J Am Geriatr Soc* 43:871–876, 1995.

Tinetti ME: Preventing falls in elderly persons. *N Engl J Med* 348:42–49, 2003.

CHAPTER 10

IMMOBILITY

Immobility is a common pathway by which a host of diseases and problems in older individuals produce further disability. Immobility often cannot be prevented, but many of its adverse effects can be. Improvements in mobility are almost always possible, even in the most immobile older patients. Relatively small improvements in mobility can decrease the incidence and severity of complications, improve the patient's well-being, and make life easier for caregivers.

This chapter outlines the common causes and complications of immobility and reviews the principles of management for some of the more common conditions associated with immobility in the older population.

CAUSES

Many physical, psychological, and environmental factors can cause immobility in older persons (Table 10-1). The most common causes are musculoskeletal, neurological, and cardiovascular disorders. Pain is a common pathway by which these disorders result in immobility, and its management is highlighted in this chapter.

Degenerative joint disease (especially those involving the weight-bearing joints), osteoporosis, and hip fractures are probably the most prevalent conditions that predispose to immobility among older adults. Podiatric problems such as bunions, calluses, and onychomycoses frequently cause pain and reluctance or inability to walk.

The incidence of several neurological disorders that can cause immobility increases with age. About half of the individuals who suffer a stroke have residual deficits for which they require assistance; most of these deficits involve immobility. Parkinson's disease, especially in its later stages, causes severe limitations in mobility. Early and active management of these patients can improve their mobility and help to avoid complications.

Severe congestive heart failure, coronary artery disease with frequent angina, peripheral vascular disease with frequent claudication, and severe chronic lung disease can restrict activity and mobility in many elderly patients. Peripheral vascular disease, especially in older diabetics, can cause claudication, limit ambulation, and eventually result in lower extremity amputations, which can restrict mobility further.

TABLE 10-1   COMMON CAUSES OF IMMOBILITY IN OLDER ADULTS

Musculoskeletal disorders
  Arthritides
  Osteoporosis
  Fractures (especially hip and femur)
  Podiatric problems
  Other (e.g., Paget's disease)
Neurological disorders
  Stroke
  Parkinson's disease
  Other (cerebellar dysfunction, neuropathies)
Cardiovascular disease
  Congestive heart failure (severe)
  Coronary artery disease (frequent angina)
  Peripheral vascular disease (frequent claudication)
Pulmonary disease
  Chronic obstructive lung disease (severe)
Sensory factors
  Impairment of vision
  Fear (from instability and fear of falling)
Environmental causes
  Forced immobility (in hospitals and nursing homes)
  Inadequate aids for mobility
Acute and chronic pain
Other
  Deconditioning (after prolonged bed rest from acute illness)
  Malnutrition
  Severe systemic illness (e.g., widespread malignancy)
  Depression
  Drug side effects (e.g., antipsychotic-induced rigidity)

Psychological and environmental factors can play an important role in immobility. Decreased mobility (i.e., taking to bed) is a common manifestation of depression. Fear of falling, especially among those with a history of instability and previous falls or with impaired vision, can lead to a bed-and-chair existence. Older patients with instability, impaired vision, and acute illnesses are often inappropriately restricted to bed or chair in acute care hospitals and nursing homes. Lack of mobility aids (e.g., canes, walkers, and appropriately placed railings) also contributes to immobility in acute care hospitals and home settings.

Drug side effects may cause immobility. Sedatives and hypnotics, by causing drowsiness and ataxia, can impair mobility. Antipsychotic drugs (especially the phenothiazine-like agents) have prominent extrapyramidal effects and can cause muscle rigidity and diminished mobility (see Chap. 14).

COMPLICATIONS

Immobility can lead to complications in almost every major organ system (Table 10-2). Prolonged inactivity or bed rest has adverse physical and psychological consequences. Metabolic effects include negative nitrogen and calcium balance and impaired glucose tolerance; diminished plasma volume and altered drug pharmacokinetics can result. Immobilized older patients often become depressed, are deprived of environmental stimulation, and, in some instances, become delirious. Deconditioning can occur rapidly, especially among older people with little physiological reserve.

The skin and musculoskeletal system often bear the brunt of immobility. Pressure sores are all too common. Muscle weakness, atrophy, and contractures can lead to prolonged disability and dysfunction. Bone density decreases in immobile patients, predisposing to fractures when the patient is mobilized. Cardiopulmonary complications of immobility are probably the most serious and life-threatening. Prolonged immobility results in cardiovascular deconditioning; the combination of deconditioned cardiovascular reflexes and diminished plasma volume can lead to postural hypotension. Postural hypotension may not only impair rehabilitative efforts but also predispose to falls and serious cardiovascular events such as stroke and myocardial infarction. Deep venous thrombosis and pulmonary embolism are well-known complications. Immobility, especially bed rest, also impairs pulmonary function. Tidal volume is diminished; atelectasis may occur, and, when combined with the supine position, predisposes to the development of aspiration pneumonia.

Gastrointestinal and genitourinary problems are among the most bothersome consequences of immobility to the patient and can lead to further complications. Immobility slows down both the gastrointestinal tract and urine flow. This predisposes to constipation, fecal impaction, urinary tract stones and infection, and fecal and urinary incontinence. These conditions and their management are discussed in Chap. 8.

ASSESSING IMMOBILE PATIENTS

Several aspects of the history and physical examination are important in the assessment of immobile patients (Table 10-3). Useful historical information includes the extent and duration of disabilities causing immobility, the underlying

TABLE 10-2   COMPLICATIONS OF IMMOBILITY

Skin
    Pressure ulcers

Musculoskeletal
    Muscular deconditioning and atrophy
    Contractures
    Bone loss (osteoporosis)

Cardiovascular
    Deconditioning
    Orthostatic hypotension
    Venous thrombosis, embolism

Pulmonary
    Decreased ventilation
    Atelectasis
    Aspiration pneumonia

Gastrointestinal
    Anorexia
    Constipation
    Fecal impaction, incontinence

Genitourinary
    Urinary infection
    Urinary retention
    Bladder calculi
    Incontinence

Metabolic
    Altered body composition (e.g., decreased plasma volume)
    Negative nitrogen balance
    Impaired glucose tolerance
    Altered drug pharmacokinetics

Psychological
    Sensory deprivation
    Delirium
    Depression

TABLE 10-3   ASSESSMENT OF IMMOBILE OLDER PATIENTS

History
    Nature and duration of disabilities causing immobility
    Medical conditions contributing to immobility
    Pain
    Drugs that can affect mobility
    Motivation and other psychological factors
    Environment

Physical examination
    Skin
    Cardiopulmonary status

Musculoskeletal assessment
    Muscle tone and strength (see Table 10-4)
    Joint range of motion
    Foot deformities and lesions

Neurological deficits
    Focal weakness
    Sensory and perceptual evaluation

Levels of mobility
    Bed mobility
    Ability to transfer (bed to chair)
    Wheelchair mobility
    Standing balance
    Gait (see Chap. 9)
    Pain with movement

medical conditions that influence mobility, and a review of medications in order to eliminate iatrogenic problems contributing to immobility. Pain should be routinely assessed as it may be a major contributing factor. Standardized pain assessment tools have been recommended for this purpose (AGS Panel on Persistent Pain in Older Persons, 2002). Psychological factors, such as depression and fear, may contribute to immobility and may make recovery difficult. They should, therefore, receive special attention. An assessment of the environment is important in determining measures that may improve the patient's mobility, such as an overhead triangle, bedside commode, railing, and other environmental manipulations.

When immobile patients are being examined, the skin should be inspected repeatedly to identify early pressure sores. Cardiopulmonary status, especially intravascular volume, and postural changes in blood pressure and pulse are important to the process of treatment. A detailed musculoskeletal examination—including evaluation of muscle tone and strength and testing of joint range of motion—and a search for potentially remediable podiatric problems should be carried out. Standardized and repeated measures of muscle strength can be helpful in gauging a patient's progress (Table 10-4). The neurological examination should identify focal weakness, as well as sensory and perceptual problems, that can impair mobility and frustrate rehabilitative efforts. Hemianopsia, or neglect of and inattention to one side of the body (usually the left side is ignored in patients with nondominant hemisphere lesions), and various apraxias are common after strokes.

Most importantly, the patient's mobility should be assessed and reassessed on an ongoing basis. There are several levels of mobility (see Table 10-3) as well as important distinctions within each level. For example, a patient may be bedbound but may be able to sit up without help, or the patient may be able to transfer independently into a wheelchair, but be unable to propel the wheelchair. Pain should also be assessed during mobility because patients may deny pain at rest but experience considerable pain with movement. Rehabilitation therapists are skilled in making these detailed evaluations of mobility and should be involved in the care of immobile patients.

MANAGEMENT OF IMMOBILITY

Optimal management of immobile older patients necessitates a thorough assessment, specific diagnoses, and multimodal treatment directed at specific dis-

TABLE 10-4   EXAMPLE OF A GRADING SYSTEM FOR MUSCLE STRENGTH IN IMMOBILE OLDER PATIENTS

	GRADE	OBSERVED STRENGTH
Normal	5	
Good	4	Muscle produces movements against gravity and can overcome some resistance
Fair	3	Muscle produces movements against gravity but cannot overcome any resistance
Poor	2	Muscle produces movements but not against gravity
Trace	1	Muscle tightens but cannot produce movement, even after gravity is eliminated
None	0	Muscle does not contract at all

eases and disabilities. This process generally involves a team of health professionals. Physical and occupational therapists can be especially helpful in the assessment and management of immobility and associated functional disabilities, and they should be consulted as early as possible when the problem of an immobile patient presents itself. In many patients, mobility cannot be completely restored and intensive rehabilitative efforts will not be cost-effective. Specific goals must be individualized, and in some patients these goals will involve preventing complications of immobility and adapting the environment to the individual (and vice versa).

It is beyond the scope of this text to detail the management of all conditions associated with immobility in older adults; important general principles of the management of some of the most common of these conditions are reviewed. Brief sections at the end of the chapter provide an overview of key principles in the management of pain and the rehabilitation of geriatric patients.

▓ Arthritis

Several different rheumatological disorders occur in the older persons. They can usually be distinguished from each other by clinical features, radiographic abnormalities, synovial fluid analysis, and selected laboratory studies (Table 10-5).

Specific diagnoses for these conditions should be made whenever possible, because the most appropriate treatment(s) of the primary disorders, as well as associated abnormalities, may differ. For example, polymyalgia rheumatica is a common condition in elderly women; its clinical features are often nonspecific—fatigue, malaise, muscle aches. Because this disorder necessitates treatment with systemic steroids and is highly associated with temporal arteritis (a disease that can rapidly lead to blindness if appropriate treatment is not instituted), it is essential to make this diagnosis. Older patients with fatigue and symmetrical muscle aches (especially in the shoulders) should be tested for sedimentation rate, which will generally be markedly elevated (approximately 75 percent of patients have values greater than 40 mm/h in polymyalgia rheumatica [Goodwin, 1992]). Any symptoms suggestive of involvement of the temporal artery—headache, jaw claudication, recent changes in vision—especially when the sedimentation rate is very high (greater than 75 mm/h) should prompt consideration of temporal artery biopsy because treatment of temporal arteritis requires higher doses of steroids than does the treatment of polymyalgia alone. Patients with polymyalgia are generally treated with 10 to 20 mg of prednisone in a single dose, whereas patients with temporal arteritis are treated with 40 to 80 mg of prednisone daily in divided doses.

Another example of the importance of making a specific diagnosis is the carpal tunnel syndrome. This disorder may be overlooked when symptoms of pain, weakness, and paresthesias in the hand are mistaken for osteoarthritis.

TABLE 10-5   CLINICAL ASPECTS OF COMMON RHEUMATOLOGICAL DISORDERS IN OLDER PATIENTS

Disorder	Osteoarthritis	Rheumatoid Arthritis	Polymyalgia Rheumatica	Gout	Pseudogout	Carpal Tunnel Syndrome	Drug-Induced Disorder
Gradual onset	+++	+++	+++	0	+	+++	+++
Joint swelling or effusion	+++	++++	+	++++	++++	+	++
Joint pain	++++	++++	+	++++	++++	+	+++
Symmetrical involvement	+	+++	++++	+	+	++	+++
Muscle pain	+	+	+++	+	+	+	+++
Radiographic abnormalities	++++	+++	0	+	+++	0	0
Synovial fluid crystals	+	+	0	+++	+++	0	0
Elevated sedimentation rate	+	+++	++++	+	+	+	+++
Anemia	0	++	+++	0	0	0	++
Positive antinuclear antibody	0	+	+	0	0	+	++++
Positive rheumatoid factor	0	+++	+	0	0	0	+

Key: 0 = does not occur; + = occurs occasionally; ++ = occurs frequently; +++ = almost always occurs; ++++ = difficult to make diagnosis without it.
Source: After Reich, 1982.

Objective weakness, sensory deficit, and atrophy of intrinsic musculature of the hand should prompt consideration of performing nerve conduction studies and surgical therapy to relieve symptoms and prevent progressive disability. Wrist splints, generally provided by occupational therapists, are sometimes effective in relieving the discomfort of this syndrome.

The history and physical examination can be helpful in differentiating osteoarthritis from inflammatory arthritides (Table 10-6); however, other procedures are often essential. Osteoarthritis itself may be inflammatory in some instances.

Synovial fluid analysis can be especially helpful in differentiating osteoarthritis from crystal-induced arthritides such as gout and pseudogout (Table 10-5). Because clinical examination alone cannot determine whether an inflamed joint is infected and joint infections can occur in conjunction with other inflammatory joint diseases, all newly inflamed joints should be tapped, Gram stained, and cultured to rule out infection. Failure to diagnose and treat joint infections can lead to osteomyelitis, joint destruction, and permanent disability.

In addition to making specific diagnoses of rheumatological disorders whenever possible, careful physical examination can detect treatable nonarticular conditions such as tendinitis and bursitis. For example, bicipital tendinitis and trochanteric bursitis are common in geriatric patients. Dramatic relief from pain and disability from these conditions can be achieved by local treatments such as the injection of steroids.

Osteoarthritis is by far the most common rheumatological disorder afflicting older adults. A wide variety of modalities can be used to treat osteoarthritis as well as other painful musculoskeletal conditions. Optimal management often involves the use of multiple treatment modalities, and the best combination of treatments will vary from patient to patient.

TABLE 10-6   CLINICAL FEATURES OF OSTEOARTHRITIS VERSUS
INFLAMMATORY ARTHRITIDES

CLINICAL FEATURE	OSTEOARTHRITIS	INFLAMMATORY ARTHRITIDES
Duration of stiffness	Minutes	Hours
Pain	Usually with activity	Occurs even at rest and at night
Fatigue	Unusual	Common
Swelling	Common but little synovial reaction	Very common, with synovial proliferation and thickening
Erythema and warmth	Unusual	Common

In general, patients with osteoarthritis and pain from inflammatory musculoskeletal conditions should be treated with an antiinflammatory agent unless they respond to local measures alone. Some older patients with chronic pain caused by osteoarthritis will respond to acetaminophen; however, when inflammation is present, nonsteroidal antiinflammatory drugs are generally appropriate. There are many such drugs; their side effects and prices vary. Nonsteroidal antiinflammatory drugs have several potential adverse effects in geriatric patients. Although the absolute risk of a significant gastrointestinal bleed may be small, monitoring of patients on chronic nonsteroidal therapy for bleeding with periodic hemoglobin levels and/or stools for occult blood is advisable. Nonsteroidal agents can also cause sodium retention and impair renal function, especially in patients with already compromised renal function and those on loop diuretics, may interfere with the efficacy of antihypertensive therapy, and are associated with hospitalization among patients with congestive heart failure. The cyclooxygenase (COX)-2 inhibitors may have fewer adverse effects than the older agents, but definitive data in the geriatric population are lacking. Combining lower doses of these drugs with acetaminophen can sometimes improve pain relief and minimize side effects. Guidelines for the management of pain in older persons have been published (AGS Panel on Persistent Pain in Older Persons, 2002) and are discussed below.

Osteoporosis

Osteoporosis is a common disorder in the elderly and frequently leads to complications that result in pain, disability, and immobility. Approximately one third of women older than age 65 have suffered either a vertebral or hip fracture related to osteoporosis; by age 80, approximately half of women have evidence of vertebral fractures, and close to 30 percent will have suffered a hip fracture. Thus, osteoporosis is a major health problem in the older adult population, resulting in substantial morbidity and cost. The US Preventive Services Task Force now recommends routine screening for osteoporosis among women age 65 and older (Nelson et al., 2002). (See Chap. 5)

Osteoporosis is a generalized bone disorder in which bone mass is diminished but the relative composition (i.e., the ratio of mineral to organic matrix content) is not changed. This is in contrast to osteomalacia, in which the ratio of mineral to matrix is diminished. Aging is associated with a decrease in bone mass. White women lose the greatest proportion of bone mass with increasing age; the bone loss accelerates after menopause, and as much as 40 percent of bone mass may be lost by age 90. A working group of the World Health Organization has defined osteoporosis as a bone mineral density that is 2.5 SD (standard deviations) below the mean peak value in young adults. Values between 1.0 and 2.5 SD below the mean are defined as osteopenia.

Two major types of age-related osteoporosis have been defined (Table 10-7). Type I (postmenopausal) osteoporosis affects mainly trabecular bone and is related to accelerated bone loss in women during the first two decades after menopause. Type II (senile) osteoporosis affects both trabecular and cortical bone and is related to impaired production of 1,25-dihydroxy vitamin D. Several factors are associated with increased risk of osteoporosis among women (Table 10-8); many of them (e.g., gastric resection, steroid or anticonvulsant use, immobility) are also risk factors among men.

The most useful technique for measuring bone density is dual-energy x-ray absorptiometry (DEXA). It is helpful in making decisions for treatment when therapy might not otherwise be started, and in monitoring therapeutic response. Bone density of the hip is most helpful in predicting hip fractures, and bone density of the spine is helpful for monitoring therapy (Eastell, 1998).

Laboratory studies in uncomplicated osteoporosis should be normal, including serum calcium, phosphorus, magnesium, alkaline phosphatase, and parathyroid and thyroid hormones. Some older patients with senile osteoporosis have elevated parathyroid hormone, presumably related to a primary decrease in 1,25-dihydroxy vitamin D levels. Vitamin D blood levels and 24-hour urinary calcium excretion (which should be greater than 100 mg/24 h) should be measured if malabsorption is suspected.

The presenting manifestations of osteoporosis most often relate to a fracture of the hip (discussed below), the wrist (Colles fracture), or the lower thoracic and

TABLE 10-7   TWO BASIC TYPES OF AGE-RELATED OSTEOPOROSIS

	TYPE I (POSTMENOPAUSAL)	TYPE II (SENILE)
Age (years)	51–75	>70
Sex ratio (F:M)	6:1	2:1
Type of bone loss	Mainly trabecular	Trabecular and cortical
Rate of bone loss	Accelerated	Not accelerated
Fracture sites	Vertebrae (crush) and distal radius	Vertebrae (multiple wedge) and hip
Parathyroid function	Decreased	Increased
Calcium absorption	Decreased	Decreased
Metabolism of 25-OH-D to 1,25-dihydroxy vitamin D	Secondary decrease	Primary decrease

Source: After Riggs and Melton, 1986.

TABLE 10-8   FACTORS ASSOCIATED WITH AN INCREASED RISK OF
OSTEOPOROSIS AMONG WOMEN*

Postmenopausal (within 20 years after menopause)
White or Asian
Premature menopause
Positive family history
Short stature and small bones
Leanness
Low calcium intake
Inactivity or immobility
Early menopause (before age 45)
Previous amenorrhea
Malabsorption syndromes
Long-term glucocorticoid therapy
Long-term use of anticonvulsants
Hyperparathyroidism
Thyrotoxicosis
Cushing's syndrome
Smoking
Heavy alcohol use

* Several of these factors also increase risk among men.
Source: After Riggs and Melton, 1986.

upper lumbar vertebrae. Vertebral compression fractures can be asymptomatic
and cause progressive kyphosis and loss of height. They may also be excruciat-
ingly painful and be precipitated by relatively minor stress, such as sitting down
quickly. The pain is exacerbated by twisting and increases in intraabdominal pressure (e.g., from coughing or straining to have a bowel movement). The pain can
radiate around the thoracic cavity and mimic cardiac pain. Diagnosing a new
compression fracture can be difficult, especially when old radiographs are not
available. The combination of the new onset of characteristic pain and radiographic evidence of a compression fracture in a compatible location should be
treated with bed rest (for as short a period as possible), heat, and analgesics.
Posterior wedging of the fracture, fractures above the midthoracic vertebrae, and
irregular-appearing vertebral bodies should raise the suspicion of a metastatic
malignancy or plasmacytoma.

Several treatments are available for osteoporosis, including exercise, supplemental dietary calcium, vitamin D, bisphosphonates, fluoride, calcitonin, estrogen, and selective estrogen-receptor modulators (Eastell, 1998; Nelson et al.,
2002). The most effective treatment for the different types of osteoporosis

remains somewhat controversial and is influenced by a number of patient-related factors. Preventive approaches are clearly the most effective; but to be effective in preventing fractures and associated morbidity later in life, treatment should be initiated soon after the menopause and continued for 10 to 20 years. Exercise probably has modest beneficial effects on bone mass and has other potential beneficial effects on muscle strength and agility (which may help prevent falls) and cardiovascular status. Thus, prescribing an exercise program suitable to the individual's preferences is certainly reasonable. Calcium supplementation of 1000 to 1500 mg/d is recommended as a preventive measure. Routine vitamin D supplementation of 400 to 800 IU per day is also recommended because it may help reduce the incidence of vertebral and hip fractures. Sodium fluoride can increase bone mass, particularly vertebral bone mass, but data on its effectiveness in preventing vertebral and hip fractures are conflicting. There is also a high incidence of gastrointestinal toxicity from fluoride, which is reduced with lower doses and simultaneous ingestion of calcium. Calcitonin therapy results in an increase in bone mineral density and a decrease in the rate of vertebral fractures, but it is expensive and can cause nausea, diarrhea, and flushing. Nasal calcitonin has fewer side effects, but has a small effect on reducing vertebral fractures in older women. Both forms of calcitonin have analgesic effects on bone pain of new vertebral fractures.

Bisphosphonate therapy results in increased bone mineral density and a decreased fracture rate. The two drugs commonly used in the United States are alendronate and risedronate. Both drugs have been shown, largely in industry sponsored trials, to prevent vertebral and nonvertebral fractures (Nelson et al., 2002; McClung et al., 2001; Harris et al., 1999). Both are available in daily and weekly dosages, and must be taken carefully (after an overnight fast with 6 to 8 ounces of water in an upright position) in order to avoid esophageal irritation.

Estrogen is also an effective treatment for preventing postmenopausal bone loss and subsequent fractures. Despite the benefits of estrogens, side effects and risks of its use must be considered in deciding whether to choose estrogen as therapy for osteoporosis in a postmenopausal woman. In women who are at high risk for osteoporosis (see Table 10-8) and who do not have a uterus, contraindications to estrogen treatment would be a history of breast cancer or recurrent thromboembolic disease. In women who have a uterus, the risk of endometrial cancer is reduced by the addition of a progestational agent to the estrogen. Cyclical estrogen-progestogen treatment can result in withdrawal bleeding, which some postmenopausal women may find unacceptable. Recent data suggest that combined estrogen-progesterone therapy is associated with an increase risk of cardiovascular events. These data make the decision about the use of postmenopausal estrogen even more complex.

The selective estrogen-receptor modulators (SERMs) have been developed to take advantage of estrogen's benefits and to minimize the side effects and risks. Raloxifene increases bone density without stimulating the endometrium. It also decreases total and low-density lipoprotein cholesterol, but its effect on reducing ischemic heart disease is not known. In short-term studies, it is also reported to decrease the incidence of breast cancer. Its beneficial effect on bone density is less than that of estrogen, and studies on reduction of fractures are still ongoing. New SERMs may take greater advantage of estrogen's benefits and further lower the risks.

Hip Fracture

Fractures of the hip and femoral neck, especially when associated with osteo-porosis, are among the major causes of immobility, disability, and health care expenditures in older adults. Fear of hip fracture because of a prior fracture or its occurrence in a friend or relative is a common concern that contributes to limitation of mobility in many elderly persons. This fear is realistic: there are more than 250,000 hip fractures in the United States every year, with the incidence increasing dramatically with advanced age. The mortality rate in the year after hip fracture can be as high as 30 percent, and as many as one-third of hip fracture patients remain in a nursing home 1 year after the fracture. There is also a high rate of decline in ability to ambulate and perform activities of daily living in the 6 to 12 months after fracture. Thus, the prevention and optimal management of hip fractures are critical to the health of our older population. The assessment and management of falls, the major cause of hip fracture, is discussed in Chap. 9.

The degree of immobility and disability caused by a hip fracture depends on several factors, including coexisting medical conditions, patient motivation, the nature of the fracture, and the techniques of management. Many older patients with hip fracture already have impaired mobility, and there is a high incidence of medical illnesses that necessitate treatment (e.g., infection, heart failure, anemia, dehydration) at the time of hip fracture. Patients with these underlying conditions and those with dementia are at especially high risk for poor functional recovery. The location of the fracture is especially important in determining the most appropriate management and the outcome of treatment (Table 10-9 and Fig. 10-1). Subcapital fractures (which are inside the joint capsule) disrupt the blood supply to the proximal femoral head, thus resulting in a higher probability of necrosis of the femoral head and nonunion of the fracture. Replacement of the femoral head is often warranted in these cases. Inter- and subtrochanteric fractures generally do not disrupt the blood supply to the femoral head; open reduction and pinning are usually successful.

In general, it takes 12 weeks for a hip fracture to heal. Surgical techniques such as a femoral head prosthesis and certain compression screws allow for almost immediate ambulation in many patients. Like almost all acute conditions in elderly patients, early mobilization is critical to the outcome. When combined with good rehabilitation and patient motivation, early mobilization can minimize disability and immobility from hip fracture. The current standard of care is for

TABLE 10-9   CHARACTERISTICS OF SELECTED TREATMENTS FOR HIP
FRACTURE

Type of Fracture	Surgical technique	Comments
Displaced subcapital	Femoral head endoprosthesis (e.g., Austin-Moore)	Allows almost immediate ambulation
Non- or minimally displaced subcapital	Closed reduction with multiple pinnings	Protected weight bearing for 8–12 weeks or until fracture heals
Intertrochanteric and low subcapital	Open reduction with compression screw and side plate	Allows early ambulation
Subtrochanteric	Open reduction with Zickel nail and intramedullary rod	Protected weight bearing until fracture heals

patients to receive prophylactic anticoagulation to prevent thromboembolic complications. Subcutaneous injection of low-molecular-weight heparin is an effective method of prophylaxis in patients with hip fractures. Intermittent pneumatic compression is of value, but the equipment is costly and the need to apply and remove the device limits its usefulness. The long-term outcome of older patients with hip fracture depends on many factors besides the type of fracture and patient motivation. Many hip fracture patients have functional disabilities prior to the fracture, as well as active medical conditions at the time of the fracture, and they may suffer complications while in the acute care hospital. Intensive interdisciplinary rehabilitation programs may improve outcome in this patient population. Such programs should begin in the acute hospital and can be completed in subacute rehabilitation facilities, nursing homes, or at home.

Parkinson's Disease

The first step in successful management of Parkinson's disease is to recognize its presence. Although many parkinsonian patients have the classic triad of resting tremor, rigidity, and bradykinesia, many others do not. Early in the disease, the symptoms and signs can be subtle and sometimes unilateral. Many elderly patients, especially in long-term care institutions, have undiagnosed and treatable forms of parkinsonism. Many patients have drug-induced parkinsonism resulting

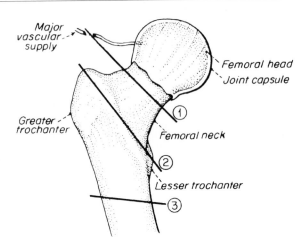

TYPE OF FRACTURE	ANATOMY	IMPLICATIONS
① Subcapital (Intra-capsular)	Disrupts blood supply to femoral head	Higher incidence of non-union and necrosis of femoral head
② Intertrochanteric ③ Subtrochanteric	Blood supply to femoral head intact	Lower incidence of non-union and necrosis of femoral head

— FIGURE 10-1 — *Characteristics of different types of hip fractures.*

from the extrapyramidal side effects of antipsychotics (see Chap. 14). Left untreated, parkinsonian patients eventually become immobile and can develop flexion contractures, pressure sores, malnutrition, and aspiration pneumonia.

Because Parkinson's disease often responds to treatment, especially early in its course, there should be a high index of suspicion for this diagnosis. Patients with more advanced Parkinson's disease frequently appear depressed or demented (sometimes both); in fact, many parkinsonian patients become depressed and develop cognitive dysfunction. Experienced neurologists or psychiatrists should be consulted when the diagnosis is in question and when the clinical picture is complicated by dementia and/or depression.

Pharmacological treatment of Parkinson's disease is based on an attempt to increase the ratio of dopamine to acetylcholine in the central nervous system, specifically the nigrostriatal system. Several drugs can be used, sometimes in combination (Table 10-10). Carbidopa/levodopa remains the mainstay of therapy. All of the antiparkinsonian drugs must be used carefully; treatment should begin with small doses that are gradually increased. Clinical response may take several weeks. Side effects are common and often limit pharmacological treatment. Wide variations in response can also occur, including morning akinesia, peak dose dyskinesias, and freezing episodes (sometimes referred to as the "on–off phenomenon"). Excessive dopamine can also cause sleep disturbances, delirium, and psychosis. These patients may require hospitalization to determine the cause(s) of their symptoms and readjustment of therapy.

Patients who are difficult to manage or who do not respond should be referred to an experienced neurologist. Some of these patients may benefit from neurosurgical procedures, such as deep brain stimulation. Parkinsonian patients with more advanced disease will also benefit from rehabilitation therapy and an ongoing program of exercise and activity in order to maintain strength and functional capabilities and to prevent complications of immobility.

Stroke

To prevent disability from immobility and its complications, patients with completed strokes should receive prompt and intensive rehabilitative therapy. In many elderly patients, coexisting medical conditions (e.g., cardiovascular disease) limit the intensity of rehabilitation treatment that can be tolerated in order to qualify for Medicare coverage in an inpatient or skilled nursing facility. However, all patients should be evaluated and managed as actively as possible during the first several weeks after a stroke. Although all stroke patients deserve an assessment and consideration for intensive rehabilitation, the cost-effectiveness of various approaches to stroke rehabilitation is controversial. Whether the rehabilitative efforts occur in the acute care hospital, special rehabilitation unit, nursing home, or at home these efforts should involve a multidisciplinary rehabilitation team, and the basic principles remain the same (see "Rehabilitation" below).

Despite the lack of data from controlled trials, even some of the most severely affected stroke patients can achieve meaningful improvements in functional status by early rehabilitative efforts. Although complete functional recovery occurs in less than half of stroke patients, immobility and its attendant complications can almost always be prevented or minimized. Development of realistic goals for individual patients is essential. Intensive efforts directed at functional recovery are probably not appropriate for patients with large or bilateral strokes causing flaccid paralysis or severe perceptual deficits or for patients with severe underlying medical conditions or dementia. The goals in these latter patients should be to prevent complications and adapt the environment. The management of older patients with cerebrovascular disease is discussed further in Chap. 11.

Pressure Ulcers

Pressure ulcers are among the most preventable and treatable conditions associated with immobility in older adults. Four factors contribute to the development

TABLE 10-10 DRUGS USED TO TREAT PARKINSON'S DISEASE

DRUG (BRAND NAME)	USUAL DOSAGES	MECHANISM OF ACTION	POTENTIAL SIDE EFFECTS
Carbidopa, levodopa (Sinemet)	40/ 400 to 200/2000 mg/d in divided doses*	Increases dopamine availability and decreases peripheral dopamine metabolism	Nausea, vomiting, anorexia Dyskinesias Orthostatic hypotension Behavioral disturbances Vivid dreams and hallucinations
Amantadine (Symmetrel)	100–300 mg/ d †	Increases dopamine release	Delirium and hallucinations
Bromocriptine (Parlodel)	1–1.5 mg tid or qid (initial); gradually increase to maximum of 30–40 mg in divided doses	Directly activates dopaminergic receptors	Behavioral changes Hypotension Nausea
Pramipexole (Mirapex)	0.5–1.5 mg tid	Dopamine agonist	Hallucinations Nausea Somnolence
Ropinirole (Requip)	3–8 mg tid	Dopamine agonist	Orthostatic hypotension Syncope Nausea Somnolence

Drug	Dosage	Action	Side effects
Anticholinergic agents, ‡ trihexyphenidyl (Artane, Tremin)	2–20 mg/d in divided doses	Decreases effects of acetylcholine and helps to restore balance between cholinergic and dopaminergic systems	Dry mouth Constipation Urinary retention Blurred vision Exacerbation of glaucoma Tachycardia Confusion Behavioral changes
Benztropine mesylate (Cogentin)	0.5–8 mg/d in divided doses		As above
Selegiline (Eldepryl)	10 mg/d in one dose	Inhibits type B monoamine oxidase	Nausea Confusion Agitation Insomnia Involuntary movements
Entacapone (Comtan)	200 mg with each dose of levodopa	Inhibits catechol methyltransferase	Nausea Dyskinesias Orthostatic hypotension Diarrhea
Tolcapone (Tasmar)	100–200 mg tid		Liver dysfunction §

* Top number represents carbidopa; bottom number, levodopa.
† Eliminated by kidney; dosages should be adjusted when renal function is diminished.
‡ Several other anticholinergic agents are available.
§ Liver function tests should be done every 6 weeks for first 6 months of treatment.

of pressure sores: pressure, shearing forces, friction, and moisture. As the name implies, pressure ulcers develop because areas of the body (most often overlying bony prominences) are exposed to prolonged pressure. The amount of pressure necessary to occlude blood supply to the skin (and thus predispose to irreversible tissue damage) is small and is generated in normal sitting and supine positions. Irreversible tissue damage can occur (especially in aging skin) after only 2 hours of continuous pressure that exceeds capillary pressure.

Shearing forces (such as those created when the head of a bed is elevated and the torso slides down and transmits pressure to the sacral area) contribute to the stretching and angulation of subcutaneous tissues. Friction, caused by the repeated movement of skin across surfaces such as bed sheets or clothing, increases the shearing force. This can eventually lead to thrombosis of small blood vessels, thus undermining and then destroying skin. Shearing forces and friction are worsened by loose, folded skin, which is common in the elderly because of loss of subcutaneous tissue and/or dehydration. Moisture from bathing, sweat, urine, and feces compounds the damage. Other risk factors for pressure ulcers include those that exacerbate oxygen transport (e.g., anemia) or impede healing (e.g., malnutrition) (Bergstrom and Braden, 1992). Hospitalized patients with fractures, fecal incontinence, and hypoalbuminemia are at especially high risk (Allman et al., 1986). The Agency for Health Care Policy and Research (AHCPR, now the Agency for Healthcare Research and Quality) has published clinical practice guidelines for the prevention of pressure ulcers (AHCPR, 1992).

Pressure ulcers can be classified into four stages, depending on their clinical appearance and extent (Table 10-11). The area of damage below the pressure ulcer can be much larger than the ulcer itself. This is caused by the manner in which pressure and shearing forces are transmitted to subcutaneous tissues. More than 90 percent of pressure ulcer occur in the lower body—mainly in the sacral and coccygeal areas, at the ischial tuberosities, and in the greater trochanter area.

The cornerstone of management of the skin in immobile patients is prevention of pressure ulcers (Table 10-12). Once a stage I or II pressure ulcer develops, all preventive measures listed in Table 10-12 should be used to avoid progression of the ulcer, and intensive local skin care must be instituted. Many techniques have been advocated for local skin care; none is more successful than the others. The most important factor in all these techniques is the attention (and thus the relief from pressure) that the skin gets. Almost any technique that involves removing pressure from the area and regularly cleansing and drying the skin will work.

The management of stages III and IV pressure ulcers is more complicated. Débridement of necrotic tissue and frequent irrigation (two to three times daily), cleansing (with saline or peroxide), and dressing of the wound are essential. Eschars should be undermined and removed if they are suspected of hiding large amounts of necrotic and infected tissue. Chemical débriding agents can be helpful. The role of wound cultures and antimicrobials in the management of stage III pressure ulcers is controversial. Topical antimicrobials may be useful, especially

TABLE 10-11   CLINICAL CHARACTERISTICS OF PRESSURE SORES

Stage I
  Acute inflammatory response limited to epidermis
  Presents as irregular area of erythema, induration, and/or superficial
    ulceration
  Often over a bony prominence
Stage II
  Extension of acute inflammatory response through dermis to the junction
    of subcutaneous fat
  Appears as a blister, abrasion, or shallow ulcer with more distinct edges
  Early fibrosis and pigment changes occur
Stage III
  Full-thickness skin ulcer extending through subcutaneous fat, limited by
    deep fascia
  Skin undermined
  Base of ulcer infected, often with necrotic, foul-smelling tissue
Stage IV
  Extension of ulcer through deep fascia, so that bone is visible at base of
    ulcer
  Osteomyelitis and septic arthritis can be present

when bacterial colony counts are high, but they are generally not recommended. Systemic antimicrobials should not be used because they do not reach sufficient concentrations in the area of the ulcer; topical therapy will be more effective unless cellulitis is present. Routine wound cultures are probably not warranted for stage III lesions because they almost always grow several different organisms and do not detect anaerobic bacteria, which are often pathogenic. Results of such cultures generally reflect colonization rather than infection. Once a lesion has progressed to stage IV, systemic antimicrobials are often necessary. Routine and anaerobic cultures of tissue or bone are most helpful in directing antimicrobial therapy. Patients with large pressure ulcers who become septic should be treated with broad-spectrum antimicrobials that will cover anaerobes, gram-negative organisms, and *Staphylococcus aureus.* In selected instances, consideration of plastic surgery for stage IV lesions is warranted. Air-fluidized and low-air-loss beds are being used with increasing frequency for the management of patients with stage III and IV pressure ulcers, as well as to prevent deep ulcers in high-risk patients. Although these beds are expensive, they may be helpful in accelerating the healing of pressure ulcers in selected patients in hospital and nursing home settings (Allman et al., 1987; Ferrell et al., 1992).

TABLE 10-12   PRINCIPLES OF SKIN CARE IN IMMOBILE OLDER PATIENTS

Preventive
  Identify patients at risk
  Decrease pressure, friction, and skin folding
  Keep skin clean and dry
  Avoid excessive bed rest
  Avoid oversedation
  Provide adequate nutrition and hydration

Stages I and II pressure sores
  Avoid pressure and moisture
  Prevent further injury
  Provide intensive local skin care*

Stage III pressure sores
  Débride necrotic tissue
  Cleanse and dress wound*
  Culture wound †
  Use topical antimicrobials †

Stage IV pressure sores
  Take tissue biopsy for culture
  Use systemic antimicrobials for cellulitis and/or osteomyelitis
  Have surgical consultation to consider surgical repair

* Many techniques are effective (see text).
† Cultures and topical antimicrobials should not be used routinely (see text).

PAIN MANAGEMENT

Pain is a major factor in causing immobility in older adults. Immobility, in turn, can exacerbate painful conditions and create a vicious cycle of pain, decreased mobility, and worsened pain. The American Geriatrics Society has published recommendations of an expert panel for the management of persistent pain in older adults, and readers are referred to this publication for more details (AGS Panel on Persistent Pain in Older Persons, 2002). Pain is also discussed in Chap. 3 of this text.

Pain in older persons is commonly underdiagnosed and undertreated despite the availability of many effective therapeutic interventions. Pain is now viewed as a "fifth vital sign," and acute hospital staff and other health professionals are increasingly routinely inquiring about pain. When pain is identified, it should be carefully characterized. In addition to the standard questions about location, timing, aggravating factors, and the like, a simple standardized pain scale can be helpful in rating the severity of pain and following response to therapy. Several such scales are available (AGS Panel on Persistent Pain in Older Persons, 2002; see Chap. 3). The degree to which pain interferes with activities of daily living and sleep is especially important to explore. Recurrent or persistent pain can result in complications such as a predisposition to falling (as a consequence of musculoskeletal pain that occurs with specific movements), depression, and the use of expensive and unproven treatments for poorly managed pain. Pain may be difficult to assess in patients with moderate or advanced dementia. In this patient population, caregivers must be observant for more subtle clues to the presence of pain, such as facial expressions and changes in activities, behavior, or mental status.

Pain is generally best treated when a specific cause for the pain is identified. A careful physical examination can supplement the history in order to help pinpoint the source(s) of pain. In many situations, however, such as visceral pain, back pain, and referred pain, the cause may not be clear. In these situations careful consideration must be given to the use of selected diagnostic tests and imaging to make a specific diagnosis. The decision about whether to pursue expensive and potentially uncomfortable diagnostic procedures, such as magnetic resonance imaging and nerve conduction studies, must be individualized, weighing the potential risks and costs versus the importance of identifying the precise etiology of the pain.

Pain management usually includes both nonpharmacological and pharmacological approaches. The former include patient and caregiver education, a program of physical activity to help avoid disability from immobility, and a variety of therapeutic modalities including heat, ice, stretching, massage, ultrasonography, acupuncture and other techniques. A regular program of exercise is recommended for older patients with pain related to osteoarthritis (American Geriatrics Society Panel on Exercise and Osteoarthritis, 2001). Physical therapists should be involved in these nonpharmacological management techniques. Local injections to trigger points or joint space injections of steroids under fluoroscopy can provide dramatic relief from pain in some patients. Topical application of capsaicin, lidocaine, and other local analgesics is sometime helpful for brief periods.

The mainstay of pain management is drug therapy. Table 10-13 lists drugs that can be helpful in managing pain in older adults. For persistent pain, most experts recommend initiating treatment with acetaminophen. The chronic use of nonsteroidal antiinflammatory agents (NSAIDs) and COX-2 inhibitors can be very effective, but there are risks of these drugs with long-term use. The higher costs of the COX-2 inhibitors must be weighed against their benefits. Older patients with renal insufficiency and/or congestive heart failure are especially vulnerable to the effects of NSAIDs and COX-2 inhibitors on the kidney and fluid retention. Acetaminophen or an NSAID with an opioid can be helpful for episodic and breakthrough type pain. Severe persistent pain often requires opioid therapy, which can be given alone or in combination with one of a number of adjuvant drugs (see Table 10-13). There are many subtleties in

TABLE 10-13   DRUG THERAPY FOR PAIN MANAGEMENT

DRUG	STARTING DOSE	USUAL EFFECTIVE DOSE (MAXIMUM DOSE)	COMMENTS
Acetaminophen (Tylenol)	325 mg q4h– 500 mg q6h	2–4 g/24 h (4 g/24 h)	Reduce maximum dose 50–75% in patients with liver disease or alcohol abuse
Choline magnesium trisalicylate (Tricosal, trilisate)	500–750 mg q8h	2000–3000 mg/24 h (same)	Long half-life may allow qd or bid dosing after steady state is reached
Salsalate (e.g., Disalcid, Mono-Gesic, Salflex)	500–750 mg q12h	1500–3000 mg/24 h (3000 mg/24 h)	Salicylate levels may be helpful in patients with diminished hepatic or renal function
Celecoxib (Celebrex)	100 mg bid or 200 qd	200 mg/24 h (400 mg/24 h)	Higher doses may be associated with a higher incidence of GI side effects; patients with indications for cardioprotective ASA require aspirin supplement
Rofecoxib (Vioxx)	12.5 mg qd	25 mg/24 h (50 mg/24 h)	As for celecoxib
Valdecoxib (Bextra)	10 mg	20 mg/24 h	As for celocoxib
Corticosteroids (prednisone)	5.0 mg qd	Variable (NA)	Use lowest possible doses to prevent chronic steroid effects

Drug	Starting dose	Usual dose	Comments
Tricyclic antidepressants: Desipramine (Norpramin) Nortriptyline (Aventyl, Pamelor)	10 mg hs	25–100 mg hs (variable)	Significant risk of adverse effects in older patients; anticholinergic effects
Anticonvulsants			
-Carbamazepine (Tegretol)	100 mg qd	800–1200 mg/24 h (2400 mg/d)	Monitor complete blood cell count, electrolytes, liver and renal function
-Clonazepam (Klonopin)	0.25–0.5 mg hs	0.05–0.2 mg/kg/d (20 mg)	Monitor sedation, memory, complete blood cell count
-Gabapentin (Neurontin)	100 mg hs	300–900 mg tid (3500 mg)	Monitor sedation, ataxia, edema
Mexiletine (Mexitil)	150 mg	150 mg tid-qid (variable)	Avoid use in patients with conduction block, bradyarrhythmia; monitor electrocardiogram
Baclofen (Lioresal)	5 mg	5–20 mg bid-tid (200 mg)	Monitor muscle weakness: avoid abrupt discontinuation because of central nervous system irritability
Tramadol (Ultram)	25 mg q4-6h	50–100 mg (300 mg/24 h)	Monitor for opioid side effects, including drowsiness and nausea; may rarely precipitate seizures
Hydrocodone (e.g., Lorcet, Lortab, Vicodin, Vicoprofen)	5 mg q4-6h	5–10 mg	Daily dose limited by fixed dose combinations with acetaminophen or nonsteroidal antiinflammatory drugs
Oxycodone, immediate release (OxyIR)	5 mg q4-6h	5–10 mg	As for hydrocodone

TABLE 10-13 DRUG THERAPY FOR PAIN MANAGEMENT (*Continued*)

DRUG	STARTING DOSE	USUAL EFFECTIVE DOSE (MAXIMUM DOSE)	COMMENTS
Oxycodone, sustained release (OxyContin)	10 mg q12h	Variable (variable)	Usually started after initial dose determined by effects of immediate-release opioid
Morphine, immediate release (e.g., MSIR, Roxanol)	2.5–10 mg q4h	Variable (variable)	Oral liquid concentrate recommended for breakthrough pain
Morphine, sustained release (e.g., MSContin, Kadian)	15 mg q12h	Variable (variable)	Usually started after initial dose determined by effects of immediate-release opioid; toxic metabolites of morphine may limit usefulness in patients with renal insufficiency or when high-dose therapy is required
Hydromorphone (Dilaudid, Hydrostat)	2 mg q3–4h	Variable (variable)	For breakthrough pain or for around-the-clock dosing
Transdermal fentanyl (Duragesic)	25 mg/h patch q72h	Variable (variable)	Usually started after initial dose determined by effects of immediate-release opioid; currently available lowest dose patch (25 $\mu g/h$) recommended for patients who require 60 mg per 24-h oral morphine equivalents; peak effects of first dose takes 18–24 h. Duration of effect is usually 3 days, but may range from 48 to 96 h

Source: After AGS Panel on Persistent Pain in Older Adults, 2002.

the effective drug treatment of pain and the avoidance of bothersome and potentially dangerous complications. The reader is referred to the AGS recommendations as well as other more comprehensive textbooks for more specific information on pain management.

EXERCISE

Exercise is a critical intervention for preventing immobility and its complications, and is also discussed in Chapter 5 of this text. The development of musculoskeletal disability with age frequently decreases quality of life. Musculoskeletal disability among older adults is commonly linked to osteoarthritis, deconditioning, soft-tissue changes, and other chronic diseases. Smoking, body mass index, and exercise patterns in midlife and late adulthood are predictors of subsequent disability (Vita et al., 1998). Persons with better health habits not only survive longer but their disability is postponed. In a longitudinal study, older persons who engaged in vigorous running had slower development of disability than the general population (Fries et al., 1994). Maximal cardiac output and aerobic exercise capacity decline with advancing age and physical inactivity. Endurance exercise training induces adaptations that can counteract some of the deleterious effects of aging, including an increase in maximal oxygen uptake and enhancement of cardiac function. Another potential benefit of exercise is maintenance of the bone mineral density of the lumbar spine in postmenopausal women (Kelley, 1998).

Strength training also is feasible and effective in both community-dwelling older adults and in frail nursing home residents (Ades et al., 1996; Fiatarone et al., 1994; Hunter et al., 1995). Training improves strength, walking endurance, and ability to carry out daily tasks. Many studies have demonstrated that exercise programs, both for endurance and strength, can be initiated in older adults with safety and with resultant benefit in delaying disability and improving function (American Geriatrics Society Panel on Exercise and Osteoarthritis, 2001). Walking is cheap and safe, and strength training can be done with inexpensive devices. The program should be tailored with specific goals for the exercise and outcomes.

REHABILITATION

The goal of rehabilitation is to restore function and prevent further disability. It is therefore a core element of geriatric practice, especially for immobile elderly patients, and usually necessitates a team effort. Physiatrists can be very helpful in developing appropriate and optimal rehabilitation plans for geriatric patients with complicated rehabilitation needs. It is beyond the scope of this text to provide a detailed discussion of rehabilitation in the older adult. Table 10-14

TABLE 10-14   BASIC PRINCIPLES OF REHABILITATION IN OLDER PATIENTS

Optimize the treatment of underlying diseases

Prevent secondary disabilities and complications of immobility

Treat primary disabilities

Set realistic, individualized goals

Emphasize functional independence
   Set measurable goals related to functional performance
   Enhance residual functional capacities
   Provide adaptive tools to maximize function
   Adapt the environment to the patient's functional disabilities when feasible

Attend to motivation and other psychological factors of both patients and
   caregivers

Use a team approach

outlines some of the key principles. Careful assessment of a patient's function, the setting of realistic goals, prevention of secondary disabilities and complications of immobility, repeated measures of functional abilities that are relevant to the patient's environment, and adapting the environment to the patients' abilities (and vice versa) are all essential elements of the rehabilitation process.

Physical and occupational therapists can be extremely valuable in assessing, treating, motivating, and monitoring patients whose mobility is impaired. Physical therapists generally attend to the relief of pain, muscle strength and endurance, joint range of motion, and gait. They use a variety of treatment modalities (Table 10-15). Occupational therapists focus on functional abilities, especially as they relate to activities of daily living. They make detailed assessments of mobility and help patients improve or adapt to their abilities to perform basic and instrumental activities of daily living. Even when mobility and function remain impaired, occupational therapists can make life easier for these patients by performing environmental assessments and recommending modifications and assistive devices that will improve the patient's ability to function independently (Table 10-16). Speech therapists are helpful in assessing and implementing rehabilitation for disorders of communication and swallowing.

Although these basic principles of geriatric rehabilitation are essential in providing optimal care for the growing populations of geriatric patients who may need rehabilitation, the cost-effectiveness of various approaches to rehabilitation in the elderly remains controversial. Most of the data on the effectiveness of rehabilitation for older adults come from studies of geriatric assessment units, where

TABLE 10-15   PHYSICAL THERAPY IN THE MANAGEMENT OF IMMOBILE
               OLDER PATIENTS

Objectives
    Relieve pain
    Evaluate, maintain, and improve joint range of motion
    Evaluate and improve strength, endurance, motor skills, and coordination
    Evaluate and improve gait and stability
    Assess the need for and teach the use of assistive devices for ambulation
        (wheelchairs, walkers, canes)

Treatment modalities

Exercise
    Active (isometric and isotonic)
    Passive

Heat
    Hot packs
    Paraffin
    Diathermy

Hydrotherapy

Ultrasound

Transcutaneous electrical nerve stimulation

short-term rehabilitation is a major component of the intervention. Most geriatric assessment units described to date have been in either acute care hospitals or ambulatory settings. The effectiveness of such units was summarized in Chap. 3. It is clear that targeting rehabilitative efforts to patients who are most likely to benefit is critical to cost-effectiveness. The decision to admit an older patient to a specialized inpatient acute rehabilitation or stroke unit as opposed to a skilled nursing facility depends on many factors including the patient's potential for benefit and ability to tolerate intensive therapy, as well as the nature and extent of medical comorbidities. More data are needed to accurately predict which geriatric patients will benefit most from specific types of rehabilitative efforts. Until these data are available, geriatricians should work closely with experienced rehabilitation therapists in setting *realistic* and *individualized* goals for their patients. The goals should be compatible with the patients' preferences and socioeconomic environment, and should be directed toward the maximum functional outcome realistic for that patient. Ongoing assessment of progress and the prevention of medical and psychological complications are also fundamental to the rehabilitative process.

TABLE 10-16   OCCUPATIONAL THERAPY IN THE MANAGEMENT OF
IMMOBILE OLDER PATIENTS

Objectives
  Restore, maintain, and improve ability to function independently
  Evaluate and improve sensory and perceptual motor function
  Evaluate and improve ability to perform activities of daily living (ADL)
  Fabricate and fit splints for upper extremities
  Improve coping and problem-solving skills
  Improve use of leisure time

Modalities
  Assessment of mobility
    Bed mobility
    Transfers
    Wheelchair propulsion
  Assessment of other ADL using actual or simulated environments
    Dressing
    Toileting
    Bathing and personal hygiene
    Cooking and cleaning

Visit home for environmental assessment and recommendations for adaptation

Provide task-oriented activities (e.g., crafts, projects)

Recommend and teach use of assistive devices (e.g., long-handled reachers,
  special eating and cooking utensils, sock aids)

Recommend and teach use of safety devices (e.g., grab bars and railing,
  raised toilet seats, shower chairs)

References

Ades PA, Ballor DL, Ashikaga T, et al: Weight training improves walking endurance in
  healthy elderly persons. *Ann Intern Med* 124:568–572, 1996.

AGS Panel on Persistent Pain in Older Persons: The management of persistent pain in older persons. *J Am Geriatr Soc* 50:S205–S224, 2002.

AHCPR: *Pressure Ulcers in Adults: Prediction and Prevention*. AHCPR Publication No.
  92–0047. Rockville, MD, Agency for Health Care Policy and Research, 1992.

Allman RM, Laprade CA, Noel LB, et al: Pressure sores among hospitalized patients. *Ann
  Intern Med* 105:337–342, 1986.

Allman RM, Walker JM, Hart MK, et al: Air-fluidized beds or conventional therapy for
  pressure sores: a randomized trial. *Ann Intern Med* 107:641–648, 1987.

American Geriatrics Society Panel on Exercise and Osteoarthritis: Exercise prescription for older adults with osteoarthritis pain: consensus practice recommendations. A supplement to the AGS Clinical Practice Guidelines on the management of chronic pain in older adults. *J Am Geriatr Soc* 49:808–823, 2001.

Bergstrom N, Braden B: A prospective study of pressure sore risk among institutionalized elderly. *J Am Geriatr Soc* 40:747–758, 1992.

Eastell R: Treatment of postmenopausal osteoporosis. *N Engl J Med* 338:736–746, 1998.

Ferrell BA, Osterweil D, Christenson P: A randomized trial of low-air-loss beds for treatment of pressure ulcers. *JAMA* 269:494–497, 1992.

Fiatarone MA, O'Neill EF, Ryan ND, et al: Exercise training and nutritional supplementation for physical frailty in very elderly people. *N Engl J Med* 330:1769–1775, 1994.

Fries JF, Singh G, Morfeld D, et al: Running and the development of disability with age. *Ann Intern Med* 121:502–509, 1994.

Goodwin JS: Progress in gerontology: polymyalgia rheumatica and temporal arteritis. *J Am Geriatr Soc* 40:515–525, 1992.

Harris ST, Watts NB, Genant HK, et al: Effects of risedronate treatment on vertebral and nonvertebral fractures in women with postmenopausal osteoporosis. *JAMA* 282:1344–1352, 1999.

Hunter GR, Treuth MS, Weinsier RL, et al: The effects of strength conditioning on older women's ability to perform daily tasks. *J Am Geriatr Soc* 43:756–760, 1995.

Kelley G: Aerobic exercise and lumbar spine bone mineral density in postmenopausal women: a meta-analysis. *J Am Geriatr Soc* 46:143–152, 1998.

McClung MR, Geusens P, Miller PD, et al: Effect of risedronate on the risk of hip fracture in elderly women. *N Engl J Med* 344:333–340, 2001.

Nelson HD, Helfand M, Woolf SH, et al: Screening for postmenopausal osteoporosis: a review of the evidence for the US Preventive Services Task Force. *Ann Intern Med* 137:529–541, 2002.

Reich ML: Arthritis: avoiding diagnostic pitfalls. *Geriatrics* 37:46–54, 1982.

Riggs BL, Melton JL: Involutional osteoporosis. *N Engl J Med* 314:1676–1684, 1986.

Vita AJ, Terry RB, Hubert HB, Fries JF: Aging, health risks, and cumulative disability. *N Engl J Med* 338:1035–1041, 1998.

Suggested Readings

Immobility, General

Gill TM, Desai MM, Gahbauer EA, et al: Restricted activity among community-living older persons: incidence, precipitants, and health care utilization. *Ann Intern Med* 135:313–321, 2001.

Harper CM, Lyles YM: Physiology and complications of bed rest. *J Am Geriatr Soc* 36:1047–1054, 1988.

Musculoskeletal Disorders

Borenstein DG, Burton JR: Lumbar spine disease in the elderly. *J Am Geriatr Soc* 41:167–175, 1993.

Felson DT, Lawrence RC, Dieppe PA, et al: Osteoarthritis: new insights. Part I: the disease and its risk factors. *Ann Intern Med* 133:635–646, 2000.

Felson DT, Lawrence RC, Hochberg MC, et al: Osteoarthritis: new insights. Part II: treatment approaches. *Ann Intern Med* 133:726–737, 2000.

Osteoporosis and Hip Fracture

Cummings SR, Bates D, Black DM: Clinical use of bone densitometry. *JAMA* 288:1889–1897, 2002.

Hannan EL, Magaziner J, Wang JJ, et al: Mortality and locomotion 6 months after hospitalization for hip fracture: risk factors and risk-adjusted hospital outcomes. *JAMA* 285:2736–2742, 2001.

Kannus P, Parkkari J, Niemi S, et al: Prevention of hip fracture in elderly people with use of a hip protector. *N Engl J Med* 343:1506–1513, 2000.

Marottoli RA, Berkman LF, Leo-Summers L, Cooney LM Jr: Predictors of mortality and institutionalization after hip fracture: the New Haven EPESE cohort. *Am J Public Health* 84:1807–1812, 1994.

NIH Consensus Development Panel on Osteoporosis Prevention, Diagnosis, and Therapy: Osteoporosis prevention, diagnosis, and therapy. *JAMA* 285:785–795, 2001.

US Preventive Services Task Force: Screening for osteoporosis in postmenopausal women: recommendations and rationale. *Ann Intern Med* 137:526–528, 2002.

Zuckerman JD: Hip fracture. *N Engl J Med* 334:1519–1525, 1996.

Parkinson's Disease

Lang AE, Lozano AM: Parkinson's disease: first of two parts. *N Engl J Med* 339:1044–1053, 1998.

Lang AE, Lozano AM: Parkinson's disease: second of two parts. *N Engl J Med* 339:1130–1143, 1998.

Pressure Ulcers

Agency for Health Care Policy and Research, Panel for the Prediction and Prevention of Pressure Ulcers in Adults: *Pressure Ulcers in Adults: Prediction and Prevention.* Clinical Practice Guideline, Number 3, AHCPR Publication No. 92–0047. Rockville, MD, ACPHR, May 1992.

Ouslander JG, Osterweil D, Morley J: *Medical Care in the Nursing Home.* New York, McGraw-Hill, 1991, pp 147–164.

Rehabilitation

Gill TM, Baker DI, Gottschalk M, et al: A program to prevent functional decline in physically frail, elderly persons who live at home. *N Engl J Med* 347:1068–1074, 2002.

Hoenig H, Nusbaum N, Brummel-Smith K: Geriatric rehabilitation: state of the art. *J Am Geriatr Soc* 45:1371–1381, 1997.

Wasson JH, Gall V, McDonald R, Liang MH: The prescription of assistive devices for the elderly: practical considerations. *J Gen Intern Med* 5:46–54, 1990.

Stroke

Brott T, Bogousslavsky J: Treatment of acute ischemic stroke. *N Engl J Med* 343:710–722, 2000.

Straus SE, Majumdar SR, McAlister FA: New evidence for stroke prevention. *JAMA* 288:1388–1395, 2002.

PART III

GENERAL MANAGEMENT STRATEGIES

CHAPTER 11

CARDIOVASCULAR DISORDERS

In older adults, heart disease is the leading cause of death worldwide and is the most common cause for hospitalization. Physiological changes of the cardiovascular system in aging may modify the presentation of cardiac disease.

PHYSIOLOGICAL CHANGES

In reviewing data on physiological changes of the cardiovascular system, it is important to recognize the selection criteria of the population studied. Because the prevalence of coronary artery disease may be 50 percent in the eighth and ninth decades of life, screening for exclusion of occult cardiovascular disease may modify findings.

In a population screened for occult coronary artery disease, there is no change in cardiac output at rest over the third to eighth decades (Gerstenblith et al., 1987) (Table 11-1). There is a slight decrease in heart rate and a compensatory slight increase in stroke volume. This is in contrast to studies in unscreened individuals, where cardiac output falls from the second to the ninth decades. During maximal exercise, however, other changes are manifest even in the screened population (Table 11-2). Heart rate response to exercise is decreased in older adults, as compared to younger individuals, reflecting a diminished ß-adrenergic responsiveness in aging. Cardiac output is decreased, slightly. Cardiac output is maintained by increasing cardiac volumes—increasing end-diastolic and end-systolic volumes. With this increase in workload and the work of pumping blood against less-compliant arteries and a higher blood pressure, cardiac hypertrophy occurs even in the screened elderly population.

Because myocardial reserve mechanisms are used to maintain normal function in aging, older persons are more vulnerable to development of dysfunction when disease is superimposed.

Diastolic dysfunction—retarded left ventricular filling and higher left ventricular diastolic pressure—is present both at rest and during exercise in older persons. Older persons are more dependent on atrial contraction, as opposed to ventricular relaxation, for left ventricular filling, and thus are more likely to develop heart

TABLE 11-1   RESTING CARDIAC FUNCTION IN PATIENTS AGED 30 TO 80 YEARS COMPARED WITH THAT IN 30-YEAR-OLDS

	UNSCREENED FOR OCCULT CAD	SCREENED FOR OCCULT CAD
Heart rate	−	−
Stroke volume	− −	+
Stroke volume index	− −	0
Cardiac output	− −	0
Cardiac index	− −	0
Peripheral vascular resistance	+ +	0
Peak systolic blood pressure	+ +	+ +
Diastolic pressure	0	0

Key: CAD, coronary artery disease; +, slight increase; + +, increase; −, slight decrease; − −, decrease; 0, no difference.

TABLE 11-2   PERFORMANCE AT MAXIMUM EXERCISE IN SAMPLE SCREENED FOR CORONARY ARTERY DISEASE, AGE 30 TO 80 YEARS

	COMPARED WITH 30-YEAR-OLDS
Heart rate	− −
End-diastolic volume	+ +
Stroke volume	+ +
Cardiac output	−
End-systolic volume	+ +
Ejection fraction	− −
Total peripheral vascular resistance	0
Systolic blood pressure	0

Key: + +, increase; −, slight decrease; − −, decrease; 0, no difference.

failure if atrial fibrillation ensues. Heart failure may occur in the absence of systolic dysfunction or valvular disease.

HYPERTENSION

Hypertension is the major risk factor for stroke, heart failure, and coronary artery disease in older adults; all are important contributors to mortality and functional disability. Because hypertension is remediable and its control may reduce the incidence of coronary heart disease and stroke, increased efforts at detection and treatment of high blood pressure are indicated.

Hypertension is defined as a systolic blood pressure of 140 mmHg or greater and/or a diastolic blood pressure of 90 mmHg or greater. Isolated systolic hypertension is defined as a systolic pressure of 140 mmHg or greater with a diastolic pressure of less than 90 mmHg. With these definitions, as many as 40 to 50 percent of individuals older than age 65 may be hypertensive.

Despite the high prevalence of hypertension in older adults, it should not be considered a normal consequence of aging. Hypertension is the major risk factor for cardiovascular disease in older adults and that risk increases with each decade. Elevation of systolic blood pressure and of pulse pressure are both better predicators of adverse events than diastolic pressure. This is particularly relevant to older individuals who frequently have isolated systolic hypertension.

Evaluation

The diagnosis should be made on serial blood pressures. In patients with labile hypertension, blood pressure should be averaged to make the diagnosis, because these patients are at no less risk than those patients with stable hypertension. The history and physical examination should be directed toward assessing the duration, severity, treatment, and complications of the hypertension (Table 11-3). Atherosclerosis may interfere with occlusion of the brachial artery by a blood pressure cuff, leading to erroneously elevated blood pressure determinations, or "pseudohypertension." Such an effect can be determined by the Osler maneuver. The cuff pressure is raised above systolic blood pressure. If the radial artery remains palpable at this pressure, significant atherosclerosis is probably present and may account for a 10- to 15-mmHg pressure error. Standing blood pressure should also be determined. Initial laboratory evaluation should include urinalysis, complete blood cell count; measurements of blood electrolytes, creatinine, fasting glucose, and lipids; and 12-lead electrocardiogram.

Secondary forms of hypertension are uncommon in older adults, but should be considered in treatment-resistant patients and in those with diastolic pressures >115 mmHg (Table 11-4). Pheochromocytoma is uncommon in older adults and

TABLE 11-3   INITIAL EVALUATION OF HYPERTENSION IN OLDER ADULTS

History
    Duration
    Severity
    Treatment
    Complications
    Other risk factors

Physical examination
    Blood pressure, including Osler maneuver and standing determinations
    Weight
    Funduscopic, vascular, and cardiac examination for end-organ damage
    Abdominal bruit
    Neurological examination for focal deficits

Laboratory tests
    Urinalysis
    Electrolytes
    Creatinine
    Calcium
    Chest radiograph
    Electrocardiogram

is particularly unusual in those older than age 75. Atherosclerotic renovascular hypertension and primary hyperaldosteronism may occur more frequently in older persons. With the use of automated calcium determinations, the frequency of diagnosis of primary hyperparathyroidism is increasing, particularly in postmenopausal women. Because there is a causal link between this disorder and hypertension, the diagnosis and treatment of hyperparathyroidism may ameliorate the elevated blood pressure.

Estrogen therapy in the postmenopausal woman may be associated with hypertension. Such an association can be assessed by withdrawing estrogen therapy for several months and following the blood pressure response.

Treatment

The issue of treatment of systolic/diastolic or isolated systolic hypertension in older individuals has been resolved. Multiple large trials have demonstrated that treating hypertension in older adults decreases morbidity and mortality from coronary artery disease and stroke (reviewed in Joint National Committee, 1997).

TABLE 11-4   SECONDARY HYPERTENSION IN OLDER PERSONS

Renovascular disease (atherosclerotic)

Primary hyperaldosteronism

Hyperparathyroidism (calcium)

Estrogen administration

Renal disease (decreased creatinine clearance)

Although there has been concern about the hazard of treating individuals with cerebrovascular disease, the evidence suggests that the presence of cerebrovascular disease is an indication for, rather than a contraindication to, hypertensive therapy.

Some of the treatment trials that have included individuals to age 84 years suggest that there should be no age cutoff above which high blood pressure is not treated. Relatively healthy older persons at any age should be treated unless they have severe comorbid disease that clearly will limit their life expectancy or unless the toxicity of treatment is so great that it outweighs potential benefits. The treatment goal for uncomplicated hypertension is a blood pressure <140/90 mmHg.

Specific Therapy

Lifestyle changes are not easily accomplished but should be attempted, including maintaining ideal body weight, limiting dietary sodium intake, eating fruits and vegetables and low fat dairy products, reducing saturated and total fats, and engaging in aerobic exercise (reviewed in August, 2003). Foods rich in potassium, calcium, and magnesium should be consumed. Other risk factors, such as smoking, dyslipidemia, and diabetes mellitus, should also be modified.

If dietary measures fail to control blood pressure, drug therapy should be considered. Physiological and pathological changes of aging should be considered in individualizing the therapy. Changes in volumes of distribution and hepatic and renal metabolism may alter pharmacokinetics (see Chap. 14). Changes in vessel elasticity and baroreceptor sensitivity may alter responses to posture and drug-induced falls in blood pressure.

Thiazide diuretics are usually the initial step in therapy, especially in older patients with isolated systolic hypertension. They are well tolerated, are relatively inexpensive, and can be given once a day (Table 11-5). Many older hypertensives can be treated with diuretics as the only medication. Low-dose thiazides, for example, 12.5 to 25 mg of chlorthalidone, are efficacious in lowering blood pressure,

TABLE 11-5   THIAZIDE DIURETICS FOR ANTIHYPERTENSIVE THERAPY

ADVANTAGES	ADVERSE EFFECTS
Well tolerated	Hypokalemia
No central nervous system side effects	Volume depletion
Relatively inexpensive	Hyponatremia
Infrequent dosing	Hyperglycemia
Good response rate	Hyperuricemia
Orthostatic hypotension uncommon	Impotence
Can be used in conjunction with other agents	
Effective in advanced age	
Effective in systolic hypertension	

while minimizing metabolic side effects. Higher doses have a minimal additional effect on blood pressure with a more marked effect on hypokalemia. Thiazides are contraindicated in patients with gout. Postural hypotension is uncommon, but serum potassium should be monitored. Diabetics may have increased requirements for insulin or oral hypoglycemic agents.

Although beta blockers are also recommended as initial-step therapy, two meta-analyses have called this into question (Psaty et al., 1997; Messerli et al., 1998). In these analyses beta blockers were shown to reduce stroke and congestive heart failure but not coronary heart disease, cardiovascular mortality, or all-cause mortality in older adults. When compared to each other, thiazides are superior to beta blockers in older adults (MRC Working Party, 1992). In ALL-HAT, thiazides were superior to angiotensin-converting enzyme (ACE) inhibitors in reducing cardiovascular disease, stroke, and heart failure (ALLHAT Collaborative Research Group, 2002). However, another trial suggests that ACE inhibitors are superior in older subjects, particularly men, in reducing cardiovascular events and mortality, but not stroke (Wing et al., 2003). Beta-blocking agents may be used as the initial drug when another indication for their use exists, such as coronary heart disease, tachyarrhythmias, or essential tremor.

If thiazides alone do not control blood pressure, a second agent is added (Table 11-6) or a thiazide is added if one of the other agents has failed. The choice should be individualized and usually selected from among beta blockers, calcium-channel antagonists, angiotensin-converting enzyme (ACE) inhibitors, or angiotensin-receptor antagonists (ARBs) (The Medical Letter, 2001). Beta blockers are indicated for treatment of angina, heart failure, previous myocardial infarction, and tachyarrhythmias in association with hypertension. These agents

TABLE 11-6 ANTIHYPERTENSIVE MEDICATIONS

AGENT*	ADVANTAGES	DISADVANTAGES
Beta-blockers	Useful in angina, previous myocardial infraction, heart failure Water-soluble agents have fewer central nervous system side effects Must be withdrawn slowly in presence of coronary artery disease	Contraindicated in cardiac conduction defects and reactive airways disease May cause bronchospasm, bradycardia, impaired peripheral circulation, fatigue, and decreased exercise tolerance
Calcium channel blockers	Peripheral vasodilator Coronary blood flow maintained Potency increased with age or in systolic hypertension	Headaches Sodium retention Negative inotropic effect Conduction abnormality
Angiotensin-converting enzyme inhibitors	Preload and afterload reduction Use in congestive heart failure, diabetes mellitus, other nephropathy with proteinuria	Hyperkalemia Hypotension Decreased renal function Cough Angioedema
Angiotensin-receptor antagonists	Use in angiotensin-converting enzyme inhibitor–induced cough, congestive heart failure, diabetes mellitus, other nephropathy with proteinuria	Hyperkalemia Angioedema (rare)
Clonidine	Increased renal perfusion	Somnolence, depression Dry mouth, constipation Rarely, withdrawal hypertensive crisis
Alpha–blockers	Useful in benign prostatic hypertrophy	Orthostatic hypotension
Hydralazine	May be useful in systolic hypertension	Reflex tachycardia, aggravation of angina Lupus-like syndrome at high dosage

* With all these agents, initiation with low dosage and careful titration may minimize side effects.

are contraindicated in patients with cardiac conduction deficits, bradyarrhyth-mias, and reactive airways disease. The more water-soluble beta blockers may be well suited for the geriatric population because they enter the central nervous system less readily and thus have fewer of the central nervous system side effects such as somnolence and depression; this would be a particular advantage in the elderly. However, if cardiac output is decreased, renal perfusion and glomerular filtration rate may be affected. One concern with beta blockers is the production of bradycardia with reduced cardiac output. One simple test to monitor for this side effect is the patient's response to mild exercise after each dosage increase; a failure to increase pulse by at least 10 beats per minute is an indication to reduce the dosage. If a patient is to be taken off a beta-blocking agent, with-drawal should be done slowly over a period of several days to avoid rebound of original symptoms.

Calcium-channel antagonists are peripheral vasodilators with the advantage of maintaining coronary blood flow. These agents appear to have increased potency with age, possibly as a result of the decreased reflex tachycardia and myocardial contractility in older adults as compared with younger individuals. Headache, sodium retention, negative inotropic effects—especially in combination with beta blockers—and conduction abnormalities may limit their use. Calcium-channel antagonists are effective in reducing stroke incidence in older patients with iso-lated systolic hypertension (Staessen et al., 1997). However, these drugs do not significantly reduce the risk of heart failure (Blood Pressure Lowering Treatment Trialists' Collaboration, 2000).

ACE inhibitors are effective and well tolerated for treatment of hypertension. They are both preload and afterload reducers and thus are particularly useful in the face of congestive heart failure. They prolong survival in patients with heart failure or left ventricular dysfunction after a myocardial infarction. Long-acting agents may have an advantage in adherence. Renal function, which may deteriorate on adminis-tration of these agents, must be monitored carefully. These agents may also induce hyperkalemia and should generally not be used with a potassium-sparing diuretic. Older adults are also more vulnerable to the hypotensive effects of these drugs.

ARBs are effective in lowering blood pressure without causing cough. They and ACE inhibitors are appropriate initial therapy in patients with diabetes melli-tus, renal disease, or congestive heart failure (August, 2003). ARBs are superior to beta blockers in the treatment of patients with isolated systolic hypertension and left ventricular hypertrophy (Kjeldsen et al., 2002).

Clonidine may cause somnolence and depression, but it increases renal per-fusion. The clonidine transdermal patch may lessen some of these adverse effects. However, local skin reactions may occur in about 15 percent of users. The once-per-week application of the patch may be an asset in improving adherence.

The major side effect of alpha blockers is orthostatic hypotension; this is especially problematic with initial doses of prazosin. Newer agents with lesser hypotensive effects are now being used to treat symptomatic benign prostatic hypertrophy. In ALLHAT, the alpha-blocker arm was stopped early because of a higher incidence of congestive heart failure. Consequently, alpha blockers are not recommended as monotherapy for hypertension.

Although hydralazine is usually a third-step drug, it may occasionally be used as a second-step drug in older adults because reflex tachycardia rarely occurs. If used with diuretics alone, it should be initiated in low dosages, which should be increased slowly. It should not be used in the absence of a beta blocker if coronary artery disease is present.

With the newer, more effective agents, drug-resistant hypertension is unusual. In such cases, drug adherence should be monitored and sodium intake assessed. If such factors are not contributing to drug resistance, secondary causes of hypertension should be considered, especially renovascular disease and primary hyperaldosteronism.

STROKE AND TRANSIENT ISCHEMIC ATTACKS

Although the incidence of stroke is declining, it is still a major medical problem affecting approximately 50,000 individuals in the United States every year. It is the third leading cause of death and is also a major cause of morbidity, long-term disability, and hospital admissions. Stroke is clearly a disease of older adults; approximately 75 percent of strokes occur in those older than age 65 years. The incidence of stroke rises steeply with age, being 10 times greater in the 75- to 84-year-old age group than in the 55- to 64-year-old age group.

Table 11-7 lists the types and outcomes of stroke. In cerebral infarct, thrombosis, usually arteriosclerotic, is the commonest cause, with embolization from an ulcerated plaque or myocardial thrombosis less frequent. Table 11-8 lists outcomes for survivors.

Table 11-9 lists the modifiable risk factors for ischemic stroke. Hypertension is the major risk factor. Systolic hypertension is associated with a three- to five-

TABLE 11-7   STROKE

Cause	Relative frequency %	Mortality rate %
Subarachnoid hemorrhage	10	50
Intracerebral hemorrhage	15	80
Cerebral infarction (thrombosis and embolism)	75	40

TABLE 11-8   OUTCOME FOR SURVIVORS OF STROKE

OUTCOME	PERCENT
No dysfunction	10
Mild dysfunction	40
Significant dysfunction	40
Institutional care	10

TABLE 11-9   MODIFIABLE RISK FACTORS FOR ISCHEMIC STROKE

Alcohol consumption (>5 drinks/d)

Asymptomatic carotid stenosis (>50%)

Atrial fibrillation

Elevated total cholesterol level

Hypertension

Obesity

Physical inactivity

Smoking

Modified from Straus et al., 2002.

fold increased risk for stroke. Hypertension accelerates the formation of atheromatous plaques and damages the integrity of vessel walls, predisposing to thrombotic occlusion and cerebral infarction. Hypertension also promotes growth of microaneurysms in segments of small intracranial arteries. Those lesions are sites of intracranial hemorrhage and lacunar infarcts.

Whether diabetes mellitus is a modifiable risk factor remains an unresolved issue. Tight glycemic control trials in type 2 diabetes have not shown improved outcomes for stroke.

Patients with a history of transient ischemic attacks (TIAs) are at substantial risk for subsequent stroke, particularly within the first few days. Completed stroke as a sequel of TIA is reported to occur in 12 to 60 percent or more of untreated TIA patients. In retrospective studies of patients with completed stroke, previous TIA is reported to have occurred in 50 to 75 percent of patients.

The keystone to the diagnosis of stroke is a clear history of sudden, acute neurological deficit. When the history is not clear, especially if the deficit could have had a gradual onset, consideration should be given to a mass lesion. In such cases, brain scanning with computed tomography is indicated. Electroencephalography is only occasionally helpful in the differential diagnosis. Lumbar puncture is indicated in stroke patients if hemorrhage is suspected, but not if there is evidence of increased intracranial pressure. An electrocardiogram should be performed routinely in cases of TIA or stroke because it may relate the episode to myocardial infarction or cardiac arrhythmia. Invasive techniques are usually unnecessary in stroke patients.

In older adults, symptoms acceptable as evidence of cerebral ischemia are often misinterpreted. Table 11-10 lists the presenting symptoms for TIA in the carotid and vertebral–basilar systems.

▨ Treatment

The FDA has approved and committees of the American Heart Association and the American Academy of Neurology have published guidelines endorsing the use of tissue plasminogen activator within 3 hours of onset of ischemic stroke. Thrombolytic therapy increases the risk for early death and intracranial hemorrhage but decreases the combined end point of death or dependency at 3 to 6 months. Despite the use of thrombolytics, treatment of stroke leads to little improvement in outcomes. Thus, intervention is directed toward prevention of stroke.

For primary prevention of stroke, adequate blood pressure reduction, and treatment of hyperlipidemia, use of antithrombotic therapy in patients with atrial fibrillation, and of antiplatelet therapy in patients with myocardial infarction are effective and supported by evidence from several randomized trials (Straus et al., 2002). These same strategies are effective in secondary prevention of stroke, as is carotid endarterectomy in patients with severe carotid artery stenosis.

Lowering blood pressure in hypertensive individuals is effective in the prevention of hemorrhagic and ischemic stroke. The benefits of antihypertensive treatment extends to patients older than age 80 years (Gueyffier et al., 1999). Thiazide diuretics, beta blockers, ACE inhibitors, and long-acting calcium channel blockers reduce the incidence of stroke. Selection of a specific class of drugs is discussed earlier in this chapter.

Patients with atrial fibrillation have a mortality rate double that of age- and sex-matched controls without atrial fibrillation. The risk of stroke with non-rheumatic atrial fibrillation is approximately 5 percent a year. Adjusted-dose warfarin and aspirin reduce stroke in patients with atrial fibrillation, and warfarin is substantially more efficacious than aspirin (Hart et al., 1999; Segal et al., 2000). Major extracranial hemorrhage is minimally increased in warfarin-treated patients. Excess bleeding risk with warfarin in elderly patients can be similar to the low

TABLE 11-10   TIA: PRESENTING SYMPTOMS

SYMPTOM	CAROTID	VERTEBROBASILAR
Paresis	+ + +	+ +
Paresthesia	+ + +	+ + +
Binocular vision	0	+ + +
Vertigo	0	+ + +
Diplopia	0	+ +
Ataxia	0	+ +
Dizziness	0	+ +
Monocular vision	+ +	0
Headache	+	+
Dysphasia	+	0
Dysarthria	+	+
Nausea and vomiting	0	+
Loss of consciousness	0	0
Visual hallucinations	0	0
Tinnitus	0	0
Mental change	0	0
Drop attacks	0	0
Drowsiness	0	0
Light-headedness	0	0
Hyperacusia	0	0
Weakness (generalized)	0	0
Convulsion	0	0

Key: + + +, most frequent; 0, least frequent.

rates achieved in the randomized trials (Caro et al., 1999). Strokes that occur in patients receiving warfarin or aspirin are not more severe than those occurring in placebo-treated patients. Stroke risks and benefits of antithrombotic therapy are similar for patients with paroxysmal or chronic atrial fibrillation (Hart et al., 2000).

Although aspirin may be beneficial in the primary prevention of myocardial infarction, it is not efficacious for the primary prevention of stroke. The risk of ischemic stroke is increased after a myocardial infarction, particularly in the first month. Aspirin reduces the risk of nonfatal stroke in patients who have experienced a myocardial infarction (Antiplatelet Trialists' Collaboration, 2002). Aspirin decreases the risk of stroke in patients with previous TIA or stroke, and there appears to be no dose-response relationship in doses of 50 to 1500 mg/d. Clopidogrel and ticlopidine are modestly more effective than aspirin in decreasing risk of the combined endpoint of stroke myocardial infarction or vascular death (Straus et al., 2002).

Carotid endarterectomy decreases the risk of stroke or death in patients with symptomatic carotid disease and severe carotid artery stenosis (70 to 99 percent). In patients with symptomatic moderate carotid artery stenosis (50 to 69 percent) benefits were more marginal. Patients with lesser degrees of stenosis (<50 percent) may be harmed by surgery. For people with asymptomatic carotid disease, the optimal therapy is unclear. However, identifying carotid artery stenosis in asymptomatic individuals can involve expensive and invasive diagnostic procedures. The costs of screening large numbers of asymptomatic people outweighs the benefits to the number of individuals screening would identify.

Stroke Rehabilitation

Table 11-11 presents factors in the prognosis for rehabilitation of elderly stroke patients. Although the benefit of stroke rehabilitation is controversial, it should be initiated early in the course if it is to be of benefit. Stroke patients fare better in rehabilitative facilities than in skilled nursing facilities (Kane et al., 1996; Schlenker et al., 1997). Generally, most neurologic return occurs during the first month after the stroke. By the end of the third month, little if any further return can be expected. Not all dysfunctions result in the same level of disability. Motor loss is often the least disabling. Perceptual and/or sensory loss, aphasia, loss of balance, hemicorporal neglect, hemianopsia, and/or cognitive damage may cause more severe and often untreatable disabilities.

TABLE 11-11   FACTORS IN PROGNOSIS FOR REHABILITATION

Availability and implementation of sound program
Mentation
Motivation
Prognosis for neurological return
Vigor

In the immediate rehabilitation stage, treatment is directed toward avoiding complications such as pressure sores, contractures, phlebitis, pulmonary embolism, aspiration pneumonia, and fecal impaction.

In the next stage of rehabilitation, treatment is directed toward reeducating muscles (affected areas) and enhancing remaining capabilities (unaffected areas). Table 11-12 describes measures to be taken during this phase.

When the patient stops making progress after intensive therapy, the goal of rehabilitation shifts to finding ways for the patient to cope with the dysfunction. At this stage, the patient is assessed for the need for braces and assistive devices for both ambulation and performance of activities of daily living. With a sound program of rehabilitation, the older patient who survives a stroke can return to the community.

CORONARY ARTERY DISEASE

The frequency of both coronary artery disease and myocardial infarction (MI) increase with age. Elderly patients have more severe disease than younger patients, and mortality rate is higher after acute MI.

Hypertension is the major risk factor for coronary artery disease in older adults. Hypercholesterolemia and cigarette smoking become less-important risk factors in this age group, although they are still significant. Risk factor reduction should include treatment of hypertension and dyslipidemia, and smoking cessation.

Angina pectoris has a similar presentation in both older adults and in younger patients, with familiar pain characteristics and radiation. Pharmacologically,

TABLE 11-12   STROKE REHABILITATION

Acute phase
    Change of patient's position at least every 2 h
    Positioning of patient's joints to prevent contractures
    Positioning of patient to prevent aspiration pneumonia
    Range-of-motion exercises

Later phase
    Activities of daily living training
    Ambulation training
    Functional activities for affected side
    Muscle reeducation exercises
    Perceptual training
    Training in transfer technique

acute episodes of angina pectoris can be treated with sublingual nitroglycerin, which should be taken in the sitting position to avoid severe orthostatic hypotension. Primary therapy for chronic stable angina is aspirin and beta blockers. Both are underused in the elderly, especially after acute MI. Secondary therapy includes long-acting nitrates and calcium-channel blockers, but their use may be limited by orthostatic hypotension in older patients.

Younger patients with chronic symptomatic coronary artery disease benefit from revascularization. Procedure-related mortality increases with age both after coronary artery bypass graft (Alexander et al., 2000) and after percutaneous coronary intervention (Batchelor et al., 2000). In those without significant comorbidity, mortality approaches that seen in younger patients. One-year outcomes in elderly patients with chronic angina are similar with regard to symptoms, quality of life, and death or nonfatal infarction with invasive versus optimized medical strategies (Pfisterer et al., 2003). Elderly patients with angina refractory to standard drug therapy have a choice between an early invasive strategy that carries a certain early intervention risk and an optimized medical strategy that carries a chance of late hospitalization and revascularization. After 1 year, quality of life outcome and survival will be similar.

The elderly patient with acute MI may present with symptoms other than chest pain (Table 11-13). Treatment of the older patient with acute myocardial infarction is similar to that of the young patient. Particular attention should be paid to avoiding drug toxicity and to beginning early mobilization when possible. Early mobilization may decrease deconditioning, orthostatic hypotension, and thrombophlebitis. No specific trials in the elderly have assessed percutaneous coronary intervention versus thrombolysis for treatment of acute MI. However, subgroup analyses indicate better outcomes with percutaneous coronary intervention. Coronary artery surgery can be performed with excellent symptomatic results in older patients, but with increased morbidity and mortality. The strongest indication for surgery is angina pectoris refractory to medical management. In patients with left main coronary artery disease, surgery significantly improves

TABLE 11-13   PRESENTING SYMPTOMS OF MYOCARDIAL INFARCTION

Chest pain

Confusion

Dyspnea

Rapid deterioration of health

Syncope

Worsening congestive heart failure

survival over medical therapy. Patients with three-vessel disease may also have improved survival. In older adults, however, improved survival must be considered in the light of the patient's projected survival and the higher operative risk.

Long-term administration of beta blockers to patients after myocardial infarction improves survival. Despite these data, physicians are reluctant to administer beta blockers to many patients, such as older patients (Krumholz et al., 1998) and those with chronic pulmonary disease, left ventricular dysfunction, or non–Q-wave myocardial infarction. However, all these subgroups benefit from beta-blocker therapy after myocardial infarction (Gottlieb et al., 1998). Given the higher mortality rates in these subgroups, the absolute reduction in mortality was similar to or greater than that among patients with no specific risk factors. Other secondary prevention interventions should include aspirin, ACE inhibitors, lipid-lowering agents, and smoking cessation.

VALVULAR HEART DISEASE

Calcific Aortic Stenosis

Pathologically, degenerative calcification of the aortic and mitral valves is common among older adults; it is found at autopsy in approximately one-third of individuals older than age 75 years. Aortic valve sclerosis is common in the elderly (29 percent in the Cardiovascular Health Study) and is associated with an increase in the risk of death from cardiovascular causes and the risk of myocardial infarction, even in the absence of hemodynamically significant obstruction of left ventricular outflow (Otto, 1999). The frequency of aortic stenosis increases with age, appearing at autopsy in approximately 4 to 6 percent of those older than age 65. Isolated aortic stenosis is more common among men than women except in those older than age 80, where women predominate. Aortic insufficiency may coexist with calcific aortic stenosis, although regurgitation is usually mild and a regurgitant murmur usually not heard.

The usual clinical presentation of aortic stenosis in older adults consists of fatigue, syncope, angina pectoris, and congestive heart failure. Because systolic murmurs are a frequent finding in older adults, differentiation of mitral regurgitation, aortic sclerosis, or aortic stenosis by auscultation is a challenge. The location of the murmur is usually along the lower left sternal border and apex and often does not radiate to the axilla or carotids. It is characteristically a crescendo-decrescendo systolic murmur ending before the second heart sound. Table 11-14 describes aspects that may help differentiate mitral regurgitation from aortic murmurs.

Differentiation of aortic stenosis from aortic sclerosis can be difficult in the elderly. The typical murmur and pulse of aortic stenosis may be modified in older

TABLE 11-14 DIFFERENTIATION OF SYSTOLIC MURMURS

	POSTPERCUTANEOUS CORONARY ANGIOPLASTY*	AMYL NITRATE	VALSALVA	SQUATTING
Aortic sclerosis	↑ [†]	↑	↓	↑
Aortic stenosis	↑	↑↓	↓	↑
Idiopathic hypertrophic subaortic stenosis	↑	↑↑	↑↑	↓↓
Mitral regurgitation	—	↓	↓	—

* Best following a premature ventricular contraction.
[†] Effect of maneuver on intensity of murmur.

adults. Systemic hypertension may shorten the systolic murmur of stenosis, giving it the characteristic of an aortic sclerosis murmur. Loss of vascular elasticity may modify the pulse pressure, so that the typical pulse contour of aortic stenosis is absent. Therefore, the physical examination alone is not reliable in diagnosing aortic stenosis in older adults. The addition of Doppler flow studies to echocardiography has improved the diagnostic accuracy of noninvasive procedures for aortic stenosis. Left ventricular catheterization remains the most reliable method of assessing aortic stenosis in older adults but should be reserved for patients who are symptomatic (angina, syncope, or dyspnea) and in whom surgery is contemplated.

Surgical mortality for valve replacement is higher in older individuals, but results have improved. Significant coexistent coronary artery disease should be treated with bypass surgery at the time of valve replacement. In general, a biological prosthetic valve is preferred.

Calcified Mitral Annulus

Mitral ring calcification is a disease of older adults and is most frequently found in patients older than age 70. It is reported in 9 percent of autopsies in individuals older than age 50 and has a striking increase with advancing age, particularly in women, in whom it rises from 3.2 percent in women younger than age 70 to 44 percent in women older than age 90.

This lesion often results in mitral insufficiency or conduction abnormalities and rarely in stenosis. It is an important contributing factor to congestive heart failure in older adults and is a site for endocarditis. As many as two-thirds of patients with mitral annulus calcification present with an apical systolic murmur of mitral regurgitation.

Echocardiography is the best technique for diagnosing mitral annulus calcification. Regurgitation is usually mild to moderate, and surgery is usually indicated only if endocarditis is superimposed. Recommendations for the prevention of bacterial endocarditis have been made by the American Heart Association (Dajani et al., 1997). There is a higher incidence of cerebral embolism in this disorder, and thus anticoagulation with Coumadin may be indicated.

Mitral Valve Prolapse

Mucoid degeneration affects mainly the mitral valve. This process allows stretching of the mitral valve leaflet under normal intracardiac pressure, with subsequent prolapse into the left atrium during systole.

Although the classic murmur is late systolic, the murmur can occur any time in systole. Mucoid degeneration of the mitral valve has been described in approximately 1 percent of autopsies on patients older than age 65 years. It is associated with mitral insufficiency; left atrial dilatation and regurgitant murmurs are common. Mitral insufficiency caused by this disorder is usually well tolerated and rarely requires surgery. Some patients with this syndrome have abnormal electrocardiograms and chest pain suggestive of coronary artery disease; sudden death has been reported.

Death directly from the valve disease is usually related to rupture of the chordae tendineae. Mucoid degeneration also predisposes to infective endocarditis. Prophylaxis for subacute bacterial endocarditis is indicated, and recommendations of the American Heart Association should be followed (Dajani et al., 1997).

Idiopathic Hypertrophic Subaortic Stenosis

In older adults, idiopathic hypertrophic subaortic stenosis (IHSS) may be misdiagnosed as aortic valve stenosis or mitral regurgitation. Presenting symptoms are similar to those of aortic stenosis or coronary artery disease. The presence of a bisferious arterial pulse in the presence of a systolic ejection murmur and in the absence of an aortic regurgitation murmur should suggest IHSS. The IHSS murmur usually does not radiate to the carotids. Squatting, which increases left ventricular filling, usually decreases the murmur of IHSS. Factors that decrease left ventricular volume (Valsalva maneuver, standing) increase the intensity of the murmur.

Documentation of IHSS is accomplished by echocardiography.

Therapy usually relies on ß-adrenergic antagonists. Symptoms may be worsened by cardiac glycosides, which increase myocardial contractility, and diuretics, which create volume depletion. Atrial fibrillation is poorly tolerated and may require cardioversion in the rapidly deteriorating patient. In patients refractory to medical therapy, surgery should be considered after cardiac catheterization to assess severity of outflow obstruction and state of coronary artery flow.

ARRHYTHMIAS

Although the prevalence of arrhythmias increases with age, most older patients without clinical heart disease are in normal sinus rhythm.

Atrial fibrillation occurs in 5 to 10 percent of asymptomatic ambulatory older adults and more frequently in hospitalized patients. It is usually associated with underlying heart disease; the causes are the same as in younger individuals. Atrial fibrillation does, however, occur more frequently in older patients with thyrotoxicosis.

Patients with recent onset atrial fibrillation and hemodynamic instability or angina should undergo urgent cardioversion (Falk, 2001). If the patient's condition is stable, heart rate should be controlled with intravenous diltiazem, beta blocker, or digoxin. If atrial fibrillation persists and onset is ≤48 hours, cardioversion may be attempted after initiation of heparin therapy. If onset is >48 hours, treatment should include 3 weeks of anticoagulation prior to cardioversion, unless a transesophageal echocardiogram reveals no atrial thrombus at presentation. Anticoagulation for persistent and intermittent atrial fibrillation was discussed in the treatment of stroke and transient ischemic attacks section of this chapter. For long-term rate control, verapamil, diltiazem, and beta blockers should be the initial drugs of choice. ß-adrenergic blockers are especially effective in the presence of thyrotoxicosis and increased sympathetic tone. Digoxin should be considered as first-line treatment only in patients with congestive heart failure secondary to impaired systolic ventricular function. In some patients, combinations of these drugs may be needed to control ventricular response. The maintenance dose of digoxin is usually lower in older adults because of decreased muscular mass and decreased renal clearance. In patients with recurrence of persistent atrial fibrillation after electrical cardioversion, rate control is not inferior to rhythm control (repeated cardioversion or antiarrhythmics) for prevention of death and morbidity from cardiovascular causes (Van Gelder et al., 2002). In drug-refractory atrial fibrillation and systolic dysfunction, ablation of the atrioventricular node and implantation of a pacemaker is a highly effective treatment. Implantable pacing/cardioversion devices can significantly decrease the incidence of atrial fibrillation and improve quality of life (Cooper et al., 2002). These devices may have an increasing role in the future.

The incidence of premature ventricular contractions increases with age and occurs in approximately 10 percent of electrocardiograms and in 30 to 40 percent of Holter monitorings. The decision to treat with antiarrhythmic therapy is difficult except in the immediate postmyocardial infarction period, when it is recommended. Criteria for therapy in older patients are the same as for therapy in younger patients. The half-life of antiarrhythmic drugs is prolonged in the elderly. Therapy should be initiated at lower doses, and blood levels should be monitored (see Chap. 14).

The sick sinus syndrome is particularly common among older patients. Diagnosis is made by Holter monitor. Table 11-15 lists the symptoms of sick sinus syndrome, which are usually related to decreased organ perfusion. There is no satisfactory medical therapy. Symptomatic patients may require pacemakers, which do not seem to decrease mortality in this syndrome but can alleviate symptoms. A pacemaker may be indicated in patients with cardiac side effects from drugs used to control tachycardias in the bradycardia-tachycardia syndrome.

CONGESTIVE HEART FAILURE

Although congestive heart failure is prevalent in older adults, it is often over-diagnosed. Pedal and pretibial edema is not sufficient to warrant the diagnosis. Venous stasis may produce a similar picture. Care is needed to establish the presence of other signs of congestive heart failure (e.g., cardiac enlargement, S3 heart sound, basilar crackles, jugular venous distention, enlarged liver). Determination of ejection fraction by two-dimensional echocardiography may assist in the diagnosis.

Greater than 75 percent of cases of overt heart failure in older patients are associated with hypertension or coronary heart disease. Diastolic dysfunction, not systolic dysfunction, is the primary cause of heart failure in older patients, and is associated with marked increases in all-cause mortality (Redfield et al., 2003).

TABLE 11-15   MANIFESTATIONS OF SICK SINUS SYNDROME

Angina pectoris
Congestive heart failure
Dizziness
Insomnia
Memory loss
Palpitations
Syncope

Diuretics should be used to treat pulmonary congestion or peripheral edema. In the absence of randomized controlled trials, ACE inhibitors, beta blockers, or calcium-channel blockers are recommended with reservation (Ahmed, 2003).

The mainstays of therapy for congestive heart failure as a result of systolic dysfunction in older patients, as in younger patients, are diuretics for fluid over-load, ACE inhibitors, beta blockers, spironolactone, and digoxin. To improve function and survival, all patients with chronic symptomatic congestive heart fail-ure that is associated with reduced systolic ejection or left ventricular remodeling should be treated with ACE inhibitors. Beta blockers also improve symptoms and survival (Hjalmarson et al., 2000). Low doses of spironolactone decrease mortal-ity in severe heart failure (The Medical Letter, 1999).

The use of digitalis preparations must be approached with caution. Patients once begun on digoxin tend to remain on it long after the indications have ceased. Subtle signs of toxicity may be missed, as the drug accumulates in the presence of decreased renal function. Because of decreases in lean body mass and glomerular filtration rate, lower doses of digoxin are generally required in the eld-erly. Initial maintenance doses should be lower; blood levels should be monitored to avoid toxic levels. Because the therapeutic window is narrowed in older adults, patients who have been on digoxin therapy for long periods of time after an acute episode of cardiac decompensation not related to arrhythmias should be consid-ered for discontinuation of digoxin. Weight should be monitored closely so that digoxin can be reinstated before congestive symptoms occur. With such evalua-tion and monitoring, some older patients on chronic digoxin therapy for other than antiarrhythmic treatment may not require digoxin therapy.

References

Ahmed A: American College of Cardiology/American Heart Association chronic heart failure evaluation and management guidelines: relevance to the geriatric practice. *J Am Geriatr Soc* 51:123–126, 2003.

Alexander KP, Anstrom KJ, Muhlbaier LH, et al: Outcomes of cardiac surgery in patients > or = 80 years: results from the National Cardiovascular Network. *J Am Coll Cardiol* 1;35:731–738, 2000.

ALLHAT Collaborative Research Group: Major outcomes in high-risk hypertensive patients randomized to angiotensin-converting enzyme inhibitor or calcium channel blocker vs diuretic. The antihypertensive and lipid-lowering treatment to prevent heart attack trial (ALLHAT). *JAMA* 288:2981–2997, 2002.

Antiplatelet Trialists' Collaboration: Collaborative meta-analysis of randomized trials of antiplatelet therapy for prevention of death, myocardial infarction and stroke in high risk patients. *BMJ* 324:71–86, 2002.

August P: Initial treatment of hypertension. *N Engl J Med* 348:610–617, 2003.

Batchelor WB, Anstrom KJ, Muhlbaier LH, et al. Contemporary outcome trends in the elderly undergoing percutaneous coronary interventions: results in 7,472 octogenarians. National Cardiovascular Network Collaboration. *J Am Coll Cardiol* 36:723–730, 2000.

Blood Pressure Lowering Treatment Trialists' Collaboration: Effects of ACE inhibitors, calcium antagonists, and other blood pressure-lowering drugs: results of prospectively designed overviews of randomized trials. *Lancet* 356:1955–1964, 2000.

Caro JJ, Flegel KM, Orejuela ME, et al: Anticoagulant prophylaxis against stroke in atrial fibrillation: effectiveness in actual practice. *CMAJ* 161:493–497, 1999.

Cohn JN: The management of chronic heart failure. *N Engl J Med* 335:490–498, 1996.

Cooper JM, Katcher MS, Orlov MV: Implantable devices for the treatment of atrial fibrillation. *N Engl J Med* 346:2062–2068, 2002.

Dajani AS, Taubert KA, Wilson JW, et al: Prevention of bacterial endocarditis. Recommendations by the American Heart Association. *JAMA* 277:1794–1801, 1997.

Falk RH: Atrial fibrillation. *N Engl J Med* 344:1067–1078, 2001.

Gerstenblith G, Renlund DG, Lakatta EG: Cardiovascular response to exercise in younger and older men. *Fed Proc* 46:1834–1839, 1987.

Gottlieb SS, McCarter RJ, Vogel RA: Effects of beta-blockade on mortality among high-risk and low-risk patients after myocardial infarction. *N Engl J Med* 339:489–497, 1998.

Gueyffier F, Bulpitt C, Borssel JP, et al: Antihypertensive drugs in very old people: a subgroup meta-analysis of randomized controlled trials. *Lancet* 353:793–796, 1999.

Hart RG, Benavente O, McBride R, et al: Antithrombotic therapy to prevent stroke in patients with atrial fibrillation: a meta-analysis. *Ann Intern Med* 131:492–501, 1999.

Hart RG, Pearce LA, Rothbart RM, et al: Stroke with intermittent atrial fibrillation: incidence and predictors during ASA therapy. *J Am Coll Cardiol* 35:183–187, 2000.

Hjalmarson A, Goldstein S, Fagerberg B, et al: Effects of controlled-release metoprolol on total mortality, hospitalizations, and well-being in patients with heart failure. The metoprolol CR/XL randomized intervention trial in congestive heart failure (MERIT-HF). *JAMA* 283:1295–1302, 2000.

Joint National Committee: *The Sixth Report of the Joint National Committee on Prevention, Detection, Evaluation, and Treatment of High Blood Pressure.* Bethesda, MD, National Institutes of Health, 1997.

Kane RL, Chen Q, Blewett LA, et al: Do rehabilitative nursing homes improve the outcomes of care? *J Am Geriatr Soc* 44:545–554, 1996.

Kjeldsen SE, Dahlof B, Devereux RB, et al: Effects of losartan on cardiovascular morbidity and mortality in patients with isolated systolic hypertension and left ventricular hypertrophy. A losartan intervention for end point reduction (LIFE) substudy. *JAMA* 288:1491–1498, 2002.

Krumholz HM, Radford MJ, Wang Y, et al: National use and effectiveness of β-blockers for the treatment of elderly patients after acute myocardial infarction. *JAMA* 280:623–629, 1998.

Messerli FH, Grossman E, Goldbourt U: Are β-blockers efficacious as first-line therapy for hypertension in the elderly? A systematic review. *JAMA* 279:1903–1907, 1998.

MRC Working Party: Medical Research Council trial of treatment of hypertension in older adults: principal results. *BMJ* 304:405–412, 1992.

Otto CM, Lind BK, Kitzman DW, et al: Association of aortic-valve sclerosis with cardiovascular mortality and morbidity in the elderly. *N Engl J Med* 341:142–147, 1999.

Pfisterer M, Buser P, Osswald S, et al: Outcome of elderly patients with chronic symptomatic coronary artery disease with an invasive vs optimized medical treatment strategy. One-year results of the randomized TIME trial. *JAMA* 289:1117–1123, 2003.

Psaty BM, Smith NL, Siscovick DS, et al: Review: low-dose diuretics, but not high-dose diuretics and β-blockers, reduce coronary heart disease and total mortality. *JAMA* 277:739–745, 1997.

Redfield MM, Jacobsen SJ, Burnett JC, et al: Burden of systolic and diastolic ventricular dysfunction in the community. Appreciating the scope of the heart failure epidemic. *JAMA* 289:194–202, 2003.

Schlenker RE, Kramer AM, Hrincevich CA, et al: Rehabilitation costs: implications for prospective payment. *Health Serv Res* 32:651–668, 1997.

Segal JB, McNamara RL, Miller MR, et al: Prevention of thromboembolism in atrial fibrillation. A meta-analysis of trials of anticoagulants and antiplatelet drugs. *J Gen Intern Med* 15:56–67, 2000.

Staessen JA, Fagard R, Thijs L, et al: Morbidity and mortality in the placebo-controlled European trial on isolated systolic hypertension in the elderly. *Lancet* 350:757–764, 1997.

Straus SE, Majumdar SR, McAlister FA: New evidence for stroke prevention. Scientific review. *JAMA* 288:1388–1395, 2002.

The Medical Letter: Spironolactone for heart failure. *Med Lett Drugs Ther* 41:81–84, 1999.

The Medical Letter: Drugs for hypertension. *Med Lett Drugs Ther* 43:17–22, 2001.

Van Gelder IC, Hagens VE, Bosker HA, et al: A comparison of rate control and rhythm control in patients with recurrent persistent atrial fibrillation. *N Engl J Med* 347:1834–1840, 2002.

Wing LMH, Reid CM, Ryan P, et al: A comparison of outcomes with angiotensin-converting-enzyme inhibitors and diuretics for hypertension in the elderly. *N Engl J Med* 348:583–592, 2003.

Suggested Readings

Carabello BA: Aortic stenosis. *N Engl J Med* 346:677–682, 2002.

Ezekowitz MD, Levine JA: Preventing stroke in patients with atrial fibrillation. *JAMA* 281:1830–1835, 1999.

Frohlich ED: Treating hypertension—what are we to believe? *N Engl J Med* 348:639–641, 2003.

Gage BF, Fihn SD, White RH: Warfarin therapy for an octogenarian who has atrial fibrillation. *Ann Intern Med* 134:465–474, 2001.

Haider AW, Larson MG, Franklin SS, et al: Systolic blood pressure, diastolic blood pressure, and pulse pressure as predictors of risk for congestive heart failure in the Framingham heart study. *Ann Intern Med* 138:10–16, 2003.

Hart RG, Halperin JL: Atrial fibrillation and thromboembolism: a decade of progress in stroke prevention. *Ann Intern Med* 131:688–695, 1999.

Kitzman DW, Little WC, Brubaker PH, et al: Pathophysiological characterization of isolated diastolic heart failure in comparison to systolic heart failure. *JAMA* 288:2144–2150, 2002.

Man-Son-Hing M, Nichol G, Lau A, et al: Choosing antithrombotic therapy for elderly patients with atrial fibrillation who are at risk for falls. *Arch Intern Med* 159:677–685, 1999.

Rich MW: Epidemiology, pathophysiology, and etiology of congestive heart failure in older adults. *J Am Geriatr Soc* 45:968–974, 1997.

Weber KT: Aldosterone in congestive heart failure. *N Engl J Med* 345:1689–1697, 2001.

CHAPTER 12

DECREASED VITALITY

Among older adults, decreased vitality is a common complaint; it has a host of underlying causes. This chapter deals with metabolic factors that may lead to decreased energy in the older adults: endocrine disease, anemia, poor nutrition, lack of exercise, and infection.

ENDOCRINE DISEASE

Carbohydrate Metabolism

Of the elderly population, approximately 50 percent have glucose intolerance with normal fasting blood sugar levels. Although poor diet, obesity, and lack of exercise may account for some of these findings, aging itself is associated with deteriorating glucose tolerance. Most data suggest a change in peripheral glucose utilization as the major factor in this phenomenon, although beta-cell dysfunction and decreased insulin secretion are also contributing factors. Glucose intolerance should not be diagnosed as diabetes mellitus. However, such individuals are at increased risk of developing diabetes mellitus. Lifestyle-modification, including weight loss and exercise, prevents or forestalls the development of type 2 diabetes in individuals with glucose intolerance (Diabetes Prevention Program Research Group, 2002). Both the US Preventive Services Task Force (USPSTF) and the American Diabetes Association (ADA) recommend these interventions for patients at risk for diabetes (US Preventive Services Task Force, 2003).

By the age of 75 years, approximately 20 percent of the population has developed diabetes mellitus (Meneilly and Tessier, 2001). At least half of these patients are unaware that they have the disease. The USPSTF concludes that the evidence is insufficient to recommend for or against routinely screening asymptomatic adults for type 2 diabetes, except that those with hypertension or hyperlipidemia should be screened as an approach to reducing cardiovascular risk. The ADA recommends that screening begin at age 45 years at 3-year intervals, but at shorter intervals in high-risk patients. The diagnosis of diabetes should be made on the basis of a fasting plasma glucose of 126 mg/dL or greater on at least two occasions.

The therapeutic goal for most older diabetic patients is the same as that in younger patients: normal fasting plasma glucose without hypoglycemia. However, in those with short life expectancies, the therapeutic goal may be modified to eliminate symptoms associated with hyperglycemia. This can be accomplished by lowering the blood sugar to levels that avoid glycosuria. The age at which tight control is no longer indicated has not been defined; however, studies that demonstrated benefit of tight control were 4 to 6 years in duration.

Several groups of oral hypoglycemic agents, each with a different mechanism of action, are now available. Sulfonylureas act primarily by increasing beta-cell insulin secretion. They increase circulating insulin levels and are frequently associated with weight gain. Although package inserts carry a warning on the increased risk of cardiovascular disease, the UK Prospective Diabetes Study (UKPDS) Group reported no adverse cardiovascular outcomes in sulfonylureas treated patients (UK Prospective Diabetes Study Group, 1998a). Acarbose reduces postprandial plasma glucose by inhibiting small intestine brush-border ß-glucosidases. It has a small effect on metabolic control and causes frequent gastrointestinal distress with bloating and flatulence. Metformin, a biguanide, exerts its major metabolic effect by inhibiting hepatic glucose production. It leads to significant improvement in glucose control when used alone or in combination with a sulfonylurea (Inzucchi et al., 1998). Unlike sulfonylureas, which often lead to weight gain, metformin therapy is associated with weight loss, a benefit to most type 2 diabetic patients. Weight should be monitored closely in thin diabetic patients.

A serious side effect of metformin is lactic acidosis. It should not be used in patients with renal insufficiency or congestive heart failure. In patients 80 years old or older, creatinine clearance should be measured before therapy is initiated. Metformin should be discontinued during illnesses associated with volume depletion and prior to surgery. Thiazolidinediones lower blood sugar by improving target-cell insulin sensitivity. Besides the potential for hepatic toxicity, which requires frequent liver function testing, thiazolidinedione therapy may be associated with marked weight gain. Fluid retention occurs more frequently in combination with insulin and in congestive heart failure, making these conditions contraindications for the use of these agents. Table 12-1 presents a step-care approach to the treatment of type 2 diabetes.

Because of the results of the UKPDS study, close control of blood glucose in type 2 diabetes is now in vogue. Intensive blood-glucose control with sulfonylureas or insulin decreased the risk of microvascular complications, but not macrovascular disease. Intensive treatment did increase the risk of hypoglycemia. Intensive blood-glucose control with metformin in overweight patients decreased the risk of both microvascular and macrovascular complications, and was associated with less weight gain and fewer hypoglycemic attacks

TABLE 12-1 STEP-CARE APPROACH TO THE TREATMENT OF TYPE 2 DIABETES

STEP	CRITERIA AND RECOMMENDATION	MONITORING
Step 1: Evaluation and nonpharmacologic approaches	Newly diagnosed or current therapy ineffective: initiate or reinforce diet, exercise, home blood glucose monitoring, formal diabetes education. Current therapy effective: continue therapy.	Success: continue step 1. Failure after 2–3 months: go to step 2.*
Step 2: Oral monotherapy	Obese or dyslipidemic: first line— metformin; second line—thiazolidinedione or acarbose. Nonobese: first line— sulfonylurea or metformin; second line— acarbose.	Success: continue step 2. Failure: go to step 3.
Step 3: Oral combination therapy	Previously on metformin: add sulfonylurea. Previously on sulfonylurea: add metformin or thiazolidinedione. Previously on thiazolidinedione: add sulfonylurea. Previously on acarbose, obese: add metformin. Previously on acarbose, nonobese: add sulfonylurea.	Success: continue step 3. Failure: go to step 4.
Step 4: Insulin initiation or insulin + oral therapy	FBG <200–240: eliminate one drug and always thiazolidinedione, start bedtime glargine. FBG >200–240: eliminate one drug, start bedtime glargine and preprandial lispro.†	Success: continue step 4. Failure: consult specialist.

* Severe hyperglycemia (fasting blood glucose >300) may require initiation of insulin therapy.
† Other long-acting soluble insulin may be substituted for glargine for basal control. Other rapid-acting insulin may be substituted for lispro for prandial control.

than insulin and sulfonylureas (UK Prospective Diabetes Study Group, 1998b). Metformin is recommended as the first-line pharmacological therapy in overweight patients. It is important to observe patients closely for hypoglycemic reactions and their ability to respond to this stress as any of these regimens is prescribed. Although each agent is effective as monotherapy, the majority of patients need multiple therapies to attain glycemic target levels in the longer term (Turner et al., 1999).

Because most patients with adult-onset diabetes are obese, weight reduction should be attempted, although only approximately 10 percent will maintain a prolonged weight loss. Dietary fats should be reduced. Aerobic exercise is of benefit in both delaying the onset of type 2 diabetes mellitus and in improving insulin resistance in individuals with established disease.

Other atherosclerotic risk factors such as smoking, dyslipidemia, and hypertension should be eliminated or treated. Tight blood pressure control reduces both micro- and macrovascular complications in type 2 diabetes (UK Prospective Diabetes Study Group, 1998c). A meta-analysis of cholesterol lowering and blood pressure lowering trials demonstrated large, significant effects on reducing macrovascular disease in type 2 diabetes (Huang et al., 2001). The goal blood pressure for patients with diabetes is 130/85 mmHg or lower. Angiotensin-converting enzyme (ACE) inhibitors and angiotensin-receptor blockers (ARBs) attenuate progression of nephropathy in both type 1 and type 2 diabetic patients with hypertension and in normotensives with microalbuminuria. They also attenuate decline in renal function in normotensive, normoalbuminuric type 2 diabetic patients (Ravid et al., 1998). The antihypertensive regimen of diabetics should include an ACE inhibitor or ARB, and such therapy should be initiated in normotensive albuminuric patients.

The goals for glycemic control are less-well established for hospitalized than for ambulatory patients. However, data suggest that maintaining blood glucose at 80 to 110 mg/dL in critically ill patients reduces mortality, and hyperglycemia adversely effects wound healing and increases the risk for infection. Although sliding scale insulin regimens are frequently used in hospitalized patients with diabetes, it is the opinion of the authors that they should not be used. The University of Washington has developed an algorithm to replace sliding scale insulin orders (Fig. 12-1).

Older adults have an increased incidence of hyperosmolar nonketotic (HNK) coma. Characteristic symptoms and signs help the physician distinguish this syndrome from diabetic ketoacidotic (DKA) coma. Table 12-2 compares HNK and DKA. Whereas DKA frequently develops over hours, HNK typically develops over days to weeks. Focal or generalized seizures are common in HNK and unusual in uncomplicated DKA. The fluid deficit is greater in HNK, thus leading to a higher serum sodium and more marked rise in blood urea nitrogen. Therapy in HNK must therefore address the volume and hyperosmolar state of the patient. Because these patients may be quite sensitive to insulin, lowering of glucose should be done cautiously. Volume replacement should be initiated with normal saline. This therapy alone may reduce blood glucose levels, as renal perfusion is enhanced and glucose is lost in the urine. If, after 1 hour of volume repletion, blood glucose levels are not reduced, a bolus of 20 U of regular insulin should be administered intravenously. If glucose levels do not respond, an insulin drip may be started. Such an approach should allow repletion of volume without lowering serum osmolarity too rapidly.

Thyroid

Although thyroid function is generally normal in aging, the physician should be aware of the norms for thyroid function tests for this age group (Table 12-3). The majority of data indicate that T_4 levels are normal. T_3 levels may be lower in healthy older people when compared to younger individuals, but are still in the normal range. It has been suggested that the lower T_3 levels reported in several studies are caused by undiagnosed illness and the low-T_3 syndrome described below. Thyroid-stimulating hormone (TSH) levels are also normal, while the TSH response to thyroid-releasing hormone (TRH) is decreased in males and normal in females. Thus, the TRH test is less valuable in older males. Metabolic clearance of thyroid hormones is decreased in aging. With intact feedback loops, normal thyroid function is maintained despite this change. However, with exogenous replacement of thyroid hormone, such regulatory mechanisms are not maintained; thyroid replacement doses in older adults should be lower to take into account the lower metabolic clearance. Laboratory evaluation tests most useful in thyroid disease are summarized in Table 12-4.

Hypothyroidism   Hypothyroidism is primarily a disease of those age 50 to 70 years. Goiter is rarely seen with hypothyroidism in the elderly except when it is iodide-induced. Diagnosis is usually made by a low free T_4 and an elevated TSH. Because total T_4 levels may be depressed in seriously ill patients, diagnosis of hypothyroidism should not be made on the basis of low T_4 levels alone. Table 12-5 lists laboratory characteristics of the low-T_4 syndrome associated with nonthyroidal illness. Not all free-T_4 methods distinguish the low-T_4 syndrome from hypothyroidism; physicians should be aware of the type of determination and interpretation used in their laboratory. Because the T_3 level may be in the normal range in hypothyroidism, this is not a helpful test. The low T_3 level associated with a host of acute and chronic nonthyroidal illnesses also contributes to the poor specificity of this test in hypothyroidism. Approximately 75 percent of circulating T_3 is derived from peripheral conversion from T_4. The enzymes that convert T_4 to T_3 or reverse T_3 are under metabolic control. During illness, more T_4 is converted to reverse T_3, leading to the characteristic laboratory findings of the low-T_3 syndrome.

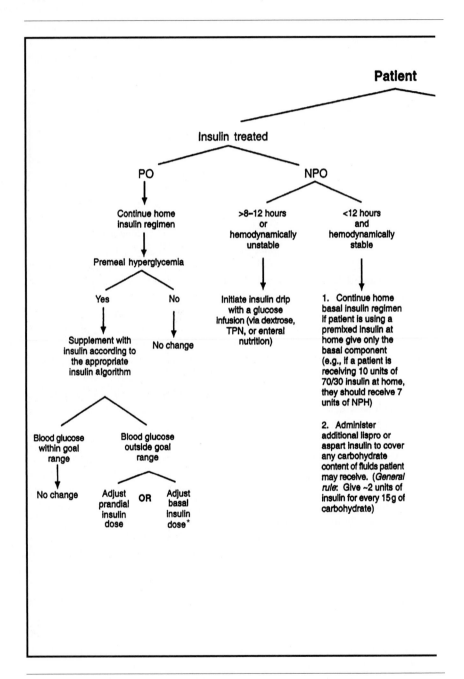

— FIGURE 12-1 — *Flow diagram for treatment of hospitalized (non-intensive care unit) patients with type 2 diabetes mellitus. CHF = congestive heart failure; NPH = neutral*

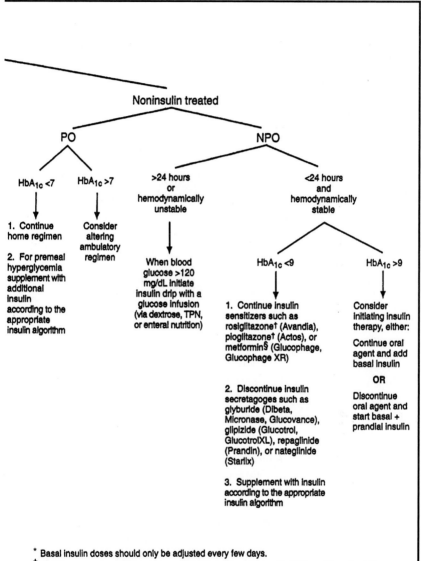

protamine Hagedorn (insulin); NPO = nothing by mouth; PO = by mouth; TPN = total
parenteral nutrition. (From Ku, 2002.)

TABLE 12-2　HYPEROSMOLAR NONKETOTIC (HNK) COMA AND
DIABETIC KETOACIDOSIS (DKA)

	HNK*	DKA
Time of development	Days to weeks	Hours
Seizures	Common	Uncommon
Fluid deficit	Marked	Present
Serum sodium	↑↑	↑
Blood urea nitrogen	↑↑	↑

* Double arrow signifies a higher increase than for a single arrow. Correction factor for sodium: 100 mg/dL of glucose = 1.6 meq/L of sodium.

TABLE 12-3　THYROID FUNCTION IN THE NORMAL ELDERLY

NORMAL	DECREASED
T_4	TSH response to TRH in males
Free T_4	Thyroid hormone production rate
T_3	Metabolic clearance rate of thyroid hormone
TSH	

Abbreviations: TRH = thyroid-releasing hormone; TSH = thyroid-stimulating hormone.

The radioactive iodine uptake is also not helpful because normal values are so low that they overlap with hypothyroidism. The TRH stimulation test can be used in females, but decreased responsiveness to TRH in older males does not allow this test to distinguish normal from pathological states. In males, a TSH stimulation test may help to confirm the presence of hypothyroidism.

Hypothyroidism may be accompanied by other laboratory abnormalities. Creatine phosphokinase (CPK) levels, including CPK hypothyroidism, may be elevated. A normocytic, normochromic anemia, which responds to thyroid hormone replacement, may be present. There is an increased incidence of pernicious anemia in hypothyroidism, but the microcytic anemia of iron deficiency remains the commonest anemia associated with hypothyroidism.

The symptoms and signs of hypothyroidism may be overlooked when such complaints as fatigue, memory loss, and decreased hearing are ascribed to aging without further investigation. The prevalence of undiagnosed hypothyroidism in healthy

TABLE 12-4   LABORATORY EVALUATION OF THYROID DISEASE IN THE ELDERLY

	HYPOTHYROIDISM	HYPERTHYROIDISM
T_4	E	E
TSH	E	E
Free T_4	E	E
T_3	O	D
Radioactive iodine uptake	O	D
TRH test	D (Females)	D (Females)
	O (Males)	O (Males)
Reverse T_3	D	D
TSH stimulation	D	O
T_3 suppression	O	O

Abbreviations: E = test for initial evaluation; D = helpful in confirming diagnosis or in differentiation of difficult cases; O = not helpful in diagnosis or not indicated; TRH = thyroid-releasing hormone; TSH = thyroid-stimulating hormone.

TABLE 12-5   THYROID-FUNCTION TESTS IN NONTHYROIDAL ILLNESS

	LOW-T_4 SYNDROME	LOW-T_3 SYNDROME
T_4	Decreased	Normal
Free T_4	Normal or increased	Normal
T_3	Decreased	Decreased
Reverse T_3	Normal or increased	Normal or increased
Thyroid-stimulating hormone	Normal	Normal

older people has varied from 0.5 to 2 percent in multiple studies; consequently, a general screening program is not cost-effective. The prevalence among older adults who are ill, however, is sufficient to support screening for hypothyroidism in this population, comprising individuals who have already presented themselves for care.

Therapy for hypothyroidism should be started at 0.025 to 0.05 mg of L-levothyroxine per day and increased by the same dose at 1- to 3-week intervals.

The decreased metabolic clearance rate of thyroid hormone in aging may lead to a lower maintenance dose of T_4. The physician should monitor heart rate response and symptoms of angina and, in the laboratory, the TSH level. When indicated for symptomatic cardiovascular disease, a beta blocker may be added to the T_4 regimen. In patients with coronary artery disease, therapy can be initiated with triiodothyronine 5 µg/d and increased by 5 µg at weekly intervals to a level of 25 µg/d, at which time the patient can be converted to T_4 therapy. Because T_3 has a shorter half-life than T_4, symptoms will remit more rapidly after discontinuance of therapy if the patient develops cardiovascular complications. A beta blocker can also be added to the T_3 regimen.

Subclinical Hypothyroidism   Subclinical hypothyroidism is characterized by increased serum TSH concentrations with normal free T_4 and free T_3 levels. It occurs in 10 to 15 percent of the general population. The presentation is nonspecific and symptoms are usually subtle. In a prospective follow-up study, based on the initial TSH level (4 to 6/>6 to 12/>12) the incidence of overt hypothyroidism after 10 years was 0 percent, 42.8 percent, and 76.9 percent, respectively (Huber et al., 2002). The incidence of overt disease was increased in those with positive microsomal antibodies. Subclinical hypothyroidism is an independent risk factor for atherosclerosis and myocardial infarction (Hak et al., 2000), and is associated with left ventricular diastolic dysfunction that is improved with T_4 therapy (Biondi et al., 1999). The decision to treat patients remains controversial. However, an algorithm for the management of subclinical hypothyroidism has been proposed (Fig. 12-2).

Myxedema Coma   Most patients with myxedema coma are older than age 60 (Table 12-6). In approximately 50 percent of the cases, the coma is induced in the hospital by treating hypothyroid patients with hypnotics. A neck scar, from previous thyroid surgery, is a clue to the cause of coma. Because patients with this disorder die of respiratory failure, hypercapnia requires prompt attention. These patients should be treated in an intensive care setting, with intubation and respiratory assistance instituted at the first sign of respiratory failure. The cerebrospinal fluid protein level is often over 100 mg/dL and should not in itself be used as an indicator of other central nervous system pathology. Therapy includes a large initial dose (200 to 300 µg) of T_4 intravenously. Although studies have not been done to demonstrate the efficacy of glucocorticoids in this syndrome, it is generally recommended that these patients receive 50 mg of hydrocortisone every 6 hours for the first 1 or 2 days. Patients with concomitant adrenal insufficiency will require continued steroid therapy.

Hyperthyroidism   Approximately 20 percent of hyperthyroid patients are older adults; 75 percent have classic signs and symptoms. Ophthalmopathy is infrequent. Approximately one-third have no goiter. Toxic multinodular goiter is more frequent than in the young. Severe nonthyroidal disease may disguise thyrotoxicosis

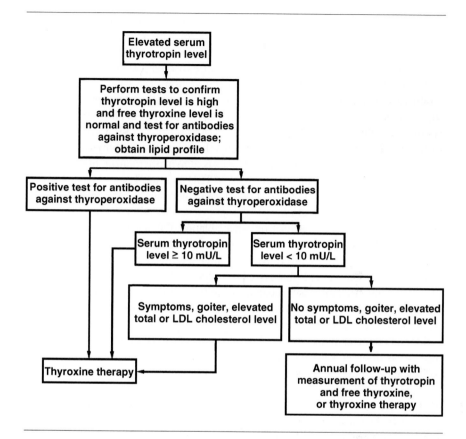

— FIGURE 12-2 — *An algorithm for the management of subclinical hypothyroidism. LDL = low-density lipoprotein.* (From Cooper, 2001.)

TABLE 12-6 MYXEDEMA COMA

Usually older than age 60 years

50 percent induced by hypnotics

Neck scar

Hypothermia

Delayed relaxation of tendon reflex

Respiratory failure and apnea

(apathetic hyperthyroidism). Congestive heart failure, stroke, and infection are common disorders associated with masked hyperthyroidism. There should be a high threshold of suspicion for hyperthyroidism in older adults. Unexplained heart failure or tachyarrhythmia, recent onset of a psychiatric disorder, or profound myopathy should raise questions about masked hyperthyroidism. The triad of weight loss, anorexia, and constipation, which may raise the possibility of neoplastic disease, occurs in 15 percent of older thyrotoxic patients. Diagnosis is made by T_4, T_3, and/or radioactive iodine uptake (see Table 12-4). The ultrasensitive TSH assays can differentiate hyperthyroidism from normal. In the absence of acute nonthyroidal disease, this test alone may confirm the clinical diagnosis of hyperthyroidism. In the presence of acute illness, concomitant determination of TSH and free T_4 may be more appropriate. A T_3 suppression test should not be done in older adults because of the risk of angina or myocardial infarction.

Therapy is usually by radioactive iodine ablation. Often patients are first treated with antithyroid medications to control hyperthyroidism and deplete the thyroid gland of hormone prior to the radioactive iodine treatment. Surgery is reserved for patients with thyroid glands that are causing local obstructive symptoms.

Severe thyrotoxicosis is treated with antithyroid drugs (preferably propylthiouracil because it blocks conversion of T_4 to T_3) to inhibit new hormone synthesis, iodides to block thyroid hormone secretion, and beta blockers to decrease the peripheral manifestations of thyroid hormone action. In older adults with underlying cardiac disease, beta-blocker therapy may be a problem; thus the cardiovascular response must be closely monitored. In patients allergic to antithyroid medications or where beta blockers are contraindicated, calcium ipodate (Oragrafin), 3 g every 3 days, can be used because it inhibits peripheral conversion of T_4 to T_3. Dexamethasone 2 mg every 6 hours inhibits peripheral conversion of T_4 to T_3 and may be added to any of the above regimens.

Subclinical Hyperthyroidism　　Subclinical hyperthyroidism is defined as a combination of undetectable serum TSH and normal serum T_3 and T_4. Subclinical hyperthyroidism caused by multinodular goiter often progresses to overt hyperthyroidism, and ablative therapy with iodine-131 is usually recommended (Toft, 2001). In older patients with atrial fibrillation or osteoporosis that may be related to the mild excess of thyroid hormone, ablative therapy is also the best initial option. In patients with subtle, nonspecific symptoms in the absence of a multinodular goiter, an antithyroidal medication should be tried for a 6-month period. If symptoms improve, ablative therapy should be considered.

▮ Hyperparathyroidism

One-third of patients with hyperparathyroidism are older than age 60. Symptoms are the same in older adults as in those who are younger, but may be overlooked.

Bone demineralization, weakness, and joint complaints may be ascribed to aging when they may actually indicate parathyroid disease. Parathyroidectomy should generally be recommended for patients with a secure diagnosis of primary hyperparathyroidism, even in the absence of classical symptoms (Silverberg et al., 1999).

Table 12-7 contrasts some of the basic patterns of the common laboratory tests in hyperparathyroidism with those of other metabolic bone diseases that are common in older adults.

Vasopressin Secretion

Basal vasopressin levels are unaltered in normal older individuals. Infusion of hypertonic saline, however, leads to a greater increase in plasma vasopressin in older as compared with younger persons. In contrast to the response to the hyperosmolar challenge, volume changes related to the assumption of upright posture are associated with less of a vasopressin response in older subjects as compared with the young. Both these findings might be explained by impaired baroreceptor input to the supraoptic nucleus. Volume expansion decreases osmoreceptor sensitivity. Hypertonic saline infusion results in volume expansion and thus decreases osmoreceptor sensitivity. If baroreceptor input is impaired in older adults, volume expansion would lead to a lesser dampening effect, and thus the vasopressin response to hyperosmolar stimuli would be increased.

Hyponatremia is a serious and often overlooked problem of the older patient. This syndrome is often associated with one of three general causes: (1) decreased renal blood flow with a decreased ability to excrete a water load; (2) diuretic administration leading to water intoxication (this condition is rapidly corrected by discontinuing diuretics); and (3) excess vasopressin secretion. Although a host of pulmonary disorders (e.g., pneumonia, tuberculosis, tumor) and central nervous

TABLE 12-7   LABORATORY FINDINGS IN METABOLIC BONE DISEASE

DISEASE	CA	P	ALK	PTH
Hyperparathyroidism	High	Low/normal	High/normal	High
Osteomalacia	Low/normal	Low	High/normal	High
Hyperthyroidism	High	High	High/normal	Low
Osteoporosis	Normal	Normal	Normal	Normal/high
Paget's disease	Normal/high	Normal/high	High	Normal

Abbreviations: Alk = alkaline phosphatase; Ca = calcium; P = phosphorus; PTH = parathyroid hormone.

system disorders (e.g., stroke, meningitis, subdural hematoma) are associated with the syndrome of inappropriate secretion of antidiuretic hormone (SIADH) in any age group, older adults seem more prone to develop this complication. Certain drugs such as chlorpropamide and barbiturates may cause this syndrome more frequently in older individuals.

In addition to treatment directed at correcting the underlying cause, water restriction and hypertonic saline are indicated when the patient is symptomatic or the sodium level is below 120 mEq/L. Demethylchlortetracycline therapy may be needed in resistant patients with SIADH. This agent induces a partial nephrogenic diabetes insipidus and thus corrects the hyponatremia. Serum creatinine and blood urea nitrogen should be closely monitored.

Anabolic Hormones

Aging is associated with a decline in anabolic hormones (Lamberts et al., 1997). The declining activity of the growth hormone insulin-like growth factor-1 (IGF-1) axis with advancing age may contribute to the decrease in lean body mass and the increase in mass of adipose tissue that occur with aging. Increased lean body mass and decreased fat mass have been demonstrated to occur in men and women with growth hormone treatment. Men had marginal improvement of muscle strength and maximum oxygen consumption (VO_2max), but women had no significant change. Adverse effects were frequent, including glucose intolerance and diabetes (Blackman et al., 2002).

Normal male aging is accompanied by a decline in testicular function, including a fall in serum levels of total testosterone and bioavailable testosterone. Only some men become hypogonadal. Androgens have many important physiological actions, including effects on muscle, bone, and bone marrow. However, little is known about the effects of the age-related decline in testicular function on androgen target organs. Studies of testosterone supplementation in older males demonstrate significant increases in lean body mass and significant decreases in biochemical parameters of bone resorption with testosterone treatment. However, there was also a significant increase in hematocrit and a sustained stimulation of prostate-specific antigen (Gruenewald and Matsumoto, 2003). Based on these results, growth hormone administration and testosterone supplementation cannot be recommended at this time for older men with normal or low normal levels of these anabolic hormones.

ANEMIA

Anemia is common in older adults, but should not be attributed simply to old age. Increased weakness, fatigue, and a mild anemia should not be dismissed as a manifestation of aging. In healthy older individuals, there is generally no change in normal levels of hemoglobin from younger adult values. A low hemo-globin concentration at old age signifies disease and is associated with increased mortality (Izaks et al., 1999).

Signs and symptoms of anemia may be subtle. Table 12-8 lists some of these manifestations. Anemia should be considered in these circumstances. If anemia is present, a diagnostic evaluation is indicated to define the cause. The appearance of the peripheral blood smear along with the history and physical examination should direct the diagnostic evaluation as described below.

Iron Deficiency

Iron deficiency is the most common cause of anemia in older adults. Laboratory findings include hypochromia, microcytosis, low reticulocyte count, decreased serum iron, increased total iron-binding capacity (TIBC), low transfer-rin saturation, and absent bone marrow iron stores. A low serum iron and elevated TIBC indicate iron deficiency even in the absence of changes in red cell mor-phology. Because transferrin is reduced in many diseases, the TIBC may be nor-mal or low in older patients with iron deficiency. However, a transferrin saturation of <10 percent would suggest iron deficiency even in the presence of a low TIBC. A low serum ferritin level is valuable in confirming the diagnosis because serum ferritin levels are below 12 mg/L in iron-deficiency anemia. Because inflamma-tory disease can elevate ferritin levels and liver disease can influence ferritin lev-els in either direction, the diagnosis of iron deficiency on the basis of a ferritin level must be made with a knowledge of the clinical situation.

Once iron deficiency is identified, it should be treated, and the cause of the anemia must be identified and corrected. Poor dietary intake of iron may con-tribute to iron deficiency in older adults. A dietary evaluation is important, both for foods that contain iron and for substances such as tea, which inhibit iron absorption. However, even in the presence of poor nutrition, evaluation for a bleeding lesion must be completed.

TABLE 12-8   SIGNS AND SYMPTOMS OF ANEMIA

Weakness	Ischemic chest pain
Postural hypotension	Congestive heart failure
Syncope	Exertional dyspnea
Falls	Pallor
Confusion	Tachycardia
Worsened dementia	

The stool should be examined for occult blood. Evaluation for a gastrointestinal lesion should be carried out in a patient with unexplained iron deficiency, even if the stool is negative for occult blood. Although gastrointestinal bleeding may be caused by drugs (especially certain analgesics, steroids, and alcohol), a gastrointestinal lesion must be excluded. Diverticulosis is a common cause of bleeding. Vascular ectasia of the cecum and ascending colon is increasingly a recognized cause of bleeding in older adults.

Replacement of iron should usually be by daily oral administration. The hemoglobin should improve in 10 days and be normal in approximately 6 weeks. Normal bone marrow iron stores should occur in an additional 4 months. If the anemia does not improve, one should consider nonadherence, continued bleeding, or an incorrect diagnosis. In unreliable patients, or when oral iron is not tolerated, parenteral iron replacement with iron dextran is indicated. Tolerance should be monitored with a test dose, and the patient should be closely observed for an acute reaction. Severe reactions occur less frequently with ferric gluconate, but a test dose should be used, as well. Parenteral iron should not be used routinely but it is an important therapeutic modality in the appropriate patient.

Chronic Disease

The anemia of chronic disease may display many similarities with iron deficiency. In older adults, this anemia is frequently associated with chronic inflammatory diseases or neoplasia. There is a defect in bone marrow red cell production and a shortening of erythrocyte life span. The finding of hypochromia, low reticulocyte count, and low serum iron may lead to confusion with iron deficiency. When a high TIBC does not confirm the presence of iron deficiency, a ferritin level can differentiate the two anemias. It is low in iron deficiency and high-normal or elevated in the anemia of chronic disease. Treatment is addressed to the underlying chronic illness, because there is no specific therapy for this type of anemia.

Sideroblastic Anemia

Sideroblastic anemia should be considered in an older patient with hypochromic anemia who does not have iron deficiency or a chronic disease. Serum iron and transferrin saturation are increased. Hence, synthesis is defective, leading to increased iron stores and the diagnostic finding of ringed sideroblasts in the marrow.

In older adults, sideroblastic anemia is commonly of the acquired type. The idiopathic group is usually refractory; only a few patients have a partial response to pyridoxine, but all should have a trial of pyridoxine. Although the prognosis is fairly good, approximately 10 percent of patients develop acute myeloblastic leukemia. Secondary sideroblastic anemia may be associated with underlying diseases such as malignancies and chronic inflammatory diseases. Certain drugs and toxins can induce sideroblastic anemia (e.g., ethanol, lead, isoniazid, chloramphenicol). The drug-induced syndromes are corrected by administering pyridoxine. Table 12-9 lists the tests that will assist in the differential diagnosis of hypochromic anemias.

Vitamin B$_{12}$ and Folate Deficiency

Both vitamin B$_{12}$ and folate deficiency may occur on a nutritional basis, although folate deficiency is the more common. Older people who live alone or who are alcoholics are most likely to have poor nutrition. Poor dietary intake of fresh fruits and vegetables may lead to folate deficiency; lack of meat, poultry, fish, eggs, and dairy products may lead to vitamin B$_{12}$ deficiency. Vitamin B$_{12}$ deficiency also occurs with the loss of intrinsic factor (pernicious anemia) and in gastrointestinal disorders associated with malabsorption of vitamin B$_{12}$.

The laboratory findings are similar in the two deficiencies and include macrocytosis, hyperchromasia, hypersegmented neutrophils, and megaloblasts in the marrow. Leukopenia and thrombocytopenia may be present, and serum lactic dehydrogenase and bilirubin may be increased. The two are differentiated by measuring serum vitamin B$_{12}$ and folate levels.

Treatment is with vitamin B$_{12}$ or folic acid, as appropriate. However, because folate will correct the hematological disorder but not the neurological abnormalities of vitamin B$_{12}$ deficiency, a correct diagnosis is essential before treatment.

TABLE 12-9   DIFFERENTIAL TESTS IN HYPOCHROMIC ANEMIA

ITEM	IRON DEFICIENCY	CHRONIC DISEASE	SIDEROBLASTIC ANEMIA
Serum iron	Low	Low	High
Total iron-binding capacity	Usually increased*	Low	Normal
Transferrin saturation	Low	Low	High
Ferritin	Low	High	Normal
Bone marrow iron	Absent	Adequate	Increased ringed sideroblasts

* May be normal or even low in older adults.

NUTRITION

A discussion of nutrition and aging is limited by the lack of adequate studies, defined methods, and standards. Although it is generally accepted that intake moderately above recommended allowances is optimal, animal studies demonstrate increased longevity with lower caloric levels than recommended. In establishing nutritional requirements in humans, we must contend with the multiple factors that confound interpretation of available data, e.g., genetic factors, social environment, economic status, selection of food, and weak methods of assessing nutritional status.

Several national surveys have been performed to assess nutrition in older adults. Taken as a whole, these surveys do not indicate poor nutritional status or marked deficiency among older individuals in the United States, and suggest that intake relates more to health and poverty than to age. However, because folate and B_{12} deficiency are associated with an increased incidence of coronary artery disease, vitamin D deficiency is associated with osteoporosis, and vitamins A, C, and E have antioxidant effects that may be beneficial in prevention of certain chronic diseases, and because most people do not consume an optimal amount of all vitamins alone, some authors recommend that all adults take vitamin supplements (Fletcher and Fairfield, 2002).

Vitamins, Protein, and Calcium

Table 12-10 summarizes nutritional requirements in older adults and demonstrates that there is no general increase in vitamin requirements with age. Studies on vitamin metabolism and requirements reveal no correlation between age and the requirement for vitamins A, B_1, B_2, or C. Vitamin B_6 and vitamin B_{12} requirements also do not increase with age.

Studies on protein requirements are not in agreement. Based on nitrogen balance studies, estimates of protein requirement varied from 0.5 to more than 1.0 g/kg daily. Data on amino acid requirements are also conflicting: some data show increased requirements with age, and other data show no change.

For calcium, estimated requirements vary from 850 to 1020 mg/d, and some recommendations are as high as 1500 mg/d for postmenopausal women. Data on the correlation of dietary calcium intake and osteoporosis are conflicting. However, calcium and vitamin D supplementation do improve postmenopausal osteoporosis. It may be necessary to use calcium and vitamin D supplements to ensure adequate intake.

Nutritional Deficiency and Physiological Impairments

There is little evidence to correlate age-associated nutritional deficiency with clinical findings. In a study on the consequences of vitamin A levels, there was no

TABLE 12-10   NUTRITIONAL REQUIREMENTS IN OLDER PERSONS

Vitamins	Unchanged in older persons
Protein	0.5 to >1.0 g/kg/d
Amino acids	Unchanged to increased
Calcium	850–1020 mg/d
Calories	Declines by 12.4 cal/d per year (maturity to senescence)

significant correlation with dark adaptation, epithelial cells excreted, or percent keratinization. In other studies, there was no correlation between vitamin C levels and gingivitis or vitamin B_{12} and lactic acid, lactic dehydrogenase, or hematocrit. Older people with limited sun exposure may be at risk of vitamin D deficiency. Studies of older individuals in nursing homes suggest that these patients require 800 IU of vitamin D per day, double the usual recommended daily requirement. Data are conflicting on correlation of dietary calcium intake and osteoporosis. Problems in assessing this correlation include reduced calcium intake in older adults, altered calcium and phosphorus ratio, decreased protein intake, and acid-base balance.

Reversal of Deficiency by Supplementation

There is no impairment of vitamin or protein absorption in older adults. Data demonstrate conclusively that low vitamin levels in older adults can be reversed by administration of oral supplementation. Because these deficiencies can be corrected by dietary supplementation, they are most likely related to decreased intake.

Caloric Needs

A study of 250 individuals age 23 to 99 demonstrated an age-associated decline in total caloric intake at the rate of 12.4 cal/d for a year. A yearly decline in basal metabolic rate accounted for 5.23 cal/d, while 7.6 cal/d related to reduction in other requirements, including physical exercise.

Dietary Restriction and Food Additives

Rats, mice, *Drosophila,* and other lower organisms have demonstrated that caloric restriction delays maturation and increases life span. The mechanism, however, is not understood, but studies suggest that it may be related to decreased levels of IGF-1. Animals fed isocaloric diets but decreased protein have an increased life span. Based on the free radical theory of aging, it has been proposed that reducing agents would prolong life. Although the data are conflicting, some studies support this hypothesis. In certain animal models, caloric restriction decreases the incidence and delay onset of disease, including chronic glomerulonephritis, muscular dystrophy, and carcinogenesis. In humans, however, body weight below ideal is not associated with increased life span. In animal experiments, nutrition is maintained during caloric variation. This may not be true in humans, and thus may lead to the differing results.

Although the influence of dietary fiber on colonic carcinoma and diverticular disease is controversial, the use of dietary fiber to maintain bowel regularity has significant support, especially in older adults, where constipation may present a difficult clinical problem. When dietary intake of fiber is low, bran can be used as a supplement, particularly in cereals, breads, or as bran powder. Intake of bran can be adjusted to maintain normal bowel movements. Adequate fluid intake should also be assured.

Although the food industry is slowly responding, most canned foods still contain large amounts of added sodium and sugar. Because some of these are less expensive than fresh or frozen foods, older adults with limited incomes may use such prepared foods exclusively. When refined carbohydrates or sodium need to be restricted, these patients should be educated about the use of canned products.

INFECTIONS

Although it is proposed that alterations in host defense mechanisms predispose older adults to certain infections, there is little evidence to support this hypothesis. It may well be that environmental factors, physiological changes in other than the immune system, and specific diseases are the major elements in the increased frequency of certain infections in older adults (Table 12-11).

Because the elderly more often have acute and chronic illnesses necessitating hospitalization and have longer hospital stays, they are at greater risk for nosocomial infections. Such hospitalizations put older patients at greater risk for gram-negative and *Staphylococcus aureus* infections. Physiological alterations (Chap. 1)—such as occur in the lungs, bladder function, and the skin—and glucose homeostasis may also predispose older adults to infections.

The incidence of malignancies is increased in older adults. Many of these neoplastic disorders, especially those of the hematological system, are associated with a higher frequency of infection. Immunosuppression during therapy is also a predisposing factor. The prevalence of diabetes mellitus is higher in older adults, thus predisposing them to more frequent urinary tract, soft-tissue, and

TABLE 12-11   FACTORS PREDISPOSING TO INFECTION IN OLDER ADULTS

More frequent and longer hospital stays
   Nosocomial infections
      Gram-negative bacilli
      Staphylococcus aureus
Physiological changes
   Lung
   Bladder
   Skin
   Glucose homeostasis
Chronic disease
   Malignancy
      Multiple myeloma and leukemia
      Immunosuppression from therapy
Diabetes mellitus
   Urinary tract infection
   Soft-tissue infections
   Osteomyelitis
Prostatic hypertrophy
   Urinary tract infection
Host defenses
   Phagocytosis unaltered
   Complement unaltered
   Cellular and humoral immunity diminished

bone infections. Prostatic hypertrophy with obstruction predisposes the older male to urinary tract infections.

Phagocytic function appears to be unaltered in aging, as is the complement system. Cell-mediated immunity and, to a lesser extent, humoral immunity, is diminished in aging. The role that these changes play in predisposing older individuals to infection has not been well defined.

Many infections occur more frequently in older adults and are often associated with a higher morbidity and mortality. Atypical presentation of infection in some older patients may delay diagnosis and treatment. Underreporting of symptoms, impaired communication, coexisting diseases, and altered physiological responses to infection may contribute to altered presentations.

As an example, failure of patients to seek medical evaluation is one factor in the higher morbidity and mortality of appendicitis in the elderly. Difficulties in communication may also alter presentation. Infections not directly involving the central nervous system may cause confusion in the elderly, particularly in individuals with preexisting dementia. The mechanism by which this occurs has not been defined. Acute unexplained functional deterioration should also alert the physician to a potential acute infectious process.

Existing chronic disease may mask an acute infection. Septic arthritis usually occurs in a previously abnormal joint. It may be difficult to distinguish clinically between exacerbation of the underlying arthritis and acute infection. Therefore, the physician should not be hesitant to examine synovial fluid in elderly patients with acute exacerbation of joint disease.

Febrile response may be blunted or absent in some older individuals with bacterial infections. This may obscure diagnosis and delay therapy. A poor febrile response may also be a negative prognostic factor. Conversely, a febrile response is more likely to indicate a bacterial rather than viral illness in older patients, particularly in the very old. The absence of leukocytosis in older patients should also not exclude consideration of a bacterial infection.

Antibiotic therapy in older adults, as in the young, is directed to the specific organism isolated. However, when empiric antimicrobial therapy is initiated, consideration should be given to including a third generation cephalosporin and/or aminoglycoside because gram-negative infections are more common regardless of the site. With all antibiotics, but particularly with the aminoglycosides, renal function must be considered and monitored for toxicity. Monitoring of drug blood level and renal function is mandatory with the aminoglycosides.

The spectrum of pathogens causing common infections in the elderly is often different than that in younger adults (Table 12-12). The frequency of gram-negative bacilli increases in each category. Pneumonia is the most frequent cause of death caused by infection in geriatric patients. *Streptococcus pneumoniae* is the most common cause of pneumonia in the elderly, but gram-negative bacilli increase in prevalence, particularly in the nursing home setting (Yoshikawa, 1999). Annual immunization against influenza, and at least one pneumococcal vaccination are recommended for all persons 65 years of age and older. Nearly 50 percent of infective endocarditis cases occur in older adults. The underlying cardiac lesion is often caused by atherosclerotic and degenerative valve diseases, as well as by prosthetic valves. Bacterial meningitis is an infection primarily of early childhood and late adulthood. Mortality in the elderly ranges from 50 to 70 percent. *S. pneumoniae* is the most frequent pathogen, but older patients may be infected with *Listeria monocytogenes* or gram-negative bacilli.

The incidence of tuberculosis is on the rise again. Older persons of both sexes among all racial and ethnic groups are especially at risk for tuberculosis. This cohort has lived through a period of higher incidence of tuberculosis, has probably not been treated with isonicotinic acid hydrazide (INH) prophylaxis, and may have predisposing factors such as physiological changes, malnutrition, and underlying disease that may lead to reactivation. Older patients are also at increased risk for

TABLE 12-12   PATHOGENS OF COMMON INFECTIONS IN OLDER ADULTS

INFECTION	COMMON PATHOGENS IN ADULTS	COMMON PATHOGENS IN OLDER ADULTS
Pneumonia	*Streptococcus pneumoniae* Anaerobic bacteria	*Streptococcus pneumoniae* Anaerobic bacteria *Haemophilus influenzae* Gram-negative bacilli
Urinary tract	*Escherichia coli*	*Escherichia coli* *Proteus* sp. *Klebsiella* sp. *Enterobacter* sp. Enterococcus
Meningitis	*Streptococcus pneumoniae* *Neisseria meningitidis*	*Streptococcus pneumoniae* *Listeria monocytogenes* Gram-negative bacilli
Septic arthritis	*Neisseria gonorrhoeae* *Staphylococcus aureus*	*Staphylococcus aureus* Gram-negative bacilli

primary infection. This is particularly the case for older patients in long-term care institutions.

Tuberculosis screening programs should be implemented in long-term care facilities because of this increased risk and because of the potential to prevent active disease among patients whose skin test converts to a strongly positive reaction (see Chap. 16). The American Thoracic Society now recommends preventive therapy for certain types of patients regardless of age, including insulin-dependent diabetic patients, those on steroids and other immunosuppressive treatment, patients with end-stage renal disease, and patients who have lost a large amount of weight rapidly. A useful rule in geriatric care is to suspect tuberculosis when a patient is inexplicably failing.

Several studies suggest that bacteriuria is associated with increased mortality in the elderly. However, other studies do not confirm this finding. Most of these non-confirming studies did not differentiate between the effect of bacteriuria and age and/or concomitant disease on mortality. When adjusted for age, fatal diseases associated with bacteriuria account for the increase in mortality among older patients with bacteriuria.

Several previous studies in elderly hospitalized or institutionalized patients have not revealed antimicrobial therapy for bacteriuria to be effective because of the high rate of recurring infection. One study in older ambulatory nonhospitalized women with asymptomatic bacteriuria demonstrated that short-course antimicrobial therapy is effective in eliminating bacteriuria in most of the women for at least a 6-month period. Survival was not an outcome measure.

Bacteriuria in older persons is common and usually asymptomatic. At present, in the absence of obstructive uropathy, no evidence exists to support the routine use of antimicrobial therapy for asymptomatic bacteriuria in older persons. Among bacteriuric patients with urinary incontinence and no other symptoms of urinary tract infection, the bacteriuria should be eradicated as part of the initial assessment of the incontinence (see Chap. 8).

DISORDERS OF TEMPERATURE REGULATION

Temperature dysregulation in the elderly demonstrates the narrowing of homeostatic mechanisms that occurs with advancing age. Older persons are less able to adjust to extremes of environmental temperatures. Hypo- and hyperthermic states are predominantly disorders of older adults. Despite underreporting of these disorders, there is evidence that morbidity and mortality increase during particularly hot or cold periods, especially among ill elderly. Much of this illness is caused by an increased incidence of cardiovascular disorders (myocardial infarction and stroke) or infectious diseases (pneumonia) during these periods.

Hypothermia is a common finding among older adults during the winter, when homes are heated at less than 70°F (21°C).

Pathophysiology

Impaired temperature perception, diminished sweating in hyperthermia, and abnormal vasoconstrictor response in hypothermia are major pathophysiological mechanisms in these disorders.

Hypothermia

Hypothermia is defined as a core temperature (rectal, esophageal, tympanic) below 95°F (35°C). Essential to the diagnosis is early recognition with a low-recording thermometer.

Table 12-13 illustrates the clinical spectrum of hypothermia. Because early signs are nonspecific and subtle, a high index of suspicion must exist to allow an early diagnosis. A history of known or potential exposure is helpful, but older patients can become hypothermic at modest temperatures. Frequently the most difficult differential diagnosis in more severe hypothermia is hypothyroidism. A previous history of thyroid disease, a neck scar from previous thyroid surgery, and a delay in the relaxation phase of the deep tendon reflexes may assist in diagnosing

TABLE 12-13   CLINICAL PRESENTATION OF HYPOTHERMIA

EARLY SIGNS (89.6–95°F [32–35°C])	LATER SIGNS (82.4–86°F [28–30°C])	LATE SIGNS (<82.4°F [28°C])
Fatigue	Cold skin	Very cold skin
Weakness	Hypopnea	Rigidity
Slowness of gait	Cyanosis	Apnea
Apathy	Bradycardia	No pulse—ventricular fibrillation
Slurred speech	Atrial and ventricular arrhythmias	Areflexia
Confusion		
Shivering (±)	Hypotension	Unresponsiveness
Cool skin	Semicoma and coma	Fixed pupils
Sensation of cold (±)	Muscular rigidity	
	Generalized edema	
	Slowed reflexes	
	Poorly reactive pupils	
	Polyuria or oliguria	

hypothyroidism. Patients may sometimes be mistaken for dead. Case reports reveal patients who have survived after being discovered without respiration and pulse.

The most significant early complications are arrhythmias and cardiorespiratory arrests. Later complications involve the pulmonary, gastrointestinal, and renal systems. Electrocardiogram (ECG) abnormalities are frequent. The most specific ECG finding is the J wave (Osborn wave) following the QRS complex. This abnormality disappears as temperature returns to normal.

General supportive therapy for severe hypothermia consists of intensive care management of complicated multisystem dysfunctions. Every attempt should be made to assess and treat any contributing medical disorder (e.g., infection, hypothyroidism, hypoglycemia). Hypothermia in older patients should promptly be treated as sepsis unless proven otherwise. While patients should have continuous ECG monitoring, central lines should be avoided if possible because of myocardial irritability. Because there is delayed metabolism, most drugs have little effect on a severely hypothermic patient, but they may cause problems once the patient is rewarmed. It is preferable to stabilize the patient and immediately undertake specific rewarming techniques. Serious arrhythmias, acidosis, and fluid and electrolyte disorders will usually respond to therapy only after rewarming has been accomplished.

Passive rewarming is generally adequate for those with mild hypothermia (>89.6°F [>32°C]). Active external rewarming has been associated with increased morbidity and mortality because cold blood may suddenly be shunted to the core, further decreasing core temperature; peripheral vasodilatation can precipitate hypovolemic shock by decreasing circulatory blood volume. For more severe hypothermia (<89.6°F [<32°C]), core rewarming is necessary. Several techniques for core rewarming have been used, but positive results have been reported only from small, uncontrolled studies. Peritoneal dialysis and inhalation rewarming may be the most practical techniques in the majority of institutions.

Mortality is usually greater than 50 percent for severe hypothermia. It increases with age and is particularly related to underlying disease.

Hyperthermia

Heat stroke is defined as a failure to maintain body temperature and is characterized by a core temperature of >105°F (>40.6°C), severe central nervous system dysfunction (psychosis, delirium, coma), and anhidrosis (hot, dry skin). The two groups primarily affected are older adults who are chronically ill and the young undergoing strenuous exercise. Mortality is as high as 80 percent once this syndrome is manifest.

There are multiple predisposing factors for heat stroke in older adults, but most often there is a prolonged heat wave. The diagnosis requires a high level of suspicion. In view of the poor survival, efforts must be directed toward prevention. Older patients should be cautioned about the dangers of hot weather. For those at particularly high risk, temporary relocation to more protected environments should be considered.

Early manifestations of heat exhaustion are nonspecific (Table 12-14). Later, severe central nervous system dysfunction and anhidrosis develop.

TABLE 12-14   CLINICAL PRESENTATION OF HYPERTHERMIA

Early signs	Later signs
Dizziness	Central nervous system dysfunction
Weakness	Psychosis
Sensation of warmth	Delirium
Anorexia	Coma
Nausea	Anhidrosis
Vomiting	Hot, dry skin
Headache	
Dyspnea	

Table 12-15 lists some of the more serious complications resulting from heat damage to organ systems. Once the full syndrome has developed for any length of time, the prognosis is very poor. While management at this stage requires intense multisystem care, the key is rapid specific therapy consisting of cooling to 102°F (38.9°C) within the first hour. Ice packs and ice-water immersion are superior to convection cooling with alcohol sponge baths or electric fans.

Prevention appears to be the most appropriate approach to management of temperature dysregulation in older adults. Education of older adults to their susceptibility to hypo- and hyperthermia in extremes of environmental temperature, education as to appropriate behavior in such conditions, and close monitoring of the most vulnerable older adults should help reduce the morbidity and mortality from these disorders.

TABLE 12-15   COMPLICATIONS OF HEAT STROKE

Myocardial damage
    Congestive heart failure
    Arrhythmias
Renal failure (20–25%)
Cerebral edema
    Seizures
    Diffuse and focal findings
Hepatocellular necrosis
    Jaundice
    Liver failure
Rhabdomyolysis
    Myoglobinuria
Bleeding diathesis
    Disseminated intravascular coagulation
Electrolyte disturbances
Acid–base disturbances
    Metabolic acidosis
    Respiratory alkalosis
Infection
    Aspiration pneumonia
    Sepsis
Dehydration and shock

References

Biondi B, Fazio S, Palmieri EA, et al: Left ventricular diastolic dysfunction in patients with subclinical hypothyroidism. *J Clin Endocrinol Metab* 84:2064–2067, 1999.

Blackman MR, Sorkin JD, Munzer T, et al: Growth hormone and sex steroid administration in healthy aged women and men: a randomized controlled trial. *JAMA* 288:2282–2292, 2002.

Boulé NG, Haddad E, Kenny GP, et al: Effects of exercise on glycemic control and body mass in type 2 diabetes mellitus: a meta-analysis of controlled clinical trials. *JAMA* 286:1218–1227, 2001.

Cooper DS: Subclinical hypothyroidism. *N Engl J Med* 345:260–265, 2001.

Diabetes Prevention Program Research Group: Reduction in the incidence of type 2 diabetes with lifestyle intervention or metformin. *N Eng J Med* 346:393–403, 2002.

Fletcher RH, Fairfield KM: Vitamins for chronic disease prevention: clinical applications. *JAMA* 287:3127–3129, 2002.

Gruenewald DA, Matsumoto AM: Testosterone supplementation therapy for older men: potential benefits and risks. *J Am Geriatr Soc* 51:101–115, 2003.

Hak AE, Pols HAP, Visser TJ, et al: Subclinical hypothyroidism is an independent risk factor for atherosclerosis and myocardial infarction in elderly women: the Rotterdam study. *Ann Intern Med* 132:270–278, 2000.

Huang ES, Meigs JB, Singer DE: The effect of interventions to prevent cardiovascular disease in patients with type 2 diabetes mellitus. *Am J Med* 111:633–642, 2001.

Huber G, Staub J-J, Meier C, et al: Prospective study of the spontaneous course of subclinical hypothyroidism: prognostic value of thyrotropin, thyroid reserve, and thyroid antibodies. *J Clin Endocrinol Metabl* 87:3221–3226, 2002.

Inzucchi SE, Maggs DG, Spollett GR, et al: Efficacy and metabolic effects of metformin and troglitazone in type II diabetes mellitus. *N Engl J Med* 338:867–872, 1998.

Izaks GJ, Westendorp RG, Knook DL: The definition of anemia in older persons. *JAMA* 281:1714–1717, 1999.

Ku S: Algorithms replace sliding scale insulin orders. *Drug Ther Topics* 31:49–53, 2002.

Lamberts SWJ, van den Beld AW, van der Lely A-J: The endocrinology of aging. *Science* 278:419–424, 1997.

Meneilly GS, Tessier D: Diabetes in elderly adults. *J Gerontol A Biol Sci Med Sci* 56A:M5–M13, 2001.

Ravid M, Brosh D, Levi Z, et al: Use of enalapril to attenuate decline in renal function in normotensive, normoalbuminuric patients with type 2 diabetes mellitus. *Ann Intern Med* 128:982–988, 1998.

Silverberg SJ, Bilezikian JP, Bone HG, et al: Therapeutic controversies in primary hyperparathyroidism. *J Clin Endocrinol Metab* 84:2275–2282, 1999.

Toft AD: Subclinical hyperthyroidism. *N Engl J Med* 345:512–516, 2001.

Turner RC, Cull CA, Frighi V, et al: Glycemic control with diet, sulfonylurea, metformin, or insulin in patients with type 2 diabetes mellitus. *JAMA* 281:2005–2012, 1999.

UK Prospective Diabetes Study (UKPDS) Group: Intensive blood-glucose control with sulphonylureas or insulin compared with conventional treatment and risk of complications in patients with type 2 diabetes (UKPDS 33). *Lancet* 352:837–852, 1998a.

UK Prospective Diabetes Study (UKPDS) Group: Effect of intensive blood-glucose control with metformin on complications in overweight patients with type 2 diabetes (UKPDS 34). *Lancet* 352:854–865, 1998b.

UK Prospective Diabetes Study (UKPDS) Group: Tight blood pressure control and risk of macrovascular and microvascular complications in type 2 diabetes: UKPDS 38. *BMJ* 317:703–712, 1998c.

US Preventive Services Task Force: Screening for type 2 diabetes mellitus in adults: recommendations and rationale. *Ann Intern Med* 138:212–214, 2003.

Yoshikawa TT: State of infectious diseases health care in older persons. *Clin Geriatr Med* 7:55–58, 1999.

Suggested Readings

Anonymous: Antimicrobial prophylaxis in surgery. *Med Lett Drugs Ther* 41:75–80, 1999.

Anonymous: The choice of antibacterial drugs. *Med Lett Drugs Ther* 41:95–104, 1999.

Treatment of hypothermia. *Med Lett Drugs Ther* 28:123–124, 1986.

Bartlett JG: Antibiotic-associated diarrhea. *N Engl J Med* 346:334–339, 2002.

Belshe RB: Influenza prevention and treatment: current practices and new horizons. *Ann Intern Med* 131:621–623, 1999.

Bentley DW, Bradley S, High K, et al: Practice guideline for evaluation of fever and infection in long-term care facilities. *J Am Geriatr Soc* 49:210–222, 2001.

Bouchama A, Knochel JP: Heat Stroke. *N Engl J Med* 346:1978–1988, 2002.

Brady MA, Perron WJ: Electrocardiographic manifestations of hypothermia. *Am J Emerg Med* 20:314–326, 2002.

Chandalia M, Garg A, Lutjohann D, et al: Beneficial effects of high dietary fiber intake in patients with type 2 diabetes mellitus. *N Engl J Med* 342:1392–1398, 2000.

Davis PJ, Davis FB: Hyperthyroidism in patients over the age of 60 years. *Medicine (Baltimore)* 53:161–181, 1974.

Elia M, Ritz P, Stubbs RJ: Total energy expenditure in the elderly. *Eur J Clin Nutr* 54:S92–S103, 2000.

Federman DD: Hyperthyroidism in the geriatric population. *Hosp Pract* 26:61–76, 1991.

Gambert SR: Effect of age on thyroid hormone physiology and function. *J Am Geriatr Soc* 33:360–365, 1985.

Gress TW, Nieto J, Shahar E, et al: Hypertension and antihypertensive therapy as risk factors for type 2 diabetes mellitus. *N Engl J Med* 342:905–912, 2000.

Lipschitz DA: An overview of anemia in older patients. *Older Patient* 2:5–11, 1988.

Mahler RJ, Adler ML: Type 2 diabetes mellitus: update on diagnosis, pathophysiology, and treatment. *J Clin Endocrinol Metab* 84:1165–1171, 1999.

Morley JE, Mooradian AD, Silver AJ, et al: Nutrition in the elderly. *Ann Intern Med* 109:890–904, 1988.

Mylonakis E, Calderwood SB: Infective endocarditis in adults. *N Engl J Med* 345:1318–1330, 2001.

Sawin CT, Castelli WP, Hershman JM, et al: The aging thyroid: thyroid deficiency in the Framingham Study. *Arch Intern Med* 145:1386–1388, 1985.

Stead WW, To T, Harrison RW, et al: Benefit-risk considerations in preventive treatment for tuberculosis in elderly persons. *Ann Intern Med* 107:843–845, 1987.

Thomas FB, Mazzaferi EL, Skillman TB: Apathetic thyrotoxicosis: a distinctive clinical and laboratory entity. *Ann Intern Med* 72:679–685, 1970.

Trevino A, Bazi B, Beller BM, et al: The characteristic electrocardiogram of accidental hypothermia. *Arch Intern Med* 127:470–473, 1971.

Trivalle C, Doucet J, Chassagne P, et al: Differences in the signs and symptoms of hyperthyroidism in older and younger patients. *J Am Geriatr Soc* 44:50–53, 1996.

Tuomilehto J, Lindstrom J, Eriksson JG, et al: Prevention of type 2 diabetes mellitus by changes in lifestyle among subjects with impaired glucose tolerance. *N Engl J Med* 344:1343–1350, 2001.

UK Prospective Diabetes Study Group: Efficacy of atenolol and captopril in reducing risk of macrovascular and microvascular complications in type 2 diabetes: UKPDS 39. *BMJ* 371:713–719, 1998.

Walsh JR: Hematologic disorders in the elderly. *West J Med* 135:445–446, 1981.

Yoshikawa TT: Infectious diseases. *Clin Geriatr Med* 8:701–945, 1992.

Yoshikawa TT: Tuberculosis in aging adults. *J Am Geriatr Soc* 40:178–187, 1992.

CHAPTER 13

SENSORY IMPAIRMENT

Because as many as 75 percent of older adults have significant visual and auditory dysfunction not reported to their physicians, adequate screening for these problems is important. These disorders may limit functional activity and lead to social isolation and depression. Correction of remediable conditions may improve the ability to perform daily activities.

VISION

Physiologic and Functional Changes

The visual system undergoes many changes with age (Table 13-1). Decreases in visual acuity in old age may be caused by morphological changes in the choroid, pigment epithelium, and retina, or by decreased function of the rods, cones, and other neural elements. Older patients frequently have difficulties turning their eyes upward or sustaining convergence. Intraocular pressure slowly increases with age.

The refractive error may become either more hyperopic or more myopic. In the young, hyperopia may be overcome by the accommodative power of the ciliary muscle on the young lens. However, with age, this latent hyperopia becomes manifest because of loss of accommodative reserve.

Other older patients may show an increase in myopia with age, caused by changes within the lens. The crystalline lens increases in size with age as old lens fibers accumulate in the lens nucleus. The nucleus becomes more compact and harder (nuclear sclerosis), increasing the refractive power of the lens and worsening the myopia.

Another definitive refractive change of aging is the development of presbyopia from nuclear sclerosis of the lens and atrophy of the ciliary muscle. As a result, the closest distance at which one can see clearly slowly recedes with

TABLE 13-1   PHYSIOLOGICAL AND FUNCTIONAL CHANGES OF THE EYE

FUNCTIONAL CHANGE	PHYSIOLOGICAL CHANGE
Visual acuity	Morphological change in choroid, pigment epithelium, or retina Decreased function of rods, cones, or other neural elements
Extraocular motion	Difficulty in gazing upward and maintaining covergence
Intraocular pressure	Increased pressure
Refractive power	Increased hyperopia and myopia Presbyopia Increased lens size Nuclear sclerosis (lens) Ciliary muscle atrophy
Tear secretion	Decreased tearing Decreased lacrimal gland function Decreased goblet cell secretion
Corneal function	Loss of endothelial integrity Posterior surface pigmentation

age. At approximately age 45, the near point of accommodation is so far that comfortable reading and near work become cumbersome and difficult. Corrective lenses are then needed to enable the patient to move that point closer to the eyes.

Diminished tear secretion in many older patients, especially postmenopausal women, may lead to dryness of the eyes, which can cause irritation and discomfort. This condition may endanger the intactness of the corneal surface. The treatment consists mainly in substitution therapy, with artificial tears instilled at frequent intervals.

The corneal endothelium often undergoes degenerative changes with aging. Because these cells seldom proliferate during adult life, the cell population is decreased. This may leave an irregular surface on the anterior chamber side, where pigments may accumulate. This type of endothelial dystrophy is frequently seen in older patients, and dense pigment accumulation may slightly decrease visual acuity. In some patients, the endothelial dystrophy will spontaneously progress and lead to corneal edema. Such cases require corneal transplants.

Blindness

The prevalence of visual problems and blindness increases with age (Fig. 13-1). The most common causes of blindness are cataracts, glaucoma, macular degeneration, and diabetic retinopathy. Screening for these disorders should include testing visual acuity, performing an ophthalmoscopic evaluation, and checking intraocular pressure (Table 13-2).

Senile Cataract Opacification of the crystalline lens is a frequent complication of aging. In the Framingham Eye Study, the prevalence of cataracts was associated with age and reached 46 percent at ages 75 to 85 (Kini et al., 1978).

The cause of age-related cataracts is unknown, but the opacifications in the lens are associated with the breakdown of the g-crystalline proteins. Epidemiological data and basic research suggest that ultraviolet light may be a contributing factor in cataract development. The pathological process may occur in either the cortex or the nucleus of the lens. Cortical cataracts have various stages of development. Early in the process, opacities are in the periphery and do not decrease visual acuity. At the mature stage, opacifications are more widespread and involve the pupillary area, leading to a slow decrease in visual acuity. In the mature stage, the entire lens becomes opaque. The nuclear cataract does not have these stages of development but is a slowly progressing central opacity, which frequently shows a yellowish discoloration, therefore preventing certain colors from reaching the retina.

Cataracts of mild degree may be managed by periodic examination and optimum eyeglasses for an extended period. Ultraviolet lenses may be of benefit. When a cataract progresses to the point where it interferes with activities, cataract surgery is generally indicated. The surgeon may use several methods to remove it, and the decision regarding the best method for each patient should be made by the ophthalmologist.

In intracapsular cataract extractions, the entire cataract and surrounding capsule are removed in a single piece. This removes the entire opacity. In extracapsular cataract extractions, the cataractous lens material and a portion of the capsule are removed. The posterior capsule is left in place to hold an intraocular lens implant.

TABLE 13-2   OPHTHALMOLOGICAL SCREENING

Visual acuity	Ability to read newspaper-sized print
Lens, fundus	Ophthalmoscopic examination
Intraocular pressure	Tonometry
	Visual fields

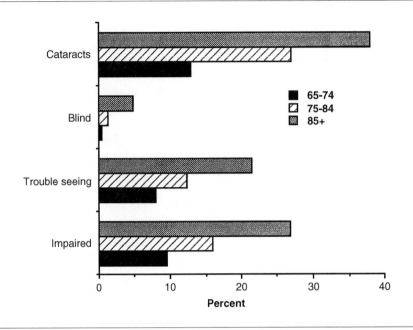

— FIGURE 13-1 — *Prevalence of vision problems in older persons, 1984.* (From Havlik, 1986.)

After cataract removal, the eye has decreased refractive power. Three methods of restoring useful vision are available: eyeglasses, contact lenses, and intraocular lenses (Table 13-3). Approximately 95 percent of those who undergo cataract surgery now receive intraocular lens implants.

Eyeglasses required after surgery are usually thick and heavy. These correct the focus of the eye and permit excellent vision through the central portion. However, they increase the apparent size of the object by approximately 25 percent, introduce optical distortion, and interfere with peripheral vision. Patients must learn to turn the head instead of the eyes to see clearly to the side. Eyeglasses can be used for patients who have had surgery on both eyes or surgery on one eye and decreased vision in the other. However, eyeglasses cannot usually be used for patients who have had surgery in one eye and have normal vision in the other eye because of the difference in image size.

Contact lenses correct the focus of the eye, permit both central and peripheral vision, and increase apparent object size by 6 percent. However, handling contact lenses is difficult for some individuals, and most lenses must be removed and inserted daily. Extended-wear contact lenses are available, and approximately 50 to 70 percent of elderly patients are able to wear them after surgery. Contacts are useful in patients who have had cataract surgery in one

TABLE 13-3   METHODS OF RESTORING VISION AFTER CATARACT
              SURGERY

EYEGLASSES

Are thick and heavy
Provide good central vision
Interfere with peripheral vision
Introduce optical distortion
Increase image size by 25%
Cannot be used after surgery on one eye if other eye is normal

CONTACT LENSES

Correct central and peripheral vision
Increase image size by 6%
Are difficult for some patients to handle
Most require daily insertion and removal
Approximately 50–70% can use extended-wear lenses
Can be used after surgery on one or both eyes
Require reading glasses

INTRAOCULAR LENSES

Correct central and peripheral vision
Increase image size by 1%
Can be used after surgery on one or both eyes
Are useful for older adults unable to wear contact lenses
Require bifocal eyeglasses
Introduce added surgical and postsurgical complications

or both eyes. The lenses correct for distant vision, but eyeglasses are required for reading.

The intraocular lens is surgically placed inside the iris and is expected to remain permanently in place. This lens corrects the focus of the eyes and permits central and peripheral vision; object size is increased by only 1 percent. It is appropriate for patients with cataracts in one or both eyes and is particularly useful for patients unable to wear a contact lens. Bifocal eyeglasses are usually required to aid distant or near vision.

Glaucoma   The glaucomas are a group of eye disorders characterized by increased intraocular pressure, progressive excavation of the optic nerve head with damage to the nerve fibers, and a specific loss in the visual field. Most cases of primary glaucoma occur in older patients. In the Framingham Eye Study, prevalence of open-angle glaucoma increased with age to 7.2 percent at ages 75 to 85, with men having much higher rates than women (Kini et al., 1978).

Angle-closure glaucoma is an acute and relatively infrequent type of glaucoma, characterized by a sudden painful attack of increased intraocular pressure accompanied by a marked loss in vision. The treatment consists of normalizing the intraocular pressure by the application of miotic eye drops or other medication (such as carbonic anhydrase inhibitors or osmotic agents). The definitive treatment, however, is surgical excision of a peripheral piece of iris or, more frequently now, by laser iridectomy, ensuring free flow of aqueous humor. Because the disease is usually bilateral, some physicians propose prophylactic iridectomy on the second eye.

Chronic open-angle glaucoma is the more frequent variety of primary glaucoma. It is characterized by an insidious onset, slow progression, and the appearance of typical defects of the visual fields. Early in the disease, intraocular pressure is only moderately elevated, and optic nerve head excavation progresses slowly and sometimes asymmetrically. While central visual acuity may remain normal for a long time, the defects in the peripheral visual field are characteristic and gradually progressive. Initially, there is a paracentral scotoma, which may coalesce. A nasal step of the visual field is another important sign. Finally, the entire field will constrict and eventually involve the visual centers.

The treatment is usually medical, with miotics of various kinds used first. Beta-blocking agents may also be used and have the advantage of not changing the diameter of the pupil. However, care should be taken because these agents may be systemically absorbed. In severe cases, combination drops may be used with systemic medications such as carbonic anhydrase inhibitors. Surgery or laser therapy is indicated only if disease progresses on maximal medical therapy.

Age-Related Macular Degeneration   The macular area of the retina lying at the posterior pole of the globe is the site of highest visual acuity. This area depends entirely on choriocapillaries for nutrition.

Any disturbance in the vessel wall of the choroidal capillaries, in the permeability or thickness of the Bruch's membrane, or in the retinal pigment epithelium may interfere with the exchange of nutrients and oxygen from the choroidal blood to the central retina. Such disturbances occur frequently in older patients. Senile degeneration of the macula is one of the most frequent causes of visual loss in older adults and is the commonest cause of legal blindness (20/200 or worse). In the Framingham Eye Study, the prevalence was 28 percent at ages 75 to 85 years, with a higher rate in women than in men (Kini et al., 1978). In addition to older age, risk factors include family history of the disorder, cigarette smoking, low dietary intake or plasma concentrations of antioxidant vitamins and zinc, and white race for "wet" lesions (Fine et al., 2000).

Ophthalmoscopic findings vary and do not always parallel loss of vision. In the "dry" form of degeneration, there are areas of depigmentation alternating with zones of hyperpigmentation caused mainly by changes in the retinal pigment epithelium. In another form, the degeneration involves the Bruch's membrane, leading to the pigmentation of well-circumscribed, roundish yellow areas.

The second type of degeneration is an exudative or "wet" type. Here there is an elevated focus in the macular area, which at first contains serous fluid but later contains blood derived from blood vessels sprouting from the choroid to the subretinal space. The blood may become organized and form a plaque.

In all these cases, central visual acuity will be markedly affected. These patients will gradually lose the ability to read or see any other details. Most macular degeneration is not treatable; however, laser treatment applied at a specific stage of exudative macular degeneration has been effective in preventing central visual loss in some patients (Macular Photocoagulation Study Group, 1993, 1994). Total blindness does not occur, as patients retain peripheral vision and therefore are able to perform activities that do not necessitate acute central vision.

Diabetic Retinopathy   In the geriatric population, a significant amount of visual loss is attributed to diabetic retinopathy. The Framingham Eye Study showed an age-associated increase in prevalence up to 7 percent at ages 75 to 85 years (Kini et al., 1978). In the adult-onset diabetic with background changes, the visual loss is usually related to vascular changes in and around the macula. Leakage of serous fluid from vessels surrounding the macula leads to macular edema and deterioration of visual acuity. This may respond to laser photocoagulation.

Hemorrhages within the macula may lead to more permanent visual loss. A loss of retinal capillaries may lead to macular ischemia and poor prognosis of visual recovery.

Recent clinical trials have demonstrated that intensive blood-glucose control and tight blood pressure control reduce the risk of microvascular disease, including retinopathy in type 2 diabetes (see Chap. 12).

General Factors

Table 13-4 summarizes the general patterns of signs and symptoms associated with common visual problems of older adults. In addition to the specific treatment discussed above, some simple techniques, such as use of a magnifying device, large-print reading material, lighting intensifiers, and reduction of glare, can help maximize visual function (see Table 13-5).

Health care providers should also be aware of the significant systemic absorption of ophthalmic medications. These agents may lead to other organ systems' dysfunction and interact with other medications (Table 13-6). The patient's other medical problems and medications should be assessed and the minimum dose to

TABLE 13-4   SIGNS AND SYMPTOMS ASSOCIATED WITH COMMON VISUAL PROBLEMS IN OLDER ADULTS

SIGNS AND SYMPTOMS	CATARACT	OPEN-ANGLE GLAUCOMA	ANGLE-CLOSURE GLAUCOMA	MACULAR DEGENERATION	TEMPORAL ARTERITIS	DIABETIC RETINOPATHY
Pain			x		x	
Red eye			x			
Fixed pupil			x			
Retinal vessel changes					x	x
Retinal exudates				x		x
Optic disk changes		x			x	
Sudden visual loss			x		x	
Loss of peripheral vision		x				
Glare intolerance	x					
Elevated intraocular pressure		x	x			
Loss of visual acuity	x			x		x

TABLE 13-5   AIDS TO MAXIMIZE VISUAL FUNCTION

Magnifying device

Lighting intensifiers without glare

Tinted glasses to reduce glare

Night light to assist in adaptation

Large-print newpapers, books, and magazines

TABLE 13-6   POTENTIAL ADVERSE EFFECTS OF OPHTHALMIC SOLUTIONS

DRUG	ORGAN SYSTEM	RESPONSES
Beta blockers (e.g., timolol)	Cardiovascular	Bradycardia, hypotension, syncope, palpitation, congestive heart failure
	Respiratory	Bronchospasm
	Neurologic	Mental confusion, depression, fatigue, lightheadedness, hallucinations, memory impairment, sexual dysfunction
	Miscellaneous	Hyperkalemia
Adrenergics (e.g., epinephrine, phenylephrine)	Cardiovascular Miscellaneous	Extrasystoles, palpitation, hypertension, myocardial infarction Trembling, paleness, sweating
Cholinergic/ anticholinesterases (e.g., pilocarpine, echothiophate)	Respiratory Gastrointestinal	Bronchospasm Salivation, nausea, vomiting, diarrhea, abdominal pain, tenesmus
	Miscellaneous	Lacrimation, sweating
Anticholinergics (e.g., atropine)	Neurologic	Ataxia, nystagmus, restlessness, mental confusion, hallucination, violent and aggressive behavior
	Miscellaneous	Insomnia, photophobia, urinary retention

Source: Anand KB and Eschmann E: Systemic effects of ophthalmic medication in the elderly. *NY State J Med* 88: 134–136, 1988.

achieve the desired effect should be used. Patients should also be monitored for systemic toxicity.

HEARING

This section covers four areas related to hearing problems in older adults: a review of the major parts of the auditory system, tests used to evaluate the hearing system, effects of aging on hearing performance, and specific pathologic disorders affecting the auditory system.

Hearing problems are common in the elderly, especially in a highly industrialized society where noise and age interact to cause hearing loss (Fig. 13-2). In the National Health and Nutrition Examination Survey, hearing loss was present in 35.1 percent of those surveyed aged 55 to 74 years (Reuben et al., 1998). Hearing loss in the elderly is usually of the sensorineural type, caused by damage of the hearing organ, the peripheral nervous system, and/or the central nervous system. These hearing problems are not usually amenable to medical or surgical

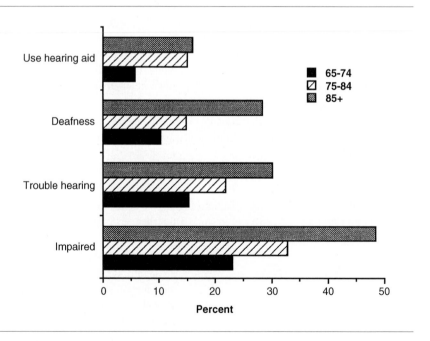

— FIGURE 13-2 — *Prevalence of hearing problems in older persons, 1984.* (From Havlik, 1986.)

intervention, and thus require hearing aids, aural rehabilitation, and understanding as the major avenues of remediation.

The Auditory System

On a functional basis, the auditory system can be divided into three major parts: peripheral, brainstem, and cortical areas (Table 13-7). Each part of the hearing system has unique functions, which combine to allow hearing and understanding of speech. Table 13-8 lists these functions.

The main functions of the peripheral auditory system are to change sound into a series of electrical impulses and to transmit those to the brainstem. The major brainstem function is binaural interaction. Binaural interaction allows localization of sound and extraction of a signal from a noisy environment. The cortex brings sound to consciousness and allows interpretation of speech and initiation of appropriate reactions to sound signals.

TABLE 13-7   PERIPHERAL AND CENTRAL AUDITORY NERVOUS SYSTEM

A. External ear and peripheral hearing mechanism
  1. Auricle
  2. Tympanic membrane
  3. Ossicular chain
  4. Eustachian tube
  5. Cochlea
    a. Bony labyrinth
    b. Membranous labyrinth
  6. Cochlear nerve
B. Auditory areas in the brainstem
  1. Entrance of the eighth cranial nerve
  2. Cochlear nucleus
  3. Superior olivary complex
  4. Lateral lemniscus
  5. Inferior colliculus
  6. Medial geniculate
  7. Auditory radiations (brainstem-to-cortex tract)
C. Auditory areas in the cortex
  1. Temporal lobe
  2. Parietal lobe
  3. Corpus callosum

TABLE 13-8   FUNCTIONAL COMPONENTS OF THE AUDITORY SYSTEM

A. Transmission of signals in the periphery
   1. Molecular motion (ear canal)
   2. Mechanical vibration (eardrum and ossicles)
   3. Hydromechanical motion (inner ear)
   4. Electrical impulse (eighth nerve)
B. Binaural interaction in the brainstrem
   1. Localization and lateralization of sound
   2. Extraction of signals from environmental noise
C. Speech processing in the cortex
   1. Conscious sensation of hearing
   2. Interpretation of speech
   3. Initiation of response to sound

▨ Assessment

Assessment of hearing function can be divided into three kinds of hearing tests: standard, binaural, and difficult speech. The standard tests are useful for evaluating the peripheral system, binaural tests for evaluating the brainstem, and difficult speech tests for evaluating cortical problems (Table 13-9). Standard tests are performed by presenting pure tones or single words at varying intensity. An audiometer (AudioScope, Welch-Allyn, Inc.) that will deliver pure tones is available for the office screening of hearing deficits.

Tympanic membrane movement is assessed with a probe. Loudness comparison assesses the individual's ability to balance intensity of sound coming from both ears; lateralization tests the individual's ability to fuse sounds from both ears; and masking level differences assesses the ability to pick out specific sounds from a background of noise. Monotic degraded tasks present difficult sounds such as noise background, filtered sound, and time-compressed speech; dichotic tasks simultaneously present sense and nonsense speech, which the individual is asked to repeat.

▨ Aging Changes

Many changes in the peripheral and central auditory system during aging have effects on the hearing mechanism (Table 13-10). These changes lead to diminished performance by older subjects (Table 13-11), including the loss of sensitivity and distortion of signals that succeed in passing to higher levels, difficulty in localizing signals and in taking advantage of two-ear listening, difficulty under-

TABLE 13-9   ASSESSMENT OF HEARING FUNCTION

A. Standard test measures
   1. Sensitivity for tones and speech
   2. Speech discrimination/understanding
   3. Movement of tympanic membrane
B. Binaural tests
   1. Loudness comparison
   2. Lateralization
   3. Masking level differences
C. Difficult speech tests
   1. Monotic degraded tasks
   2. Dichotic tasks

TABLE 13-10   EFFECTS OF AGING ON THE HEARING MECHANISM

Atrophy and disappearance of cells in the inner ear

Angiosclerosis in the inner ear

Calcification of membranes in the inner ear

Bioelectric and biomechanical imbalances in the inner ear

Degeneration and loss of ganglion cells and their fibers in the eighth cranial nerve

Eighth nerve canal closure, with destruction of nerve fibers

Atrophy and cell loss at all auditory centers in the brainstem

Reduction of cells in auditory areas of the cortex

standing speech under unfavorable listening conditions, and problems with language, especially when aging is compounded by stroke.

Three major factors enhance the progression of hearing loss with advancing age: previous middle-ear disease, vascular disease, and exposure to noise. These factors alone, however, do not account for the hearing loss of old age, called *presbycusis*. Although clinically and pathologically complex, this is a distinct progressive sensorineural hearing loss associated with aging. The deterioration is not limited to the peripheral sensory receptor. Presbycusis affects 60 percent of individuals older than age 65 in the United States. However, only a fraction of these have a functional deficit necessitating aural rehabilitation.

TABLE 13-11   HEARING PERFORMANCE IN OLDER ADULTS

A. Peripheral pathology
   1. Hearing loss for pure tones
   2. Hearing loss for speech
   3. Problems understanding speech
B. Brainstem pathology
   1. Problems localizing sounds
   2. Problems in binaural listening
C. Cortical pathology
   1. Problems with difficult speech
   2. Language problems

Sensitivity

Beginning with the third decade of life, there is a deterioration in the hearing threshold. At first, sensitivity at the high frequencies declines gradually. This age-associated loss has been confirmed in populations not exposed to high levels of noise. This gradual impairment is sensorineural and can be tested by pure-tone audiometry, which reveals useful information about the physiological condition of hearing, but does not disclose some important aspects of deterioration.

Speech

Although there is a close relationship between pure tone loss and the ability to hear speech, the audiogram does not precisely measure hearing for speech. To assess this auditory function, speech audiometry can be performed by presenting the undistorted test words above threshold intensities in the absence of background noise.

Older people with hearing impairment may have difficulty understanding speech under less-favorable conditions, as with background noise, under poor acoustic conditions, or when speech is rapid. This difficulty may be caused in part by the longer time required by higher auditory centers to identify the message. Such hearing loss may necessitate testing of desired signals with the presentation of a competing signal. This will more accurately reflect hearing of speech in social circumstances.

Speech occurring in rooms that cause long reverberations is also much less intelligible to the elderly. Auditory temporal discrimination and auditory reaction time and frequency discrimination also decline with age. Because consonant sounds are of higher frequency and shorter duration, the loss of high-frequency hearing in the elderly may affect these sounds, which encode much of speech information. Lipreading may compensate to some extent for this effect on understanding speech, but other factors of processing information still remain.

Loudness

A common auditory problem of the elderly is abnormal loudness perception. This can occur as hypersensitivity to sounds of high intensity and appears as increased "loudness recruitment," in which gradually increasing loudness, such as amplified sound, is unpleasantly harsh and difficult to tolerate. In older adults with hearing impairment, this abnormality is manifest when a speaker is asked to speak louder or the output of a hearing aid is increased. It may result from a sensorineural loss attributable to changes in the hair cells of the inner ear.

Localization

Sound localization contributes to effectiveness of signal detection and helps with discrimination. Loss of directional hearing results in greater hearing difficulty in a noisy environment. Localization is disturbed in older adults with hearing loss and may be partly caused by the aging brain's deranged processing of interaural intensity differences and time delays. A strongly asymmetrical hearing loss also disturbs localization.

Tinnitus

Tinnitus, an internal noise generated within the hearing system, occurs in many types of hearing disorders at all ages but is much more frequent in older adults. Tinnitus, however, is not necessarily associated with hearing loss and may occur in older adults without hearing impairment. Estimates of prevalence of tinnitus in the United States are about 10 percent, with the majority of persons with tinnitus being 40 to 80 years of age (Peifer et al., 1999). Treatment is generally unsatisfactory.

Other Hearing Disorders

One of the most easily treatable but too easily overlooked causes of hearing loss is cerumen that occludes the external auditory canal (Table 13-12).

TABLE 13-12   DISORDERS OF HEARING IN OLDER ADULTS

Cerumen plug
Tympanosclerosis
Otosclerosis
Paget's disease
Ototoxic medications
Sound trauma
CNS lesions
Pseudo-deafness (depression)

Cerumen usually affects low-frequency sounds and complicates existing hearing impairments.

Hearing loss in the geriatric patient may be caused by scarring of the tympanic membrane. In tympanosclerosis, there is calcification of the tympanic membrane that results in stiffening of the drumhead.

Otosclerosis may cause fixation of the ossicular chain and lead to a conduction hearing loss. The bony capsule may also be affected, leading to sensorineural loss. Paget's disease may also lead to both kinds of hearing loss and should be evaluated radiologically and by an alkaline phosphatase determination.

Ototoxic medication is an acquired cause of hearing loss producing cochlear damage. The aminoglycoside antibiotics require special caution. At high doses, ethacrynic acid and furosemide may be ototoxic.

High doses of aspirin may cause a reversible hearing impairment. Unfortunately, except for aspirin, removal of the offending drug usually does not reverse the sensorineural loss.

Sound trauma is an environmental factor with neurosensory consequences. Superimposed on the changes of aging, sound trauma can have a severe impact on a patient's communicative ability.

Vascular or mass lesions may affect hearing at one of several levels, including the middle and inner ear, auditory nerve, brainstem, and cortex.

Aural Rehabilitation

Every individual who has communication difficulties caused by a permanent hearing loss should have an ear, nose, and throat evaluation to rule out remediable disease and then an audiological evaluation to assess the roles of amplification and aural rehabilitation. Table 13-13 lists the factors that should be considered during the evaluation for a hearing aid. In the severely impaired, in addition to a hearing aid, aural rehabilitation with speech reading may be necessary.

Patient and family counseling may improve use of and satisfaction with a hearing aid. Realistic expectations should be explained to the patient. Hearing aids are most useful in one-on-one conversations and are less effective in noisy, group settings. They are also less useful in improving understanding of less-familiar accents and languages, for example, a British accent in a movie or television production. Such understanding can be improved by use of the closed caption feature on television. Facing the speaker and lipreading also improves understanding. Improvements and modifications in design and construction of hearing aids have enabled a greater proportion of the hearing-impaired population to profit from amplification. The old adage that hearing aids will not help people with sensorineural loss is simply not true. The aid can be adjusted to a specific frequency rather than all frequencies, thus decreasing loudness problems, improving discrimination, and making the aid more acceptable. Binaural aids improve sound localization and discrimination.

The hearing aid that is worn on the body provides the greatest amplification but is necessary only for patients with the most severe hearing loss. The controls are large and therefore more easily managed by some elderly persons. However, many elderly people prefer behind-the-ear or in-the-ear devices. The in-the-ear devices are small, cosmetically more acceptable, but more difficult to manipulate.

TABLE 13-13   FACTORS IN EVALUATION FOR A HEARING AID

Exclude contraindicating medical or other correctable problem

Greatest satisfaction is achieved with aid if loss is 55–80 dB; there is only partial help if loss is greater than 80 dB

Less satisfaction is achieved when poor discrimination is present

Aid is specifically designed for face-to-face conversation; patient's expectations should be realistic

Aid may need to be combined with lipreading

Loudness perception abnormalities may make aid unacceptable

More severe hearing loss requires aid worn on the body rather than behind-the-ear device

Assess for monaural or binaural aids

Assess for patient's ability to handle aid independently

Assess patient's motivation for using an aid

Although expensive, cochlear implants can restore hearing in individuals with severe hearing loss not corrected by hearing aids.

TASTE

During aging there is a significant loss of lingual papillae and an associated diminution of ability to taste. Salivary secretion also diminishes, thus decreasing solubilization of flavoring agents. Upper dentures may cover secondary taste sites and decrease taste acuity.

Olfactory bulbs also show significant atrophy with old age. In a population-based, cross-sectional study of adults aged 53 to 97, the prevalence of impaired olfaction by olfaction testing was 24.5 percent and increased with age to 62.5 percent of 80- to 97-year-olds (Murphy et al., 2002). Taste and olfactory changes together may account for the lessened interest in food shown by older adults.

POLYNEUROPATHY

Patients with polyneuropathy have impairments in balance and an increased risk for falls and falls causing injury (Richardson, 2002). Epidemiological data on polyneuropathy are relatively limited. In a study from Italy of subjects ages 55 and older, the prevalence of polyneuropathy was 11 percent. Diabetes mellitus was the most common risk factor (44 percent of patients with polyneuropathy). The next most common risk factors were alcoholism, nonalcoholic liver disease, and malignancy (Beghi and Monticelli, 1998). In a natural history study of type 2 diabetes mellitus, 42 percent of the diabetic population had nerve conduction abnormalities consistent with polyneuropathy after 10 years (Partanen et al., 1995). The prevalence of diabetes mellitus in older persons is increasing, and, therefore, the prevalence of polyneuropathy is likely to increase as well.

In chronic polyneuropathies, such as diabetes mellitus, symptoms usually begin in the lower extremities and sensory symptoms usually precede motor symptoms. In demyelinating polyneuropathies, such as Guillain-Barré syndrome, weakness rather than sensory loss is more typical. The physical examination should focus on the sensory examination including pin prick, light touch, vibration, cold, and proprioception, and on muscle strength testing and appearance of muscle wasting. Extensive diagnostic testing is usually not necessary in a patient with mild symptoms and a known underlying diagnosis such as diabetes mellitus or alcohol abuse. In patients with no clear etiology, electrodiagnostic testing should be the initial diagnostic study (Dyck et al., 1996). Rutkove has described an algorithm for a diagnostic approach to polyneuropathy

(Rutkove, 2002; see Fig. 13-3). Laboratory tests, which might include a complete blood count, erythrocyte sedimentation rate, thyroid stimulating hormone, serum and urine protein electrophoresis, blood glucose, vitamin B_{12} level, antinuclear antibody, and urinalysis, should be directed by the electrodiagnostic testing results.

Treatment should address the underlying disease process and alleviation of symptoms. Avoidance of toxins, such as alcohol or drugs, is the most important step. In patients with diabetes, tight control may help maintain nerve function (see Chap. 12). In painful neuropathies, tricyclic antidepressants are effective, as is gabapentin. In patients with weakness, physical therapy evaluation is important and use of ankle–foot orthosis, splints, and walking-assistance devices can improve function. Proper foot and nail care is important in reducing risk for foot ulcers.

ACKNOWLEDGMENT

The authors wish to thank Dr. Douglas Noffsinger for his assistance in preparing material for an earlier version of the section on hearing in this chapter.

References

Anand KB, Eschmann E: Systemic effects of ophthalmic medication in the elderly. *NY State J Med* 88:134–136, 1988.

Beghi E, Monticelli ML: Chronic symmetric symptomatic polyneuropathy in the elderly: a field screening investigation of risk factors for polyneuropathy in two Italian communities. *J Clin Epidemiol* 51:697–702, 1998.

Dyck PJ, Dyck PJB, Grant IA, et al: Ten steps in characterizing and diagnosing patients with peripheral neuropathy. *Neurology* 47:10–17, 1996.

Fine SL, Berger JW, Maguire MG, et al: Age-related macular degeneration. *N Engl J Med* 342:483–492, 2000.

Havlik RJ: Aging in the eighties, impaired senses for sound and light in persons age 65 years and over. *NCHS Advance Data*, No. 125, 1986.

Kini MM, Liebowitz HM, Colton T, et al: Prevalence of senile cataract, diabetic retinopathy, senile macular degeneration, and open-angle glaucoma in the Framingham Eye Study. *Am J Ophthalmol* 85:28–34, 1978.

Macular Photocoagulation Study Group: Laser photocoagulation for subfoveal neovascular lesions of age-related macular degeneration: updated findings from two clinical trials. *Arch Ophthalmol* 111:200–209, 1993.

Macular Photocoagulation Study Group: Laser photocoagulation for juxtafoveal choroidal neovascularization: five-year results from randomized clinical trials. *Arch Ophthalmol* 112:500–509, 1994.

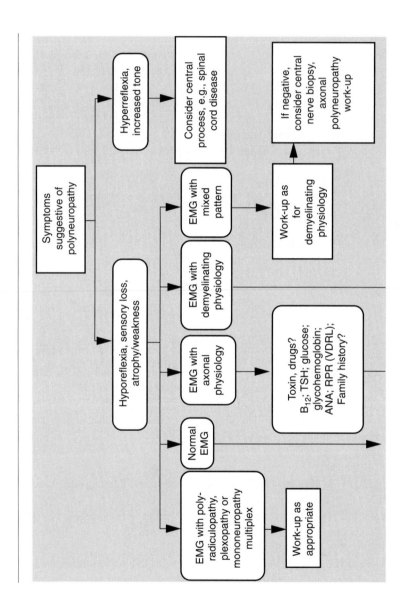

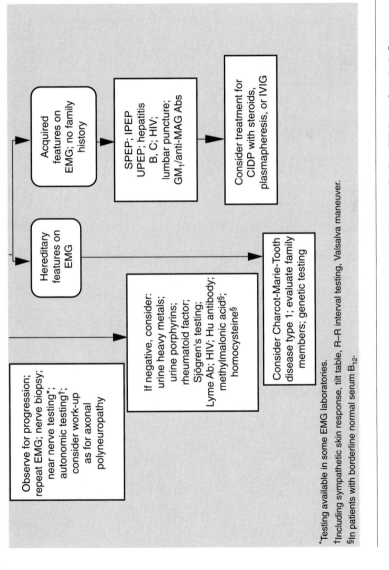

Observe for progression;
repeat EMG; nerve biopsy;
near nerve testing*;
autonomic testing†;
consider work-up
as for axonal
polyneuropathy

Hereditary
features on
EMG

Acquired
features on
EMG; no family
history

If negative, consider:
urine heavy metals;
urine porphyrins;
rheumatoid factor;
Sjögren's testing;
Lyme Ab; HIV; Hu antibody;
methylmalonic acid§;
homocysteine§

SPEP; IPEP
UPEP; hepatitis
B, C; HIV;
lumbar puncture;
GM₁/anti-MAG Abs

Consider Charcot-Marie-Tooth
disease type 1; evaluate family
members; genetic testing

Consider treatment for
CIDP with steroids,
plasmapheresis, or IVIG

*Testing available in some EMG laboratories.
†Including sympathetic skin response, tilt table, R–R interval testing, Valsalva maneuver.
§In patients with borderline normal serum B₁₂.

— FIGURE 13-3 — *Diagnostic approach to polyneuropathy. Ab = antibody; CIDP = chronic inflammatory demyelinating polyneuropathy; EMG = electromyography; GM₁ = ganglioside antibodies; Hu = human; IPEP = immunoprotein electrophoesis; IVIG = intravenous immunoglobulin; MAG = myelin-associated glycoprotein; SPEP = serum protein electrophoresis; UPEP = urine protein electrophoresis.* (From Rutkove, 2002.)

Murphy C, Schubert CR, Cruickshanks KJ, et al: Prevalence of olfactory impairment in older adults. *JAMA* 288:2307–2312, 2002.

Partanen J, Niskonen L, Lehtinen J, et al: Natural history of peripheral neuropathy in patients with non-insulin dependent diabetes mellitus. *N Engl J Med* 89:333:89–94, 1995.

Peifer KJ, Rosen GP, Rubin AM: Tinnitus: etiology and management. *Clin Geriatr Med* 15:193–204, 1999.

Reuben DB, Walshk K, Moore AA, et al: Hearing loss in community-dwelling older persons: national prevalence data and identification using simple questions. *J Am Geriatr Soc* 46:1008–1011, 1998.

Richardson JK: Factors associated with falls in older patients with diffuse polyneuropathy. *J Am Geriatr Soc* 50:1767–1773, 2002.

Rutkove SB: Overview of polyneuropathy. *UpToDate 2002, see www.uptodate.com.*

Suggested Readings

Gottlieb JL: Age-related macular degeneration. *JAMA* 288:2233–2236, 2002.

Kollarits CR, Rubin AM, Goebel JA (eds): Visual and auditory challenges. *Clin Geriatr Med* 15:1–204, 1999.

Lavizzo-Mourey RJ, Siegler EL: Hearing impairment in the elderly. *J Gen Intern Med* 7:191–198, 1992.

Mulrow CD, Lichtenstein MJ: Screening for hearing impairment in the elderly: rationale and strategy. *J Gen Intern Med* 6:249–258, 1991.

Uhlmann RF, Rees TS, Psatz BM, et al: Validity and reliability of auditory screening tests in demented and non-demented older adults. *J Gen Intern Med* 4:90–96, 1989.

CHAPTER 14

DRUG THERAPY

Geriatric patients are frequently prescribed multiple drugs in complex dosage schedules. In some instances, this is justified because of the presence of multiple chronic medical conditions, the proven efficacy of an increasing number of drugs for these conditions, and practice guidelines that recommend their use. In many instances, however, complex drug regimens are unnecessary; they are costly and predispose to noncompliance and adverse drug reactions. Many older patients are prescribed multiple drugs, take over-the-counter drugs, and are then prescribed additional drugs to treat the side effects of medications they are already taking. This scenario can result in an upward spiral in the number of drugs being taken and commonly leads to polypharmacy.

Several important considerations, some pharmacological and others nonpharmacological, influence the safety and effectiveness of drug therapy in the geriatric population. This chapter focuses on these considerations and gives practical suggestions for prescribing drugs for older patients. Drug therapy for specific geriatric conditions is discussed in several other chapters throughout this text.

NONPHARMACOLOGICAL FACTORS INFLUENCING DRUG THERAPY

Discussions of geriatric pharmacology frequently center around age-related changes in drug pharmacokinetics and pharmacodynamics. Although these changes are sometimes of clinical importance, nonpharmacological factors can play an even greater role in the safety and effectiveness of drug therapy in the geriatric population. Several steps make drug therapy safe and effective (Fig. 14-1). Many factors can interfere with this scheme in the geriatric population, and, as can be seen, most of them come into play before pharmacological considerations arise.

Effective drug therapy can be hampered by inaccurate diagnoses. Many older patients tend to underreport symptoms; complaints of other patients may be vague and multiple. Symptoms of physical diseases frequently overlap with symptoms of psychological illness. To add to this complexity, many diseases present with atypical symptoms. Consequently, making the correct diagnoses and prescribing the appropriate drugs are often difficult tasks in the geriatric population.

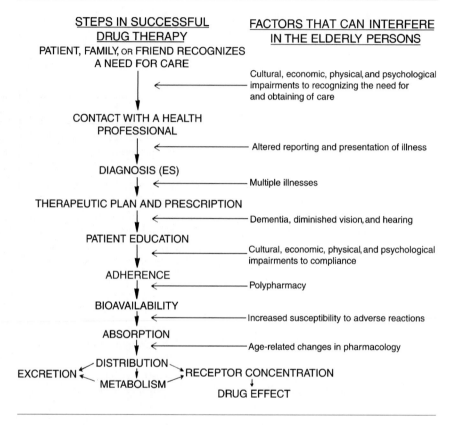

— FIGURE 14-1 — *Factors that can interfere with successful drug therapy.*

There is a tendency among health care professionals to treat symptoms with drugs rather than to evaluate the symptoms thoroughly. Because older patients tend to have multiple problems and complaints and consult several health care professionals, they often end up with prescriptions for several drugs. Moreover, older patients or their family members sometimes exert pressure on health care professionals to prescribe medication, thus adding to the tendency for polypharmacy. This pressure is increasing because of the new trend of direct-to-consumer advertising of drugs.

Frequently, neither the patients nor the health care providers have a clear picture of the total drug regimen. New patients undergoing initial geriatric assessment should be asked to empty their medicine cabinets and to bring all bottles to their first appointments. Medication records, such as the one shown in Fig. 14-2, carried by the patient and maintained as an integral part of the overall medical

NAME _____ DOCTOR _____ PHONE: ( )_____

MEDICATION NAME	REASON FOR USE	DESCRIBE OR TAPE MEDICINE HERE	WHEN TO TAKE MEDICINE				SPECIAL NOTES

<u>REMEMBER</u>

BRING THIS CHART TO ALL DOCTOR APPOINTMENTS
INCLUDE ALL THE MEDICATIONS YOU ARE TAKING
DO NOT CHANGE THE WAY YOU TAKE THE MEDICATIONS WITHOUT CALLING THE DOCTOR
DO NOT SHARE MEDICATIONS
IF YOU HAVE ANY QUESTIONS, CALL THE DOCTOR

— FIGURE 14-2 — *Example of a medication record.*

record, may help to eliminate some of the polypharmacy and noncompliance common in the geriatric population. Such records should be updated at each patient visit. Drug regimens should be simplified whenever possible and patients instructed to discard old medications.

Adherence plays a central role in the success of drug therapy in all age groups (see Fig. 14-1). In addition to the tendency for polypharmacy and complex dosage schedules, older patients face other potential barriers to adherence. The chronic nature of illness in the geriatric population can play a role in nonadherence. The consequences of these illnesses are often delayed (as opposed to the more dramatic effects of acute illnesses), and chronic illnesses necessitate ongoing prophylactic or suppressive rather than relatively short and time-limited courses of therapy. Adherence tends to be poor for these types of drug regimens. Diminished hearing, impaired vision, and poor literacy, and poor short-term memory can interfere with patient education and adherence. Problems with transportation can make getting to a pharmacy difficult. Outpatient prescriptions are not covered by Medicare (as of June, 2003), thus forcing older persons to pay for their drugs from a limited income. A Medicare prescription benefit will help, but is likely to be limited and involve substantial copayments. Some older people have "Medigap" insurance policies that cover some medication costs, and capitated programs commonly offer drug benefits (usually limited to a formulary and generic drugs when available). Even if the older person gets to the pharmacy, can afford the prescription, understands the instructions, and remembers when to take it, the use of childproof bottles and tamper-resistant packaging may hinder adherence in those with arthritic or weak hands.

Several strategies might improve adherence in the geriatric population (Table 14-1). As few drugs as possible should be prescribed, and the dosage schedule should be as simple as possible. Drugs should be given on the same dosage schedules whenever possible, and the administration should correspond to a daily routine in order to enhance the consistency of taking the drugs and compliance. For many drugs, once-daily dosing is available and should be prescribed when clinically appropriate. Relatives or other caregivers should be instructed in the drug regimen, and they, as well as others (e.g., home health aides and pharmacists), should be enlisted to help the older patient comply. Specially designed pill dispensers, dosage calendars, and other innovative techniques can be useful. Geriatric patients and their health care providers should keep an updated record of the drug regimen (see Fig. 14-2). Medications should be brought to appointments, and patients and families should show all medications to their physicians, particularly on initial visits to new primary care physicians or at a consultation with a specialist. Health care professionals should regularly inquire about other medications being taken (prescribed by other physicians or purchased over the counter) and review their patients' knowledge of and compliance with the drug regimen.

TABLE 14-1　STRATEGIES TO IMPROVE COMPLIANCE IN THE GERIATRIC POPULATION

1. Making drug regimens and instructions as simple as possible.
   a. Use the same dosage schedule whenever feasible (e.g., once or twice per day)
   b. Time the doses in conjunction with a daily routine.
2. Instruct relatives and caregivers on the drug regimen.
3. Enlist others (e.g., home health aides, pharmacists) to help ensure compliance.
4. Make sure the older patient can get to a pharmacist (or vice versa), can afford the prescriptions, and can open the container.
5. Use aids (such as special pillboxes and drug calendars) whenever appropriate.
6. Keep updated medication records (see Fig. 14-2).
7. Review knowledge of and compliance with drug regimens regularly.

ADVERSE DRUG REACTIONS AND INTERACTIONS

Primum non nocere ("first, do no harm"), a watchword phrase in the practice of medicine, is nowhere more applicable than when drugs are being prescribed for the geriatric population. Adverse drug reactions are the most common forms of iatrogenic illness (see Chap. 5). The incidence of adverse drug reactions in hospitalized patients increases from approximately 10 percent in those between 40 and 50 years of age to 25 percent in those older than age 80 (Lazarou et al., 1998). They account for between 3 and 10 percent of hospital admissions of older patients each year, and result in several billion dollars in yearly health care expenditures. Many drugs can produce distressing, and sometimes disabling or life-threatening, adverse reactions (Table 14-2). Psychotropic drugs and cardiovascular agents are common causes of serious adverse reactions in the geriatric population. In part, this is because of the narrow therapeutic:toxic ratio of many of these drugs. In some instances, age-related changes in pharmacology, such as diminished renal excretion and prolonged duration of action, predispose to adverse reactions. Some side effects can have a therapeutic benefit and may be key factors in drug selection (see below).

Because symptoms can be nonspecific or may mimic other illnesses, adverse drug reactions may be ignored or unrecognized. Patients and family members should be educated to recognize and report common and potentially serious adverse reactions. In some instances, another drug is prescribed to treat these symptoms, thus contributing to polypharmacy and increasing the likelihood of an adverse drug interaction. The problem of polypharmacy is exacerbated by visits to multiple physicians who may prescribe still more drugs and the use of multiple pharmacies. Medication records kept by the patient (see Fig. 14-2), as well as the physician's medical record, should help to prevent unnecessary polypharmacy when many physicians are involved. Several drugs commonly prescribed for the geriatric population can interact, with adverse consequences (Table 14-3). The more common types of potential adverse drug interactions are drug displacement from protein-binding sites by other highly protein-bound drugs, induction or suppression of the metabolism of other drugs, and additive effects of different drugs on blood pressure and mental function (mood, level of consciousness, etc.). In addition to the potential to interact with other drugs, several drugs can interact adversely with underlying medical conditions in the geriatric population, creating "drug–patient" interactions (Table 14-4). A good example of this problem is the increased risk of hospitalization for congestive heart failure among older patients taking diuretics who are told to take a nonsteroidal antiinflammatory drug (Heerdink et al., 1998).

Health care professionals should have a thorough knowledge of the more common drug side effects, adverse reactions to drugs, and potential drug interactions

TABLE 14-2   EXAMPLES OF COMMON AND POTENTIALLY SERIOUS
ADVERSE DRUG REACTIONS IN THE GERIATRIC POPULATION

DRUG	COMMON ADVERSE REACTIONS
ANALGESICS (SEE CHAP. 10)	
Antiinflammatory agents	Gastric irritation and ulcers
	Chronic blood loss
Narcotics	Constipation
ANTIMICROBIALS	
Aminoglycosides	Renal failure
	Hearing loss
ANTIPARKINSONIAN DRUGS (SEE CHAP. 10)	
Dopaminergic agents	Nausea
	Delirium
	Hallucinations
	Postural hypotension
Anticholinergics	Dry mouth
	Constipation
	Urinary retention
	Delirium
CARDIOVASCULAR DRUGS (SEE CHAP. 11)	
Angiotensin-converting enzyme (ACE) inhibitors	Cough
	Impaired renal function
Antiarrhythmics	Diarrhea (quinidine)
	Urinary retention (disopyramide)
Anticoagulants	Bleeding complications
Antihypertensives	Hypotension
	Sedation and/or other changes in mental function
Calcium-channel blockers	Decreased myocardial contractility
	Edema
	Constipation
Diuretics	Dehydration
	Hyponatremia
	Hypokalemia
	Incontinence

TABLE 14-2   EXAMPLES OF COMMON AND POTENTIALLY SERIOUS
             ADVERSE DRUG REACTIONS IN THE GERIATRIC POPULATION
             (*Continued*)

DRUG	COMMON ADVERSE REACTIONS
CARDIOVASCULAR DRUGS (SEE CHAP. 11)	
Digoxin	Arrhythmias
	Nausea
	Anorexia
Nitrates	Hypotension
HYPOGLYCEMIC AGENTS	
Insulin	Hypoglycemia
Oral agents	
PSYCHOTROPIC DRUGS (SEE TABLES 14-9, 10 AND 11)	
Antidepressants	(See Chap. 7)
Antipsychotics	Sedation
	Hypotension
	Extrapyramidal movement disorders
Lithium	Weakness
	Tremor
	Nausea
	Delirium
Sedative and hypnotic agents	Excessive sedation
	Delirium
	Gait disturbances and falls
OTHERS	
Alendronate, risedronate	Esophageal ulceration
Aminophylline, theophylline	Gastric irritation
	Tachyarrhythmias
Carbamazepine	Anemia
	Hyponatremia
	Neutropenia
Cimetidine	Mental status changes
Terbutaline	Tremor

TABLE 14-3   EXAMPLES OF POTENTIALLY CLINICALLY IMPORTANT DRUG–DRUG INTERACTIONS

INTERACTION	EXAMPLES	POTENTIAL EFFECTS
Interference with drug absorption	Antacids interacting with digoxin, INH, antipsychotics	Diminished drug effectiveness
	Enteral tube feedings and liquid phenytoin	
	Iron and ciprofloxacin	
Displacement from binding proteins	Warfarin, oral hypoglycemics, aspirin, chloral hydrate, other highly protein-bound drugs (see Table 14-6)	Enhanced effects and increased risk of toxicity
Altered distribution	Digoxin and quinidine	Increased risk of toxicity
Altered metabolism	Antifungals, erythromycin, clarithromycin SSRIs, with antihistamines, calcium-channel blockers, others*	Decreased metabolism, increased levels of toxicity
Altered excretion	Lithium and diuretics	Increased risk of toxicity and electrolyte imbalance
Pharmacological antagonism	Levodopa and clonidine	Decreased antiparkinsonian effects
Pharmacological synergism	Tricyclic antidepressants and antihypertensives	Increased risk of hypotension

* See text.
Abbreviations: INH = isonicotine hydrazine; SSRI = selective serotonin reuptake inhibitor.

TABLE 14-4   EXAMPLES OF POTENTIALLY CLINICALLY IMPORTANT DRUG–PATIENT INTERACTIONS

DRUG	PATIENT FACTORS	CLINICAL IMPLICATIONS
Diuretics	Diabetes	Decreased glucose tolerance
	Poor nutritional status	Increased risk of dehydration and electrolyte imbalance
	Urinary frequency, urgency	Incontinence may result
Angiotensin-converting enzyme (ACE) inhibitors	Renovascular disease (severe)	Worsening renal function
Beta blockers	Stress incontinence	Precipitate incontinence (cough)
	Diabetes	Sympathetic response to hypoglycemia may be masked
	Chronic obstructive lung disease	Increased bronchospasm
	Congestive heart failure (CHF)	Decreased myocardial contractility
	Peripheral vascular disease	Increased claudication
Narcotic analgesics	Chronic constipation	Worsening symptoms, fecal impaction
Tricyclic antidepressants	CHF, angina	Tachycardia, decreased myocardial contractility, postural hypotension exacerbating cardiovascular conditions
Tricyclic antidepressants, antihistamines, and other drugs with anticholinergic effects	Constipation, glaucoma, and other visual impairments, prostatic hyperplasia, reflux esophagitis	Worsening of symptoms
Antipsychotics	Parkinsonism	Worsening of immobility
Psychotropics	Dementia	Further impairment of cognitive function
Nonsteroidal antiinflammatory drugs	CHF, on diuretics	Increased risk of exacerbation of CHF

in the geriatric population. Electronic databases available on the World Wide Web or on personal digital assistants (PDAs) can be helpful in this regard. Careful questioning about side effects should be an important part of reviewing the drug regimen at each visit. Many institutions use computers to detect potential adverse drug interactions and to prevent their occurrence. Software programs are now available that can assist in identifying potential adverse drug interactions. Special attention should be given to the potential for any newly prescribed drug to interact with drugs already being taken or with underlying medical or psychological conditions.

AGING AND PHARMACOLOGY

Several age-related biological and physiological changes are relevant to drug pharmacology (Table 14-5). With the exception of changes in renal function, however, the effects of these age-related changes on dosages of specific drugs for individual patients are variable and difficult to predict. In general, an understanding of the physiological status of each patient (taking into account factors such as state of hydration, nutrition, and cardiac output) and how that status affects the pharmacology of a particular drug is more important to clinical efficacy than are age-related changes. New technology in drug delivery systems, such as oral sustained-release preparations and skin patches, have been developed for many medications. Such technology may be useful in designing strategies to account for the effect of aging changes on pharmacology and to make many drugs safer in the geriatric population. Given these caveats, the effects of aging on each pharmacological process are briefly discussed below.

Absorption

Several age-related changes can affect drug absorption (see Table 14-5). Most studies, however, have failed to document any clinically meaningful alterations in drug absorption with increasing age. Absorption, therefore, appears to be the pharmacological parameter least affected by increasing age.

Distribution

In contrast to absorption, clinically meaningful changes in drug distribution can occur with increasing age. Serum albumin, the major drug-binding protein, tends to decline, especially in hospitalized patients. Although the decline is numerically small, it can substantially increase the amount of free drug available for action. This effect is of particular relevance for highly protein-bound drugs,

TABLE 14-5   AGE-RELATED CHANGES RELEVANT TO DRUG
PHARMACOLOGY

PHARMACOLOGICAL PARAMETER	AGE-RELATED CHANGES

Absorption	Decreases in
	   Absorptive surface
	   Splanchnic blood flow
	   Increased gastric pH
	   Altered gastrointestinal motility

Distribution	Decreases in
	   Total body water
	   Lean body mass
	   Serum albumin
	   Increased fat
	   Altered protein binding

Metabolism	Decreases in
	   Liver blood flow
	   Enzyme activity
	   Enzyme inducibility

Excretion	Decreases in
	   Renal blood flow
	   Glomerular filtration rate
	   Tubular secretory function

Tissue sensitivity	Alterations in
	   Receptor number
	   Receptor affinity
	   Second-messenger function
	   Cellular and nuclear responses

especially when they are used simultaneously and compete for protein-binding sites (see Table 14-3).

Age-related changes in body composition can prominently affect pharmacology by altering the volume of distribution (Vd). The elimination half-life of a drug varies with the ratio Vd:drug clearance. Thus, even if the rate of clearance of a drug is unchanged with age, changes in Vd can affect a drug's half-life and duration of action.

Because total body water and lean body mass decline with increasing age, drugs that distribute in these body compartments, such as most antimicrobial agents, digoxin, lithium, and alcohol, may have a lower Vd and can, therefore, achieve higher concentrations from given amounts of drugs. On the other hand, drugs that distribute in body fat, such as many of the psychotropic agents, have a large Vd in the geriatric patients. The larger Vd will thus cause a prolongation of the half-life unless the clearance increases proportionately, which is unlikely to happen with increasing age.

Metabolism

The effects of aging on drug metabolism are complex and difficult to predict. They depend on the precise pathway of drug metabolism in the liver and on several other factors, such as gender and amount of smoking. There is evidence that the first, or preparative, phase of drug metabolism, including oxidations, reductions, and hydrolyses, declines with increasing age, and that the decline is more prominent in men than in women. In contrast, the second phase of drug metabolism (biotransformation, including acetylation and glucuronidation) appears to be less affected by age. There is also evidence that the ability of environmental factors (most importantly smoking) to induce drug-metabolizing enzymes declines with age. Even when liver function is obviously impaired, as by intrinsic liver disease or right-sided congestive heart failure, the effects of aging on the metabolism of specific drugs cannot be precisely predicted. It is *not* safe to assume, however, that geriatric patients with normal liver function tests can metabolize drugs as efficiently as can younger individuals.

The cytochrome P450 system in the liver has been extensively studied. More than 30 isoenzymes have been identified and classified into families and subfamilies. Genetic mutations in some of these enzymes, while relatively uncommon, can impair metabolism of specific drugs. Although aging may affect this system, the effects of commonly used drugs are probably more important. Ketoconazole, erythromycin, and the selective serotonin reuptake inhibitors (especially fluoxetine) can inhibit the metabolism of several drugs (see Chap. 7). Potentially fatal ventricular arrhythmias have been caused by high levels of the antihistamines terfenadine and astemizole, resulting from inhibition of these enzymes.

Excretion

Unlike those of metabolism, the effects of aging on renal functions are somewhat more predictable. The tendency for renal function to decline with increasing age can affect the pharmacokinetics of several drugs (and their active metabolites) that are eliminated predominantly by the kidney (Table 14-6). These drugs are cleared from the body more slowly, their half-lives (and duration of action) are prolonged, and there is a tendency to accumulate to higher (and potentially toxic) drug concentrations in the steady state.

TABLE 14-6   IMPORTANT CONSIDERATIONS IN GERIATRIC PRESCRIBING

DRUG	MAJOR ROUTE OF ELIMINATION	OTHER PHARMACOLOGICAL CONSIDERATIONS	OTHER CONSIDERATIONS
		ANALGESICS (SEE CHAP. 10)	
Nonnarcotic Acetaminophen	Hepatic	No substantial age-related change in kinetics Liver toxicity may occur in high doses	Analgesic effects of noninflammatory condition similar to aspirin and other antiinflammatory agents
Aspirin	Renal	Highly protein-bound Half-life may be prolonged at higher dosages	Enteric-coated preparations useful
Nonsteroidal antiinflammatory agents	Renal (naproxen, ibuprofen) Hepatic (indomethacin)	Highly protein-bound	(See Chap. 10)
Cyclooxygenase-2 (COX-2) inhibitors	Mixed		
Narcotic	Hepatic	Blood levels may be higher, pain relief longer	Lower doses generally effective for analgesia Constipation a major problem

TABLE 14-6 IMPORTANT CONSIDERATIONS IN GERIATRIC PRESCRIBING (*Continued*)

DRUG	MAJOR ROUTE OF ELIMINATION	OTHER PHARMACOLOGICAL CONSIDERATIONS	OTHER CONSIDERATIONS
		ANTIMICROBIALS	
Antibacterial			
Aminoglycosides (gentamicin, tobramycin, amikacin)	Renal	Half-life prolonged	Nephrotoxicity and ototoxicity are major problems Blood levels important
Aztreonam	Renal	Half-life prolonged	
Cephalosporins	Renal	Half-life prolonged	
Clindamycin	Hepatic		
Erythromycin	Hepatic		
Quinolones	Renal, hepatic	Relatively long half-life allows twice a day dosage	Can increase warfarin effects
Penicillins	Renal	Half-life prolonged	Carbenicillin and ticarcillin— high parenteral doses give a large sodium load
	Hepatic (nafcillin, cloxacillin)	Highly protein-bound (nafcillin, cloxacillin, oxacillin)	
Sulfonamides	Renal	Highly protein-bound	Increased effects of warfarin
Tetracyclines	Renal	Half-life prolonged	
	Hepatic (doxycycline)		
Vancomycin	Renal	Half-life prolonged	Ototoxicity, nephrotoxicity

Drug	Elimination	Comments
		Blood levels important
		Poor oral absorption makes oral preparation useful for *Clostridium difficile*–associated diarrhea
Antitubercular		
Ethambutol	Renal	
Isoniazid	Hepatic	Genetic variation in rate of metabolism; no substantial age-related change — Hepatotoxicity increases with age
Rifampin	Hepatic	
Antifungal		
Amphotericin	Nonrenal	Nephrotoxicity a major problem
ANTIPARKINSONIAN AGENTS (SEE CHAP. 10)		
Amantadine	Renal	
Bromocriptine	Hepatic	
Carbidopa-levodopa	Hepatic	Cardiovascular toxicity increased
Entacapone, tolcapone	Hepatic	
Pergolide	Hepatic	Postural hypotension may occur
Pramipexole	Renal	
Ropinirole	Hepatic	Hallucinations relatively common at higher doses
Trihexyphenidyl	Nonrenal	

TABLE 14-6 IMPORTANT CONSIDERATIONS IN GERIATRIC PRESCRIBING (*Continued*)

DRUG	MAJOR ROUTE OF ELIMINATION	OTHER PHARMACOLOGICAL CONSIDERATIONS	OTHER CONSIDERATIONS
CARDIOVASCULAR DRUGS (SEE CHAP. 11)			
Antiarrhythmic			
Disopyramide	Renal, hepatic		Can cause urinary retention
Encainide	Hepatic		
Lidocaine	Hepatic	Volume of distribution increased Half-life prolonged Clearance unchanged	Blood levels helpful
Procainamide	Renal	Clearance decreased Steady-state levels higher	Blood levels helpful
Quinidine	Nonrenal	Highly protein-bound Clearance decreased Half-life prolonged	Blood levels helpful
Tocainide	Renal, hepatic		
Verapamil	Hepatic	Clearance decreased Pharmacological effects more pronounced and prolonged	Interacts with and raises digoxin blood levels
Anticoagulant			
Heparin	Nonrenal		
Sulfinpyrazone	Renal		

Drug	Route	Characteristics	Comments
Warfarin	Hepatic	Highly protein-bound; Sensitivity to effects increased	Multiple drug interactions
Antihypertensives			See Chap. 11 for more detailed discussion of antihypertensive therapy
Atenolol	Renal		
Captopril	Renal		
Clonidine	Renal		
Diltiazem	Hepatic	Clearance decreased	Use carefully with sinus node dysfunction
Enalapril/ lisinopril	Renal	Pharmacological effects more pronounced and prolonged	
Hydralazine	Hepatic	Highly protein-bound	
Metoprolol	Hepatic	Blood levels higher	
Methyldopa	Renal		
Nadolol	Renal		
Nifedipine	Hepatic		
Propranolol	Hepatic	Highly protein-bound; Blood levels higher; Clearance decreased; Half-life prolonged; Sensitivity to effects decreased	
Prazosin	Hepatic	Highly protein-bound	
Terazosin	Renal, hepatic	Highly protein-bound	
Diuretics			
Furosemide	Renal	Highly protein-bound	Older patients predisposed to dehydration and electrolyte imbalance

TABLE 14-6 IMPORTANT CONSIDERATIONS IN GERIATRIC PRESCRIBING (*Continued*)

DRUG	MAJOR ROUTE OF ELIMINATION	OTHER PHARMACOLOGICAL CONSIDERATIONS	OTHER CONSIDERATIONS
		CARDIOVASCULAR DRUGS (SEE CHAP. 11)	
Thiazides	Renal		Potassium supplementation not always necessary
Triamterene	Hepatic		Glucose intolerance or diabetes may worsen
Digoxin	Renal (15–40 % nonrenal)	Decreased clearance Half-life prolonged	Many with heart failure and sinus rhythm may not need digoxin (see Chap. 11)
		HYPOGLYCEMIC AGENTS (SEE CHAP. 12)	
Oral Acetohexamide	Renal, hepatic	Highly protein-bound (all oral hypoglycemics)	See Chap. 12 for more detailed discussion of hypoglycemic therapy in the elderly
Glipizide	Hepatic		
Glyburide	Hepatic		
Metformin	Renal		May cause lactic acidosis Must be withheld 48 h before and after iodinated contrast media

Drug	Metabolism/Excretion	Pharmacokinetic Notes	Comments
Pioglidazone, rosiglitazone	Hepatic		Serum transaminase monitoring suggested
Tolazamide	Hepatic		
Tolbutamide	Hepatic		
Troglitazone	Hepatic		
Insulin	Renal, hepatic	Renal metabolism may be decreased Sensitivity to effects may be decreased	
PSYCHOTROPIC DRUGS (SEE TABLES 14-9, 10, AND 11)			
Antidepressants (tricyclic, tetracyclic)	Hepatic	Highly protein-bound Blood levels may be higher	See Chap. 7 for more detailed discussion on antidepressant drugs
Selective serotonin reuptake inhibitors (SSRIs)	Hepatic	Can inhibit cytochrome P450 isoenzymes	May cause inappropriate antidiuretic hormone secretion and hyponatremia
Lithium	Renal	Clearance decreased	Blood levels important
Antipsychotics	Hepatic	Highly protein-bound	See Tables 14-9 and 14-11
Sedatives and hypnotics			
Benzodiazepines	Hepatic Renal (oxazepam)	Highly protein-bound Diazepam half-life prolonged	See Tables 14-10 and 14-11
Chloral hydrate	Hepatic	Highly protein-bound	
Diphenhydramine	Hepatic	Highly protein-bound	Anticholinergic side effects may be a problem

TABLE 14-6 IMPORTANT CONSIDERATIONS IN GERIATRIC PRESCRIBING (*Continued*)

DRUG	MAJOR ROUTE OF ELIMINATION	OTHER PHARMACOLOGICAL CONSIDERATIONS	OTHER CONSIDERATIONS
		PSYCHOTROPIC DRUGS	
Zolpidem	Hepatic	Highly protein-bound	
		OTHER DRUGS	
Aminophylline, theophylline	Hepatic	Half-life prolonged	Lower doses may give therapeutic blood levels Blood levels helpful
Carbamazepine	Hepatic	Highly protein bound	Several drugs can affect metabolism Blood levels helpful
Cimetidine	Renal	Half-life prolonged Steady-state blood levels higher	Can cause mental changes at high doses
Famotidine	Renal, hepatic		
Gabapentin	Renal		
Nizatidine	Renal		
Oxybutynin	Hepatic		Prominent anticholinergic effects Blood levels helpful
Phenytoin	Hepatic	Clearance decreased	Low albumin results in higher free drug than levels indicate

Prophylthiouracil	Hepatic, renal		
Raloxifene	Hepatic		Increased risk of thromboembolism
Ranitidine	Renal		
Sildenafil	Hepatic	Half-life prolonged	
Terbutaline	Hepatic		
Thyroxine	Hepatic	Clearance decreased	Maintenance dose lower Effects can be monitored by thyroid-stimulating hormone blood levels (see Chap. 12)
Tolterodine	Hepatic	Blood levels higher	Can have anticholinergic effects

Several considerations are important in determining the effects of age on renal function and drug elimination:

1. There is wide interindividual variation in the rate of decline of renal function with increasing age. Thus, although renal function is said to decline by 50 percent between the ages of 20 and 90 years, this is an *average* decline. A 90-year-old individual may not have a creatinine clearance of only 50 percent of normal. Applying average declines to individual elderly patients can result in over- or underdosing.

2. Muscle mass declines with age; therefore, daily endogenous creatinine production declines. Because of this decline in creatinine production, serum creatinine may be normal at a time when renal function is substantially reduced. Serum creatinine, therefore, does not reflect renal function as accurately in elderly people as it does in younger persons.

3. A number of factors can affect renal clearance of drugs and are often at least as important as age-related changes. State of hydration, cardiac output, and intrinsic renal disease should be considered in addition to age-related changes in renal function.

Several formulas and nomograms have been used to estimate renal function in relation to age. Table 14-7 shows the most widely used and accepted formula. This formula is useful in *initial estimations* of creatinine clearance for the purpose of drug dosing in the geriatric population. Clinical factors (such as state of hydration and cardiac output), which vary over time, should be considered in determining drug dosages.

When drugs with narrow therapeutic:toxic ratios are being used, actual measurements of creatinine clearance and drug blood levels (when available) should be used.

Tissue Sensitivity

A proportion of the drug or its active metabolite will eventually reach its site of action. Age-related changes at this point—that is, responsiveness to given drug

TABLE 14-7   RENAL FUNCTION IN RELATION TO AGE*

$$\text{Creatinine clearance} = \frac{(140 - \text{age}) \times \text{body weight (kg)}}{72 \times \text{serum creatinine level}} \ (\times 0.85 \text{ for women})$$

* Several other factors can influence creatinine clearance (see text).
Source: From Cockcroft and Gault, 1976, with permission.

concentrations (without regard to pharmacokinetic changes)—are termed *pharmacodynamic changes*. Older persons are often said to be more sensitive to the effects of drugs. For some drugs, this appears to be true. For others, however, sensitivity to drug effects may decrease rather than increase with age. For example, older persons may be more sensitive to the sedative effects of given blood levels of benzodiazepines but less sensitive to the effects of drugs mediated by ß-adrenergic receptors. There are several possible explanations for these changes (see Table 14-5). The effects of age-related pharmacodynamic changes on dosages of specific drugs for individual geriatric patients remain largely unknown.

GERIATRIC PRESCRIBING

General Principles

Several considerations make the development of specific recommendations for geriatric drug prescribing very difficult. These include the following:

1. Multiple interacting factors influence age-related changes in drug pharmacology.
2. There is wide interindividual variation in the rate of age-related changes in physiological parameters that affect drug pharmacology. Thus, precise predictions for individual older persons are difficult to make.
3. The clinical status of each patient (including such factors as state of nutrition and hydration, cardiac output, intrinsic renal and liver disease) must be considered in addition to the effects of aging.
4. As more research studies with newer drugs are carried out in well-defined groups of older subjects, more specific recommendations will be possible.

Adherence to several general principles can make drug therapy in the geriatric population safer and more effective (Table 14-8). Cardiovascular drugs, which account for a substantial proportion of adverse drug reactions, are also discussed in Chap. 10. Because psychotropic drugs are so commonly used, they are discussed in greater detail below.

GERIATRIC PSYCHOPHARMACOLOGY

Psychotropic drugs can be broadly categorized as antidepressants (discussed in detail in Chap. 7), antipsychotics (Table 14-9), and sedatives and hypnotics (Table 14-10). These drugs are probably the most misused class of drugs in the geriatric population. Several studies show that more than half of nursing home residents are prescribed at least one psychotropic drug and that these prescriptions are changed

TABLE 14-8   GENERAL RECOMMENDATIONS FOR GERIATRIC PRESCRIBING

1. Evaluate geriatric patients thoroughly in order to identify all conditions that could (a) benefit from drug treatment; (b) be adversely affected by drug treatment; (c) influence the efficacy of drug treatment.
2. Manage medical conditions without drugs as often as possible.
3. Know the pharmacology of the drug(s) being prescribed.
4. Consider how the clinical status of each patient could influence the pharmacology of the drug(s).
5. Avoid potential adverse drug interactions.
6. For drugs or their active metabolites eliminated predominantly by the kidney, use a formula or nomogram to approximate age-related changes in renal function and adjust dosages accordingly.
7. If there is a question about drug dosage, start with smaller doses and increase gradually.
8. Drug blood concentrations can be helpful in monitoring several potentially toxic drugs used frequently in the geriatric population.
9. Help to ensure compliance by paying attention to impaired intellectual function, diminished hearing, and poor vision when instructing patients and labeling prescriptions (and by using other techniques listed in Table 14-1).
10. Monitor older patients frequently for compliance, drug effects, and toxicity.

frequently. Ironically, there is also evidence that antidepressants may be underused in nursing homes, where there is a high prevalence of depression. Other studies suggest that psychotropic drugs are commonly prescribed inappropriately in the nursing home setting. This is of special concern because of the frequency of adverse reactions to these drugs. Federal rules and regulations contained in the Omnibus Budget Reconciliation Act of 1987 (OBRA 1987) contained specific guidelines on the use of psychotropic drugs in nursing homes. The OBRA 1987 guidelines are discussed in detail elsewhere (Ouslander et al., 1997) and are currently being updated (as of June 2003). These guidelines emphasize avoiding the use of frequent "as needed" dosing for nonspecific symptoms (e.g., agitation, wandering) and the inappropriate use of these drugs as chemical restraints. The appropriate use of antipsychotics for psychosis and several behavioral symptoms associated with dementia must, however, be distinguished from their use as "chemical restraints."

Several considerations can be helpful in preventing the misuse of psychotropic drugs in the geriatric population:

TABLE 14-9   EXAMPLES OF ANTIPSYCHOTIC DRUGS*

| | | | POTENTIAL FOR SIDE EFFECTS | | |
DRUG	APPROXIMATE EQUIVALENT DOSE (MG)	GERIATRIC DAILY DOSE RANGE (MG)	RELATIVE SEDATION	HYPOTENSION	EXTRAPYRAMIDAL EFFECTS †
Chlorpromazine (Thorazine, others)	100	10–300	Very high	High	Moderate
Haloperidol (Haldol)	2	0.25–6	Low	Low	Very high
Olanzapine (Zyprexa)	—‡	2.5–10 §	Low	Low	Low
Quetiapine (Seroquel)	—‡	12.5–200 §	Low	Low	Low
Risperidone (Risperdal)	—‡	0.25–8	Low	Low	Low
Thioridazine (Mellaril)	100	10–300	High	Moderate	Low
Thiothixene (Navane)	5	1–5	Low	Low	Very high
Ziprasidone (Geodon)	80	20–40§	Low	Moderate	Low

* Other agents are also available.
† Rigidity, bradykinesia, tremor, akathisia.
‡ Not available.
§ Geriatric dosage ranges not well studied.

– 381 –

TABLE 14-10 EXAMPLES OF SEDATIVES AND HYPNOTIC AGENTS*

DRUG (BRAND NAME)	GERIATRIC DAILY DOSE RANGE (MG)	RELATIVE RAPIDITY OF EFFECT AFTER ORAL ADMINISTRATION	HALF-LIFE(H)	ACTIVE METABOLITES
		BENZODIAZEPINES		
Longer acting †				
Clonazepam (Klonopin)	0.5–5	Intermediate	20–100	No
Clorazepate (Tranxene)	7.5–15	Fast	50–100	Yes
Diazepam (Valium)	1–5	Fast	40–200	Yes
Flurazepam (Dalmane)	15	Fast	18–50	Yes
Shorter acting				
Alprazolam (Xanax)	0.25–0.75	Fast	2–5	No
Estrazolam (ProSom)	0.5–2	Intermediate	10–24	No
Lorazepam (Ativan)	1–2	Intermeidate	10–20	No
Oxazepam (Serax)	10–30	Slow	5–15	No
Temazepam (Restoril)	7.5–15	Fast	5–15	No
Triazolam (Halcion)	0.0625– 0.125	Intermediate	2–5	No

OTHERS

Chloral hydrate (Noctec, etc.)	500–1500	Fast	7–10	Yes
Buspirone (BuSpar) ‡	10–30	Fast	2–3	Yes
Zaleplon (Sonata)	10	Very fast	1	No
Zolpidem (Ambien)	5	Very fast	2–3	No

* Several other agents are also available.
† Longer-acting benzodiapines should be avoided in geriatric patients.
‡ Must be used chronically to be an effective antianxiety agent.

1. Psychological symptoms (depression, anxiety, agitation, insomnia, paranoia, disruptive behavior) are often caused or exacerbated by medical conditions in geriatric patients. A thorough medical evaluation should therefore be done before symptoms are attributed to psychiatric conditions alone and psychotropic drugs are prescribed.

2. Reports of psychiatric symptomatology such as agitation are often presented to physicians by family caregivers and nursing home personnel who are inexperienced in the description, interpretation, and differential diagnosis of these symptoms. "Agitation" or "disruptive behavior" may, in fact, have been a reasonable response to an inappropriate interaction or situation created by the caregiver. Psychotropic drugs should, therefore, be prescribed only after the physician has clarified what the symptoms are and what correctable factors might have precipitated them.

3. Psychological symptoms and signs, like physical symptoms and signs, can be nonspecific in the geriatric patient. Therefore, appropriate drug treatment often depends on an accurate psychiatric diagnosis. Psychiatrists and psychologists experienced with geriatric patients should be consulted, when available, in order to identify and help target psychotropic drug treatment to the major psychiatric problem(s).

4. Many nonpharmacological treatment modalities can either replace or be used in conjunction with psychotropic drugs in managing psychological symptoms. Behavioral modification, environmental manipulation, supportive psychotherapy, group therapy, recreational activities, and other related techniques can be useful in eliminating or diminishing the need for drug treatment.

5. Within each broad category of psychotropic drug, there are considerable differences among individual agents with regard to effects, side effects, and potential interactions with other drugs and medical conditions. Rational prescription of these drugs necessitates careful consideration of the characteristics of each drug in relation to the individual patient.

6. Because geriatric patients are, in general, more sensitive to the effects and side effects of psychotropic drugs, initial doses should be lower, increases should be gradual, and monitoring should be frequent.

7. Careful, ongoing assessment of the response of target symptoms and behaviors to psychotropic drugs is essential. In addition to reports from patients themselves, objective observations by trained and experienced professionals should be continuously evaluated in order to adjust psychotropic drug therapy.

All psychotropic drugs must be used judiciously in geriatric patients because of their potential side effects. The most common and potentially disabling side effects of psychotropic drugs fall into four general categories: changes in cognitive status (e.g., sedation, delirium, dementia) and extrapyramidal, anticholinergic, and cardiovascular effects. Research documents that psychotropic drugs can contribute to cognitive impairment (Larson et al., 1987) and are associated with hip fractures in the geriatric population (Ray et al., 1987).

Anticholinergic and cardiovascular side effects are most prominent with the tricyclic antidepressants. Antipsychotic drugs with ß-adrenergic–blocking properties, including chlorpromazine and thioridazine, also have cardiovascular side effects, most notably hypotension. Newer drugs without such effects have largely replaced these agents. Extrapyramidal side effects are most common with several antipsychotic drugs (see Table 14-9). These effects—which include pseudoparkinsonism (rigidity, bradykinesia, tremor), akathisia (restlessness), and involuntary dystonic movements (such as tardive dyskinesia)—can be severe and may cause substantial disability. Rigidity and bradykinesia can lead to immobility and the complications discussed in Chap. 10. Akathisia can make the patient appear more anxious and agitated, and can lead to the inappropriate prescription of more medication. Tardive dyskinesia can cause permanent disability as a consequence of continuous orolingual movements and difficulty with eating. In addition to side effects, many psychotropic drugs interact with each other and with other drug classes. Some of these interactions can be clinically important and can enhance the risk of toxicity (Steffens and Krishnan, 1998).

Optimal efficacy of psychotropic drugs necessitates considering the characteristics of the drugs in relation to several clinical factors in each patient (Table 14-11). In general, the antipsychotic agents should be reserved for treatment of psychoses (i.e., paranoid states, delusions, and hallucinations), which are common in dementia patients. These drugs may also be useful for severe physical and/or verbal agitation that does not respond to nonpharmacological interventions. Environmental and behavioral interventions should be attempted before psychotropic drugs are prescribed. There is no clear choice of one antipsychotic agent over another based on controlled clinical trials. Some of the newer agents, such as risperidone, olanzapine, and quetiapine, have less extrapyramidal side effects than older drugs. They are clearly the drugs of choice for psychosis that occurs in dementia of Parkinson's disease and dementia associated with Lewy bodies (see Chap. 6). In some situations, intermittent agitation, especially at night, is best treated by a short-acting benzodiazepine (see Table 14-10). When antipsychotics fail or cause side effects, and sedation is not desired, carbamazepine and valproic acid may be useful alternatives in some patients. Both of these drugs, however, have the potential for hematological and hepatic toxicity and must be used cautiously in the geriatric population. Periodic attempts to taper and discontinue the use of these drugs are required in nursing facilities, and can result in the successful removal of psychotropics for some patients (Cohen Mansfield et al., 1999).

A variety of nonpharmacological measures can be effective in geriatric patients with agitation or excessive anxiety. Specific behavioral and other nonpharmacological therapeutic approaches are described in detail in some of the

TABLE 14-11 CLINICAL CONSIDERATIONS IN PRESCRIBING PSYCHOTROPIC DRUGS

CLINICAL INDICATOR	MOST USEFUL TYPES	COMMENTS
Depression with psychomotor retardation	Less sedating antidepressant (e.g., fluoxitene, paroxetine, sertraline)	See Chap. 7
Depression with insomnia and/or weight loss	Antidepressant with sedative and weight-gaining effects (e.g., mirtazapine)	
Agitation without psychosis that occurs at night	Short-acting sedative (e.g., lorazepam) or a hypnotic (e.g., zolpidem, temazepam)	Should generally be used on an "as-needed" basis Nonpharmacologic intervention may be more appropriate
Psychoses without prominent agitation (e.g., delusions and hallucinations in patients with depression or dementia)	Less sedating antipsychotic (e.g., risperidone, olanzapine)	Extrapyramidal effects may occur Risperidone may cause postural hypotension if not titrated slowly
Severe physical or verbal agitation poorly controlled by nonpharmacological intervention	More sedating antipsychotic (e. g., quetiapine, thioridazine, loxapine)	Akathisia can make patient appear more agitated
Insomnia	Temazepam Zolpidem	Underlying cause (s) should be sought; nonpharmacological interventions often helpful

suggested readings at the end of this chapter (see also Chap. 6). These measures, however, are often unavailable, impractical, inappropriate, or unsuccessful. Patients with severe impairment of cognitive function can be especially difficult to manage with nonpharmacological measures alone, particularly when their physical and/or verbal agitation is interfering with their care (or the care of others around them). Thus, drug treatment of agitation is necessary in these patients.

Insomnia, like agitation, can be the manifestation of depression or physical illness. It is a very common complaint in geriatric patients, and causes of sleep disorders should be sought (see Chap. 7). Nonpharmacological measures (such as increasing activity during the day, diminishing nighttime noise, and ensuring cooler nighttime temperatures) are sometimes helpful. Several alternatives are available for drug treatment of insomnia (see Table 14-10). Melatonin, a naturally occurring hormone available over the counter, has gained increasing popularity as a hypnotic. Geriatric sleep disturbances are associated with changes in the melatonin cycle. Doses of 1 to 3 mg may improve the initiation and maintenance of sleep. The long-term effects of chronic hypnotic use in the geriatric population are unknown, but rebound insomnia can become a problem in patients who use hypnotics (especially benzodiazepine hypnotics and melatonin) regularly and then discontinue them. Whatever the indication, it is extremely important that after a psychotropic drug is prescribed the patient be closely monitored for the effects of the drug on the target symptoms and side effects, and that the drug regimen be adjusted accordingly.

References

Cockcroft DW, Gault MH: Predictions of creatinine clearance from serum creatinine. *Nephron* 16:31–41, 1976.

Cohen-Mansfield J, Lipson S, Werner P, et al: Withdrawal of haloperidol, thioridazine, and lorazepam in the nursing home. *Arch Intern Med* 159:1733–1740, 1999.

Heerdink ER, Leufkens HG, Herings RMC, et al: NSAIDs associated with increased risk of congestive heart failure in elderly patients taking diuretics. *Arch Intern Med* 158:1108–1112, 1998.

Larson EB, Kukull WA, Buchner D, et al: Adverse drug reactions associated with global cognitive impairment in elderly persons. *Ann Intern Med* 107:169–173, 1987.

Lazarou J, Pomeranz BH, Corey PN: Incidence of adverse drug reactions in hospitalized patients: a meta-analysis of prospective studies. *JAMA* 279:1200–1205, 1998.

Ouslander J, Morley J, Osterweil D: *Medical Care in the Nursing Home,* 2d ed. New York, McGraw-Hill, 1997.

Ray WA, Griffin MR, Schaffner W, et al: Psychotropic drug use and the risk of hip fracture. *N Engl J Med* 316:363–369, 1987.

Steffens DC, Krishnan KRR: Metabolism, bioavailability, and drug interactions. *Clin Geriatr* 14:17–32, 1998.

Suggested Readings

Anonymous: Antimicrobial prophylaxis in surgery. *Med Lett* 39:97–102, 1997.

Anonymous: Drugs for psychiatric disorders. *Med Lett* 39:33–40, 1997.

Anonymous: Drugs that may cause psychiatric symptoms. *Med Lett* 44:59–62, 2002.

Beers MH: Explicit criteria for determining potentially inappropriate medication use by the elderly. *Arch Intern Med* 157:1531–1536, 1997.

Board of Directors of the American Association for Geriatric Psychiatry, Clinical Practice Committee of the American Geriatrics Society, and Committee on Long- Term Care and Treatment for the Elderly: Psychotherapeutic medications in the nursing home. *J Am Geriatr Soc* 40:946–949, 1992.

Carlson DL, Fleming KC, Smith GE, et al: Management of dementia-related behavioral disturbances: a nonpharmacologic approach. *Mayo Clin Proc* 70:1108–1115, 1995.

Mintzer JE, Hoernig KS, Mirski DF: Treatment of agitation in patients with dementia. *Clin Geriatr Med* 14:147–175, 1998.

Selma TP, Beizer JL, Higbee MD: *Geriatric Dosage Handbook,* 5th ed. Hudson, OH, American Pharmaceutical Association and Lexi-Comp, 2000–2001.

CHAPTER 15

HEALTH SERVICES

Geriatrics can be thought of as the intersection of chronic disease care and geron-tology. The latter refers largely to the contents of this book: the syndromes asso-ciated with aging, the atypical presentations of disease, and the difficulties of managing multiple, simultaneous, interactive problems. Health care for older per-sons consists largely of addressing the problems associated with chronic illness. However, medical care continues to be practiced as though it consisted of a series of discrete encounters. What is needed is a systematic approach to chronic care that encourages clinicians to recognize the overall course expected for each patient and to manage treatment within those parameters. The clinical glide path approach (described in Chap. 4) is one way to encourage such practice.

Care for frail older persons has been impeded by an artificial dichotomy between medical and social interventions. This separation has been enhanced by the funding policies, such as the auspices of Medicare and Medicaid, but it also reflects the philosophies of the dominant professions. A prerequisite for effective coordination is shared goals. Until the differences in goals are reconciled, there is little hope for integrated care.

Medical practice has been driven by what may be termed a therapeutic model. The basic expectation from medical care is that it will make a difference. The dif-ference may not always be reflected in an improvement in the patient's status. Indeed, for many chronically ill patients decline is inevitable, but good care should at least delay that decline. Because many patients do get worse over time, it may be difficult for clinicians to see the effects of their care.

Appreciating the benefits of good care in the context of decline in function over time may require a comparison between what happens and what would have occurred in the absence of that care. In effect, the yield from good care is the dif-ference between what is observed and what is reasonable to expect; but without the expected value, the benefit may be hard to appreciate. Figure 15-1 provides a the-oretical model of these two curves. Both trajectories show decline, but the slope associated with better care is less acute. The area between them represents the effects of good care. Unfortunately, that benefit is invisible unless specific steps are taken to demonstrate the difference between the observed and expected course.

The alternative model, usually associated with social services, is compensa-tory care. Under this concept, a person is assessed to determine deficits and a plan of care is developed to address the identified deficits. Good care is defined as pro-viding services that meet the profile of dependencies and thereby allows the client

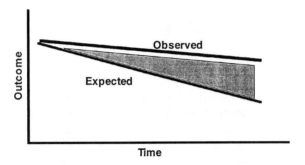

— FIGURE 15-1 — *Theoretical model of observed versus expected clinical course. The shaded area between the observed and expected outcomes represents the benefits of good care. Thus a patient's condition may deteriorate and still be considered as an indication of good care if the rate of deterioration is less than expected.*

to enjoy as normal a lifestyle as possible without incurring any adverse consequences. The two approaches should not be incompatible. Providing needed services should enhance functioning or at least slow its decline.

Care for the frail older patient requires a synthesis of medical and social attention. The medical care system has not facilitated that interaction. The new developments in managed care could provide a framework for achieving this coordination, but the track record so far does not suggest that the incentives are yet in place to produce this effect. A few notable programs have been able to merge funding and services for this frail population. Probably the best example of creative integration is seen in the Program of All-inclusive Care of the Elderly (PACE), which uses pooled capitated funding from Medicare and Medicaid to provide integrated health and social services to older persons who are deemed to be eligible for nursing home care but who are still living in the community (Kane, 1999). Another model that shows promise for demonstrating this integration is the second generation of the social health maintenance organization (SHMO) (Kane et al., 1997b). Whether managed care will achieve its potential as a vehicle for improving coordination of care for older persons remains to be seen. In any event, care for older persons will require such integration and eventually some reconciliation about what constitutes the desired goals of such care.

Geriatric care thus implies team care. This concept does not mean that everyone needs to do everything. Rather, it means that some activities can be the purview of other disciplines with special skills and training for such tasks. However, these colleagues must not be expected to operate alone. Good communication and coordination will avoid duplication of effort and lead to a better overall outcome. To play a useful role on the health care team, physicians need to appreciate what other health professions can do and know how and when to call on their skills.

PUBLIC PROGRAMS

The physician caring for elderly patients must have at least a working acquaintance with the major programs that support older people. We are accustomed to thinking about care of older people in association with Medicare. In fact, at least three parts (called *Titles*) of the Social Security Act provide important benefits for the elderly: Title XVIII (Medicare), Title XIX (Medicaid), and Social Services Block Grants (formerly Title XX). Medicare was designed to address health care, particularly acute care hospital services. The Medicare program is in flux. Changes in the payment system have been introduced to counter what some saw as abuses (certainly expansions) of the previous system. Medicare was intended to deal with long-term care only to the extent that long-term care can supplant more expensive hospital care, leaving the major funding for long-term care to Medicaid. However, the funding demarcation between acute and long-term care services became blurred. Especially with regard to home health care, Medicare began to cover more care that would be considered long-term. In 1993, approximately 60 percent of home health care visits under Medicare were delivered to persons who have received such care for at least 6 months, well beyond the traditional designation of acute care (Welch et al., 1996). As a result, a new prospective payment system was introduced for home health care under Medicare. This approach caps the amounts paid and links them to patient characteristics. Long bouts of services are discouraged.

This distinction in programmatic responsibility between Medicare and Medicaid is a very important one. Whereas Medicare is an insurance-type program to which persons are entitled after contributing a certain amount, Medicaid is a welfare program, eligibility for which depends on a combination of need and poverty. Thus, to become eligible for Medicaid, a person must not only prove illness but also exhaustion of personal resources—hardly a situation conducive to restoring autonomy.

The pattern of coverage is quite different for the various services covered. Figures 15-2 and 15-3 trace spending on health care for elderly persons by Medicare and Medicaid, respectively. Medicare is a major payer of hospital and physician care but pays for only a small portion of nursing home care, whereas just the reverse applies to Medicaid. (Medicare has played a larger role in nursing home and home health care as the role of postacute care grew, but new funding priorities have attempted to reduce that role.)

Medicare

Eligibility for Medicare differs for each of its two major parts. Part A (hospital services insurance) is available to all who are eligible for Social Security, usually

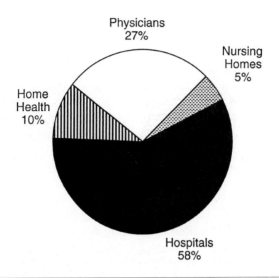

Physicians
27%

Nursing
Homes
5%

Home
Health
10%

Hospitals
58%

— FIGURE 15-2 — *Distribution of Medicare expenditures for the aged, 1995.* (From US Department of Health and Human Services, 1997a.)

by virtue of paying the Social Security tax for a sufficient number of quarters. This program is supported by a special payroll tax, which goes into the Medicare Trust Fund. Part B (medical services insurance) is offered for a monthly premium, paid by the individual but heavily subsidized by the government (which pays approximately 70 percent of the cost from general tax revenues). Almost everyone older than age 65 is automatically covered by Part A. (Federal, state, and local government employees are exceptions; until recently they were not covered by Social Security and had their own pension and medical programs.) The introduction of prospective payment for hospitals under Medicare created a new set of complications. Hospitals are paid a fixed amount per admission according to the diagnosis-related group (DRG), to which the patient is assigned on the basis of the admitting diagnosis. The rates for DRGs are, in turn, based on expected lengths of stay and intensity of care for each condition. The incentives in such an approach run almost directly contrary to most of the goals of geriatrics. Whereas geriatrics addresses the functional result of multiple interacting problems, DRGs encourage concentration on a single problem. Extra time required to make an appropriate discharge plan is discouraged. Use of ancillary personnel, such as social workers, is similarly discouraged. As a result of DRGs, hospital lengths of stay have decreased, leading to the phenomenon of "quicker and sicker" discharges. Many of these former hospital patients are now cared for through home health and nursing homes. In effect, Medicare is paying for care twice: It pays for the hospital stay regardless of length

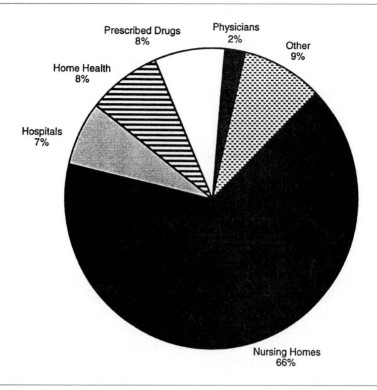

— FIGURE 15-3 — *Distribution of Medicaid expenditures for the aged, 1995.* (From US Department of Health and Human Services, 1997b.)

and then pays for the posthospital care. The rapid rise in this latter sector has led Medicare to search for solutions. Different types of Medicare prospective payment for the different types of posthospital care have been established. Nursing homes are paid on a per-diem basis, whereas home health agencies and rehabilitation units are paid on a per-episode basis. A more effective solution would be to combine the payment for hospital and posthospital care into a single bundled payment, although some fear that such a step would place too much control in the hands of hospitals. The Balanced Budget Act of 1997 (BBA) included a small step in this direction. For selected DRGs, hospital discharges to postacute care are treated as transfers. Hospitals receive a lower payment than the usual DRG payment if the length of stay is less than the median.

The payment systems now in effect create much confusion for Medicare beneficiaries. Although hospitals are paid a fixed amount per case, the patients continue to pay under a system of deductibles and copayments.

Managed care is aggressively being pursued as an option to traditional fee-for-service care. Under that arrangement, the managed care organizations receive a fixed monthly payment from Medicare in exchange for providing at least the range of services covered by Medicare. Although many managed care companies were initially attracted to this business because of the generous rates offered, subsequent reductions have made the business less attractive and many are exiting the program, leaving beneficiaries to scramble for alternative coverage, especially for the so-called Medigap policies that pay for deductibles and copayments.

The pricing system used by Medicare basically reflects the prices paid for fee-for-service care in each county. Managed care organizations are paid a fixed amount calculated on the basis of the average amount Medicare paid for its beneficiaries in that county. This adjusted average per capita cost (AAPCC) varies widely from one location to another. The BBA called for a shift to national pricing. In an effort to attract more providers into managed care, the BBA broadened the definition of what kinds of organizations can provide managed care to Medicare beneficiaries, removing many of the restrictions (especially financial surety bonding) that left managed care largely in the hands of insurance companies. Unlike managed care enrollees in the rest of the population, who are locked into health plans for a year, Medicare beneficiaries have the right to disenroll at any time. There is some evidence to suggest that Medicare beneficiaries may move in and out of managed care as they use up available benefits. The future of managed care as a Medicare venue is still unclear. The current administration continues to back this approach despite the number of managed care companies exiting from the market. Managed care participation has fallen from its high in 1998 of approximately 15 percent of Medicare beneficiaries to approximately half that number.

The likelihood of managed care achieving its potential symbiosis with geriatrics appears dim. Ideally, managed care could provide an environment where many of the principles of geriatrics could be implemented to the benefit of all; on the other hand, the performance to date suggests that managed care for Medicare beneficiaries has so far responded more to the incentives from favorable selection (recruiting healthy patients and getting paid average rates), discounted purchasing of services, and barriers to access than to the potential benefits from increased efficiency derived from a geriatric philosophy (Kane, 1998).

Although Medicare does pay for authorized posthospital services in nursing homes and through home health care, the payment for physicians does not encourage their active participation. For example, while a physician would be paid a regular consultation visit fee for daily rounds on a Medicare patient in a hospital, if the patient is discharged to a nursing home the following day, both the rate of physician reimbursement for a visit and the number of visits per week considered customary decrease dramatically. Although physician home visits are still a rarity, payment for these services has increased substantially in recent years. There are now physician groups that have made a business out of nursing home care and home health care. An interesting model of Medicare managed care directed specifically at nursing home residents is Evercare, which makes active use of nurse practitioners to increase the primary care attention residents receive. They have shown that it is possible to reduce the use of hospital care by this means (Kane, in press).

Many Medicare beneficiaries have also purchased so-called Medigap insurance. This insurance comes in a variety of forms (federal law now dictates the various components); most of this insurance covers only the gaps up to the ceilings established by Medicare (i.e., it pays deductibles and coinsurance but generally does not cover the difference between billed charges and allowable charges). An increasing number of policies cover at least some drug costs. In some cases, older persons may have purchased multiple Medigap policies under the erroneous assumption they were buying more coverage.

Medicare coverage is important but not sufficient for three basic reasons: (1) To control use, it mandates deductible and copayment charges for both Parts A and B. (2) It sets physician's fees by a complicated formula called the Resource-Based Relative Value Scale (RBRVS). The RBRVS is designed to pay physicians more closely according to the value of their services as determined both within a specialty and across specialties. Theoretically, both the value of the services provided and the investment in training are considered in setting the rates. This new payment approach was intended to increase the payment for primary care relative to surgical specialties, but early reports suggest that, ironically, many geriatric assessment services have been reimbursed at a level lower than before its introduction. Under Medicare Part B physicians are generally paid less than they would usually bill for the service. [Some physicians opt to bill the patient directly for the difference but a number of states have mandated that physicians accept "assignment" of Medicare fees, i.e., they accept the fee (plus the 20 percent copayment) as payment in full.] (3) The program does not cover several services essential to patient functioning, such as drugs, eyeglasses, hearing aids, and many preventive services (although the benefits for the latter are expanding). Medicare specifically excludes services designed to provide "custodial care"—the very services often most critical to long-term care. (However, as noted above, the boundary between acute and long-term care exclusions seems to be eroding.)

As a result of these three factors, a substantial amount of the medical bill is left to the individual. Today, elderly persons' out-of-pocket costs for health care represent more than 20 percent of their income, a figure comparable to before the passage of Medicare. In general, out-of-pocket costs are less for those in managed care.

Medicaid

Medicaid, in contrast to Medicare, is a welfare program designed to serve the poor. It is a state-run program to which the federal government contributes (50 to

78 percent of the costs, depending on the state). In some states, persons can be covered as medically indigent even if their income is above the poverty level if their medical expenses would impoverish them. As a welfare program, Medicaid has no deductibles or coinsurance (although current proposals call for modest charges to discourage excess use). It is, however, a welfare program cast in the medical model.

It is important to appreciate that the shape of the Medicaid expenditures for older people is determined largely by the gaps in Medicare. Medicaid serves primarily two distinct groups: mothers and young children under Temporary Assistance to Needy Families (TANF) and elderly persons eligible for Old Age Assistance. The other major route to eligibility for older people is the medically needy program, whereby eligibility is conferred when medical costs—usually nursing homes—exceed a fixed fraction of a person's income. Medicaid has been described as a universal health program that had a deductible of all of your assets and a copay of all of your income. The numerically larger group made up of mothers and children use less care per capita. They use some hospital care around birth and for the small group of severely ill children. A large portion of the Medicaid dollar goes to the services needed by the elderly enrollees but not covered by Medicare, namely, drugs, nursing home care, and custodial home care. (Most states automatically enroll eligible Medicaid recipients in Medicare Part B.)

Medicaid is the major source of nursing home payments. It requires physicians to certify a patient's physical limitations in order to gain the patient admittance to a nursing home. In some cases physicians may have to invent medical justifications for primarily social reasons (i.e., lack of social supports necessary to remain in the community).

Medicaid is thus important in shaping nursing home policies. It pays about half of the nursing costs but covers almost 70 percent of the residents. The discrepancy is explained by the policies that require residents to expend their own resources first. Thus Social Security payments, private pensions, and the like are used as primary sources of payment, and Medicaid picks up the remainder. However, it does not directly pay for most physician care in the nursing home; that is covered by Medicare. Medicaid would pay the deductibles and copayments and those services not covered under Medicare.

Whereas going on Medicaid was once seen as a great social embarrassment, associated with accepting public charity, there appears to be a growing sense among many older persons that they are entitled to receive Medicaid help when their health care expenses, especially their long-term care costs, are high. The stigma appears to be displaced by the idea that they paid taxes for many years and are now entitled to reap the rewards. As a result of this shift in sentiment, at least in the states with generous levels of Medicaid eligibility, there is a burgeoning industry of financial advisers to assist older persons in preparing to become Medicaid eligible. Because eligibility is usually based on both income and assets, such a step necessitates advance planning. Usually state laws require that assets transferred within two or more years of applying for Medicaid funds are considered to still be owned. (The situation is more complicated in the case of a married couple, where provisions have been made to allow the spouse to retain part of the family's assets.) This requirement means that older persons contemplating becoming eligible for Medicaid must be willing to divest themselves of their assets at least several years in advance of the time they expect to need such help. This step places them in a very dependent position, financially and psychologically. Much has been made of the "divestiture phenomenon" whereby older people scheme to divest themselves of their assets in order to qualify for Medicaid, but there is no good evidence about the scale of the phenomenon.

There is also growing enthusiasm for promoting various forms of private long-term care insurance. This coverage, in effect, protects the assets of those who might otherwise be marginally eligible for Medicaid or who simply want to preserve an inheritance for their heirs. Like any insurance linked to age-related events but to a greater degree, long-term care insurance is quite affordable when purchased at a young age (when the likelihood of needing it is very low) but becomes quite expensive as the buyer reaches age 75 or older. Thus, those most likely to consider buying it would have to pay a premium close to the average cost of long-term care itself. Only a small number of young persons have shown any interest in purchasing such coverage, especially when companies are not anxious to add it to their employee benefit packages as a free benefit. Although economic projections suggest that private long-term care insurance is not likely to save substantial money for the Medicaid program, several states have developed programs to encourage individuals to purchase the insurance by offering linked Medicaid benefits.

Other Programs

The third part of the Social Security legislation pertinent to older persons is Title XX, now administered as Social Services Block Grants. This is also a welfare program targeted especially to those on categorical welfare programs such as Temporary Assistance to Needy Families and, more germane, Supplemental Security Income. The latter is a federal program, which, as the name implies, supplements Social Security benefits to provide a minimum income. Title XX funds are administered through state and local agencies, which have a substantial amount of flexibility in how they allocate the available money across a variety of stipulated services. The state also has the option of broadening the eligibility criteria to include those just above the poverty line.

Another relevant federal program is Title III of the Older Americans Act. This program is available to all persons over age 60 regardless of income. The single largest component goes to support nutrition through congregate meal programs where elderly persons can get a subsidized hot meal, but it also provides meals-on-wheels (home-delivered meals) and a wide variety of other services. Some services duplicate or supplement those covered under Social Security programs; others are unique.

Table 15-1 summarizes these four programs and their current scope. It is important to appreciate that this summary attempts to condense and simplify a complex and ever-changing set of rules and regulations. Physicians should be familiar with the broad scope and limitations of these programs but will have to rely on others, especially social workers, who are familiar with the operating details.

LONG-TERM CARE

A proportion of older patients require substantial long-term care. There is no uniform definition for long-term care, but the following description of the term highlights the important aspects: "A range of services that addresses the health, personal care, and social needs of individuals who lack some capacity for self-care. Services may be continuous or intermittent but are delivered for sustained periods to individuals who have a demonstrated need, usually measured by some index of functional incapacity." This statement emphasizes the common thread of most discussions of long-term care: the dependence of an individual on the services of another for a substantial period. The definition is carefully vague about who provides those services or what they are. Long-term care is certainly not the exclusive purview of the medical profession; in fact, most of the long-term care in this country is not provided by professionals at all, but by a host of individuals loosely referred to as *informal support*. These persons may be family, friends, or neighbors.

Informal care has been and remains the backbone of long-term care. In many instances, the family (and often nonrelatives) is the first line of support. The ideal program would keep older people at home, relying on family care and bolstering their efforts with more formal assistance to provide professional services and occasional respite care. More than 80 percent of all the care given in the community comes from informal sources. (In truth, the proportion is higher because much of the formal care is made possible by a substrate of informal care.) Surprisingly, this figure seems to remain fairly constant in countries with more generous provision of formal long-term care. Many observers have questioned whether the informal care role, which is largely performed by women, can be sustained as more women enter the labor force and are already managing several roles. Despite dire predictions about its inevitable collapse, there is yet no evidence of serious decline in informal care. It is important to bear in mind that as the age of frailty rises, the "children" of these frail older people may themselves be in their seventh and eighth decades.

The best estimates suggest that about 15 percent of the elderly population need the help of another person to manage their daily lives. The good news is that

TABLE 15-1 SUMMARY OF MAJOR FEDERAL PROGRAMS FOR ELDERLY PATIENTS

PROGRAM	ELIGIBLE POPULATION	SERVICES COVERED	DEDUCTIBLES AND COPAYMENTS
Medicare (Title XVIII of the Social Security Act) Part A: Hospital insurance	All persons eligible for Social Security and others with chronic disabilities, such as end-stage renal disease, plus voluntary enrollees age 65+ years	Per benefit period, "reasonable cost" (DRG-based) for 90 days of hospital care plus 60 lifetime reserve days; 100 days of skilled nursing facility (SNF); home health visits (see text); hospice care*	Full coverage for hospital care after a deductible of about 1 day for days 2–60; then one-quarter day copay for days 61–90. Can use "lifetime reserve" days thereafter. 20 SNF days fully covered; one 8-day copay for days 21–100
Part B: Supplemental medical insurance	All those covered under Part A who elect coverage; participants pay a monthly premium	80% of "reasonable cost" for physicians' services; supplies and services related to physician services; outpatient, physical, and speech therapy; diagnostic tests and radiographs; mammograms; surgical dressings; prosthetics; ambulance	Deductible and 20% copayment (no copay after a limit reached)

TABLE 15-1 SUMMARY OF MAJOR FEDERAL PROGRAMS FOR ELDERLY PATIENTS (*Continued*)

PROGRAM	ELIGIBLE POPULATION	SERVICES COVERED	DEDUCTIBLES AND COPAYMENTS
Medicaid (Title XIX of the Social Security Act	Persons receiving Supplemental Security Income (SSI) (such as welfare) or receiving SSI and state supplement or meeting lower eligibility standards used for medical assistance criteria in 1972 or eligible for SSI or were in institutions and eligible for Medicaid in 1973; medically needy who do not qualify for SSI but have high medical expenses are eligible for Medicaid in some states; eligibility criteria vary from state to state	Mandatory services for categorically needy: Inpatient hospital services; outpatient services; SNF; limited home health care; laboratory tests and radiographs; family planning; early and periodic screening, diagnosis, and treatment for children through age 20 Optional services vary from state to state: Dental care; therapies; drugs; intermediate-care facilities; extended home health care; private duty nurse; eyeglasses; prostheses; personal-care services; medical transportation and home health care services (states can limit the amount and duration of services)	None, once patient spends down to eligibility level Spend-down based on income and assets

Social Services Block Grant (Title XX of the Social Security Act)	All recipients of TANF and SSI; optionally, those earning up to 115% of state median income and residents of specific geographic areas	Day care; substitute care; protective services; counseling; home-based services; employment, education, and training; health-related services; information and referral; transportation; day services; family planning; legal services; home-delivered and congregate meals	Fees are charged to those with family incomes greater than 80% of state's median income
Title III of the Older Americans Act	All persons age 60 and older; low-income, minority, and isolated older persons are special targets	Homemaker; home-delivered meals; home health aides; transportation; legal services; counseling; information and referral plus 19 others (50% of funds must go to those listed)	Some payment may be requested

* Certified hospice providers are paid a preset amount when a patient who is certified as terminal opts for this benefit in lieu of regular Medicare.

the prevalence of disability among older persons has declined about 1 percent per year over the last several decades (Cutler, 2001). As shown in Fig. 15-4, the proportion of persons who have difficulty performing one or more activities of daily living (ADL) increases with age, from approximately 8 percent at age 65 to 53 percent after age 85. If only those living in the community are examined, the proportion of persons needing help with one or more ADL in 1991–1992 was 4.1 percent of those age 65 to 74, 9.6 percent of those age 75 to 84, and 22.9 percent of those age 85 and older (Kennedy et al., 1997). Recall that for each person in a nursing home today, there are between one and three equally disabled persons living in the community. Thus, first instincts are not always best. Physicians have been trained to respond to the dependent elderly person by thinking of admission to a nursing home. Nursing home placement should be the *last* resort, not the first.

Current practice is trying to shift the balance between institutional care and home and community based services to emphasize use of the latter (Kane et al., 1998). Table 15-2 suggests a wider array of treatment choices for various types of patients. The physician, in conjunction with other health professionals (especially social workers and nurses), can do a great deal to steer patients and their families toward these resources. Although the physicians are not always actively involved in specific placement decisions, they should be. Indeed, the physician's suggestions and opinions about what should be considered can play a pivotal role. Moreover, the physician's medical certification of need is essential for establishing eligibility for long-term care services under several reimbursement programs.

Why then does our system rely so heavily on the nursing home? Several reasons can be offered. First, nursing homes are available; there are more nursing home beds than acute care hospital beds in this country. Nonetheless, there is usually a waiting list to get in, especially into a relatively good home. (That situation is beginning to change, however. With the growth in alternatives, especially assisted living, we are seeing for the first time substantial numbers of empty nursing home beds.) Second, nursing home care is cheap; it runs around $100 a day in most states, while a hospital day costs at least $1000, and even a good hotel room costs more than $100. Finally, and related to the first two points, the nursing home comes as an already assembled package of services. The programs to cover long-term care services have become a complex maze of eligibility and regulations, which has not encouraged anyone to develop innovative alternatives. The pressure for faster discharge from hospitals has created a new industry of postacute nursing home care. Although changes in Medicare payment have dampened some of the enthusiasm, this sector is still vital.

There have been periodic efforts to develop alternatives to nursing home care. Some were the results of deliberate public policies; others arose as new marketing efforts. For a period of time, great effort was expended trying to find less expensive ways of caring for people needing long-term care in the community. The upshot of these efforts was the recognition that community care is preferable

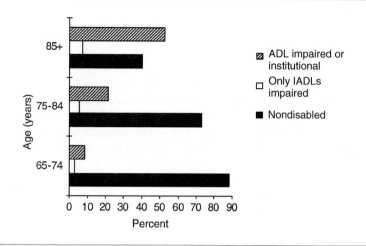

— FIGURE 15-4 — *Prevalence of chronic disability in the United States, 1994.* (From Manton et al., 1997.)

in many cases, but not always cheaper. A major difficulty in controlling the cost of this care is the potential for widespread use. Because a large number of dependent older persons live in the community, a dependency-based eligibility system will include many people who would not opt for a nursing home. This need to control entry has stimulated great interest in case management. The continuing need to improve community care has led to some innovations, including Medicaid waiver programs that allow use of nursing home funds for community care if the total long-term care budget is kept constant. As a result, there has been uneven development of community programs in different parts of the country.

The earlier emphasis on seeking community-based alternatives to nursing home care has shifted to some extent to developing other mechanisms for providing the combined housing and service functions. Among these are assisted living and adult foster care. Assisted living, in effect, renders the recipient first and foremost a tenant, who has control over her singly occupied living space (e.g., a lock on the door and determination about waking and retiring times). In addition to single occupancy, the client's autonomy is reenforced by providing modest cooking and refrigeration facilities, which allow the person to function independently without relying exclusively on the services of the institution and even to entertain modestly (Kane, 2001). However, as assisted living became a more desirable product it began to lose its identity. A variety of providers surfaced, many of whom offered very different services under that name. Today, it is hard to know just what one is getting when assisted living is cited.

TABLE 15-2 RELATIONSHIP BETWEEN TARGET GROUPS AND POSSIBLE ALTERNATIVES

TARGET GROUP NOW IN NURSING HOME	COMMUNITY ALTERNATIVES		
	INTERMEDIATE	LONG RANGE	INSTITUTIONAL BACKUP REQUIREMENT
Terminally ill	Home health Home hospice Homemaking Counseling	Narcotic law reform	Possibly a hospice
Those who might benefit from rehabilitation	Home health Day hospital		Rehabilitation hospital
Those requiring skilled nursing care	Home health Day hospital Meals-on-wheels Homemaking	Personal care attendant policy	Policy of acute care hospital service when needed

Those who are mentally ill	Halfway house Day hospital Sheltered workshops Day care	Bereavement counseling Identification of high-risk groups	Possible need for acute care hospital service
Those with social needs and minimal health problems— the frail, the very old	Sheltered housing Assisted living Day care Social programming Senior centers Primary health care	Reeducation Changed income transfer programs Employment programs	
The completely disoriented—ambulatory but needing constant supervision	Foster care		Possibility that better services can be provided through institutions

Adult foster care homes are usually limited to a small number of clients in any home (usually no more than five). Single rooms are not required; the situation is more analogous to individuals taking clients into their own homes, with small numbers of flexibly deployed nonprofessional staff. Recent trends suggest that the historic growth in nursing home use is changing. The last few years have witnessed a decline in nursing home occupancy. At least some of this effect undoubtedly comes from the growing availability of other residential models, which consumers find more attractive.

At the same time, there is concern that a preoccupation with a search for alternatives to nursing homes may distract efforts from the sorely needed work to improve the quality of nursing home care. Even in the best situation, a substantial number of older persons will continue to need such care. One scenario for the future holds that the form of nursing homes will change. Many of the residents currently cared for in nursing homes will be treated in more flexible situations, like assisted living, which emphasize living arrangements with nursing and other services brought to the residents on a more individualized basis. Those patients needing more intensive care will be treated in more medically oriented facilities.

THE NURSING HOME

The nursing home is an important part of the health care delivery system for frail older persons. Virtually without planning, it has emerged as the touchstone of long-term care. Given its origins as the stepchild of the almshouse and the hospital, it is not surprising that it has enjoyed a poor reputation. Since the passage of the Medicaid legislation in 1965, the nursing home industry has gone through growth and transformation. As a reaction to scandals during the early years, nursing homes are heavily regulated.

Today's nursing homes operate under two different principles, which complicate any attempt to describe them. For one group of clients admitted from hospitals for rehabilitation, they function as Medicare posthospital care providers, responsible for administering rehabilitative and restorative services to get these persons back into community living as soon as possible. For another stream of clients (often supported by Medicaid), they provide long-term care, which may last a lifetime.

Seen from one vantage point, the term *nursing home* is a misnomer. Although these institutions are better staffed and run than in the past, they remain generally somber places that offer their residents neither a great deal of real nursing care nor a very homelike environment.

Most nursing home residents share their rooms. There is little privacy and few opportunities to retain control over even small parts of one's life. Fire regulations often prevent residents from bringing personal furniture into the homes. The nursing home is not a miniature hospital. Nursing homes are smaller and less well staffed than hospitals. Whereas a hospital has a ratio of greater than three staff for each bed, the nursing home has only about a sixth of that number, and most of those staff are aides. Whereas the distinction whereby nursing homes were certified as being capable of caring for patients with different needs based on these levels has been abandoned, the distinction between nursing home care and that provided in purely residential facilities with little or no nursing component has been retained. But even here the boundaries are blurred. Some forms of assisted living seek to serve a population that heavily overlaps the long-term care groups served by nursing homes.

Admission to a nursing home is very much a function of age (Fig. 15-5). There is a sharp rise in the rate of nursing home use with each decade after age 65, such that only about 1 percent of people age 65 to 74 are in nursing homes, but 5 percent of those age 74 to 85 and 20 percent of those age 85 or more are in nursing homes. Because this latter portion of the population is growing rapidly, there is great fear of being inundated with nursing home users.

The residents in nursing homes are distinguishable from older persons living in the community on several basic parameters. As shown in Table 15-3, in addition to being older, they are more likely to be white, female, unmarried, and have multiple chronic problems.

Nursing home users appear to have become more disabled in the last several years (Fig. 15-6). Some attribute this change to the impact of DRGs, but the trend had begun well in advance of that change. The contemporary nursing home user is older and more disabled than in the past.

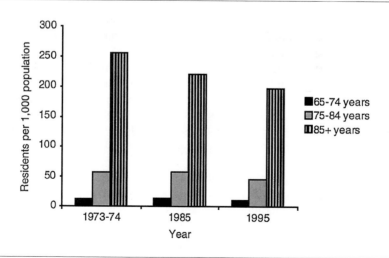

— FIGURE 15-5 — *Rate of nursing home use.* (From National Center for Health Statistics, 1997.)

TABLE 15-3   COMPARISON OF NURSING HOME RESIDENTS AND THE
NONINSTITUTIONALIZED POPULATION AGE 65+, 1995

	PERCENT OF NURSING HOME RESIDENTS*	PERCENT OF NONINSTITUTIONALIZED POPULATION[†]
Age (years)		
65–74	17.5	55.9
75–84	42.3	33.2
85+	40.2	10.8
Sex		
Male	24.7	40.8
Female	75.3	59.2
Race		
White	89.5	89.6
Black	8.5	8.1
Other	2.0	2.3
Marital status		
Married	16.5	56.9
Widowed	66.0	33.2
Divorced and/ or separated	5.5	5.7
Never married/single	11.1	4.2
Unknown	0.8	—

* From Dey, 1997.
[†] From US Census Bureau, 1996.

Any effort to describe the nursing home resident population must recognize that the nursing home plays multiple roles. It caters to a wide variety of clientele. At least five distinct groups of residents can be identified.

1. Those actively recuperating or being rehabilitated. These are largely persons discharged from hospitals and are expected to have a short course in the nursing home before returning home. This care has been called "subacute" or "transitional." The evidence of the nursing home's capacity to provide effective care of this type is mixed (Kramer et al., 1997; Kane et al., 1996).
2. Those with substantial physical dependencies. These residents need regular and usually frequent assistance during the day. Their care could be managed in the community with sufficient formal and informal support.

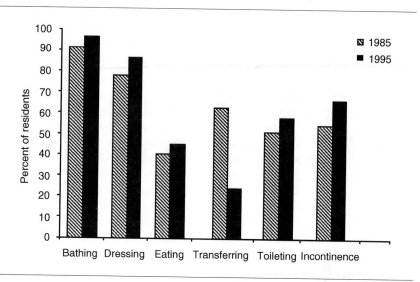

— FIGURE 15-6 — *Percent of nursing home residents older than 65 years of age who are receiving assistance with activities of daily living.* (From Dey, 1997, and Hing et al., 1989.)

3. Those with primarily severe cognitive losses. These people present special management problems because of their behavior and their propensity to wander. Some favor separate facilities for them, primarily to remove them from the environment of those who are cognitively intact. There is no evidence of improvement in the outcomes of demented residents from these "special care units."
4. Those receiving terminal care. This hospice care is directed toward making the person as comfortable as possible. Palliative care is provided but no heroic efforts are undertaken.
5. Those in a permanent vegetative state. This group is distinguished by its inability to relate to the environment. Care is primarily directed toward avoiding complications (e.g., decubitus ulcers).

For those who are sensitive to their environments and likely to be in the nursing home for some time (i.e., groups 2 and 4), quality-of-life issues will be at least as salient as traditional technical quality-of-care issues.

Especially in the wake of changing hospital practice and the rise of "subacute care," great care must be exercised in using nursing home data because of the differences in the characteristics of those entering or leaving and those resident at any point in time. The latter are more likely to have chronic problems such as dementia, whereas the former will have problems that are either rehabilitatable or fatal (e.g., hip fracture and cancer). This distinction makes it tricky to talk about nursing home patients and may explain the often contradictory data presented.

The problem with data about nursing home residents is made more confusing when different approaches to sampling are used. The characteristics of discharges are different from those of a cross-section of residents. The former have sorter lengths of stay, whereas the latter have a preponderance of dementia.

Payment for nursing home care has been increasingly based on measures that reflect the costs of providing that care. Although this type of payment is often called "prospective reimbursement," it is important to recognize that it is quite different from that used with hospitals. Nursing home prospective payment is calculated on a daily rate basis in contrast to the episode basis used for hospitals. Hence as a person's status changes, so does the payment. Medicare payments now use a daily prospective payment rate based on case mix and many states are adapting a corresponding approach for Medicaid payments, although the specific systems may use fewer categories. This form of case-mix reimbursement is largely driven by the costs of the nursing personnel who provide that care. The costs are usually calculated by estimating these costs based on a set of observed times spent by different types of personnel (nurses aides, LPNs, and RNs) for different classes of residents. In some cases, the time spent is self-reported by the staff; in other instances, it is based on observations. These data are then used to construct models that relate the cost of professional time to the characteristics of the clients. This approach has two major problems.

1. The models generally rely on looking at what kind of care is being given rather than what sort of care is actually needed; the care is not related to outcomes obtained nor is it based on any models of especially good care.
2. The logic behind this approach to estimating payments is inherently perverse. If carried to its logical extreme, this system of payment rewards nursing homes for residents becoming more dependent instead of more independent.

The most commonly used case-mix system is the Resource Utilization Groups (RUGS). Since its development for use in New York, it has been revised several times and is now linked to a form of the Minimum Data Set (MDS), which is the mandated assessment approach for nursing home care. Figure 15-7 illustrates the RUGS-III approach to classifying nursing home residents according to groups that imply different levels of staffing needs. This approach has been used by some Medicaid programs and is the basis for Medicare skilled nursing facility payments.

The physician's role in nursing home care is discussed in greater detail in Chap. 16. Suffice it to say here that the nursing home has not been an attractive place for physicians to practice. However, conditions are changing. The physician can play a critical role in setting the tone for the care of patients in the nursing home. Physicians' expectations of professional performance and their advocacy of their patients' needs can be very influential in shaping staff behavior.

New types of personnel can be used effectively to deliver primary care to nursing home patients. Nurse practitioners and physician assistants deliver high-quality care in this setting (Kane et al., in press). Medicare regulations covering

Part B were altered to allow greater use of physician assistants and nurse practitioners. Similarly, clinical pharmacists are very helpful for simplifying drug regimens and avoiding potential drug interactions.

A managed care program directed specifically at nursing home patients points to the art of the possible. Building on the prior successes of using nurse practitioners as key figures to provide primary care to nursing home residents, the Evercare program has developed Medicare managed care risk contracts specifically for long-stay nursing home patients. Under this arrangement, Evercare is responsible for all the residents' Medicare costs (both Part A and Part B) but not their nursing home costs. The underlying concept is that by providing more aggressive primary care they can prevent hospital admissions.

Evercare places nurse practitioners in each participating nursing home to work with the residents' own physicians. The nurse practitioners provide closer follow up and work closely with the nursing home staff to identify problems early. In some cases, Evercare will pay the nursing home extra to increase nursing attention for patients in order to treat that person in the nursing home rather than admitting the patient to a hospital. The theory is that the savings from avoided or shortened hospital stays will offset the added costs of more attentive primary care provided by the nurse practitioners. The apparent success of the Evercare model has spawned similar approaches.

A study by the Institute of Medicine pointed to the need for reforms, many of which were incorporated into Omnibus Budget Reconciliation Act of 1987 (OBRA 1987). The implementation of the OBRA 1987 regulations has produced a number of changes in the way nursing homes are operated. In addition to the standardized assessment mandated in the Minimum Data Set (described in Chap. 16), the emphasis in regulation has shifted more toward addressing the outcomes of patient care; but some increases in process measures have also been introduced. For example, guidelines for the use of psychoactive drugs have been mandated. All residents admitted and already living in the nursing home must be screened to determine if they are there primarily because of chronic mental illness. If so, a specific plan of care must be developed with appropriate participation from mental health professionals. Those residents who do not require skilled care are supposed to be transferred to more appropriate care settings. More training is mandated for nurses' aides and the staffing requirements overall have been upgraded.

Data elements from the MDS have been used to create a series of quality indicators, which are antedated to reflect potential areas of poor care in need of further exploration by state surveyors (Zimmerman et al., 1995). In a move to foster informed consumer choice, some of these quality indicators are now being posted on Web sites to provide consumers and their families with better information about the quality of nursing home care.

New models of nursing home care are being developed despite regulatory constraints on creativity. In some settings, large institutions are being converted into smaller living communities, where residents exert more control over their

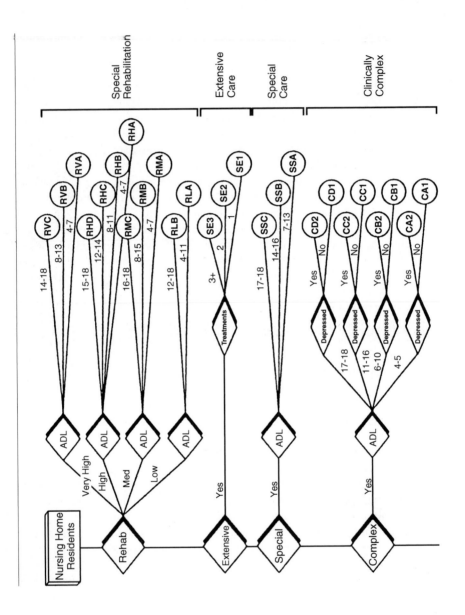

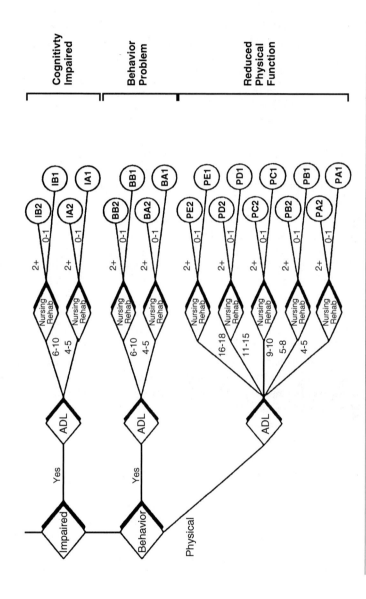

— FIGURE 15-7 — *The Resource Utilization Group (RUG-III) case-mix classification system. RUGs are generated from items in the Minimum Data Set (MDS) and used as a basis for case-mix reimbursement.* (Figures supplied by Dr. Brant Fries.)

lives. The Eden Alternative has provided a model for how to humanize nursing home care. The Wellspring Movement is trying to pursue a quality improvement agenda by empowering nursing home staff to take greater responsibility for identifying ways to improve care. Although both are attractive concepts, neither has yet been shown to produce dramatic improvements in residents' quality of care or quality of life.

ASSISTED LIVING

A new form of chronic care is emerging. "Assisted living" describes a form of care for many of those persons who currently require nursing home care. It is designed to provide services to persons as they require them, in a setting that more closely resembles a person's home. In effect, service recipients need not lose their personhood and their autonomy to get care. Residents still live in institutional settings that house many people within the same facility, thus maximizing efficiency of service delivery. They use common facilities, such as a dining room, but they also retain their privacy. Basically, each resident is treated as a tenant and has control over a living unit. At a minimum, each individually occupied dwelling unit contains space for living and sleeping, a bathroom, and at least minimal cooking facilities. (The stove can be disconnected for those for whom it might pose a serious danger.) Each unit can be locked by the occupant.

Under this approach, control is shifted toward empowering the recipient of care. In contrast to the situation in a nursing home, where residents are expected to conform to the norms of the institution, in an assisted living facility individualized care is stressed. As the tenant, the resident has control over the use of her space: care providers must be invited in; care plans must be accepted by the resident. These shifts, while subtle at one level, are fundamental at another. They imply a dramatically altered approach to care, some of which is tangible and some of which is not. The lore of nursing homes is laden with evidence of learned helplessness and enforced dependency. This approach to care is aimed at maximizing a resident's sense of self and independence as much as possible.

Especially for those chronically impaired persons who have retained an appreciation of their environment, such a philosophy of care makes great sense. Examples of such care are becoming more prevalent. Assisted living is able to serve quite disabled persons although most recipients are less impaired. The majority of assisted living exists as a privately paid service. Medicaid in most states has been slow to cover this service, and where it has, it covers only the services component, leaving Social Security and welfare payments to address the room and board costs.

The costs of assisted living are usually much less than comparable nursing home care. One reason that assisted living is less expensive and more flexible is that it has thus far been spared the heavy regulatory mantle laid on nursing homes.

Staffing patterns are not as intense or as professionally dictated. Staff performs multiple functions. If it is regulated in the same way, it will inevitably come to resemble nursing home care.

Once again, the form of care is determined by society's willingness to accept some risks. At a minimum, those who receive the care should have an opportunity to choose what kind of care they want to get.

At the same time, assisted living has come under criticisms reminiscent of those addressed at nursing homes in years past. With growth has come great variation. It is no longer clear just what is being offered by whom. Some standardized taxonomy is needed to allow consumers to make more informed choices. Concerns about quality are frequently expressed, especially with regard to the management of the more frail and medically complex residents.

HOME CARE

As already noted, we have developed a backward system of long-term care in this country that focuses on the nursing home. We tend to speak of the nursing home and alternatives to it, when we should begin with the premise that elderly people belong at home and want to be cared for at home. Institutional care will be needed in some cases, when the strain on caregivers is too great, but it should not be the resource of first resort. Our system has not evolved that way, and the resources available for home care are meager, but not so underdeveloped as to be ignored. Even today, most communities have at least some home care services, and more are likely to develop.

Home care involves at least two basic types of care: home health services; and homemaking and chore services. As shown in Table 15-4, different programs provide one or both types. Most elderly people treated at home require homemaking more than home health services.

Sometimes the differences between the two are purely arbitrary. If we consider that the homemaker replaces or supplements a family member, many of the tasks involved are extensions of home nursing (for example, supervising medication or giving baths). The definitions have emerged to fit the regulations governing a particular program. The physician will usually find that the home health agency is familiar with these regulations and how to deal with them.

The major problem at present is getting services. In response to political pressures, Medicare broadened its long-term care benefit (including waiving the former requirement that a person have a prior hospital stay of at least 3 days) and moved the program from Part B to Part A, thereby removing the copayment requirement. The subsequent enormous growth in home health care under Medicare has led to instituting prospective payment and making revisions in coverage that move part of the program back under Part B. (Home health care not related to a prior 3-day hospital stay, or visits after the 100th visit if related to a

TABLE 15-4   HOME CARE PROVIDED UNDER VARIOUS FEDERAL PROGRAMS

	Medicare	Medicaid	Title XX
Eligibility criteria	Must be homebound; need skilled care; need and expect benefit in a reasonable period; need certification by physician	State can use homebound criterion; not limited to skilled care; need certification by physician	Vary from state to state
Payment to provider	Final costs per episode based on functional status, case needs, and diagnoses	Varies with state	Three modes of payment possible: (1) direct provision by government agency; (2) contract with private agency; (3) independent provider
Services covered	Home health services, skilled nursing, physical or speech therapy as primary services; secondary services (social worker and home health aide) available *only* if primary service is provided; position of occupational therapy in service hierarchy ambiguous*	Limited home health care mandatory; expanded home care optional; personal care in home optional	Wide variety of home services allowed, including home health aide, homemaker, chore worker, meal services

* Occupational therapy is considered an "extended" secondary service, which may continue if needed after primary services are discontinued.

stay, will be covered under Part B.) Medicare covered home health care had been growing annually until the imposition of prospective payment in 1997.

Despite the growth in use, some still maintain that the criteria for eligibility for these services severely restricts their use. To get home health services for a patient, a physician must certify that the patient is homebound and that intermittent skilled care is likely to produce a benefit in a reasonable time. Thus, a large number of dependent older persons who need continuing home nursing but are "custodial" are ineligible unless the physician misrepresents their situation. *Skilled service* is defined as a skilled service offered by a nurse, a physical therapist, or a speech therapist.

If one of these establishing services is present, the patient may also receive the skilled services of an occupational therapist or medical social worker and/or the services of a home health aide if required by the plan. Medicare has begun to allow home health agencies to continue to serve clients who need case management, thus permitting some cases to remain open longer than the "intermittent" rule might otherwise imply. All reimbursed services must be given by a certified home health agency. (To be certified, the agency needs to offer nursing plus at least one of the five other services.) The requirement for using a certified agency greatly increases the costs of the services, although the assumption is that this certification assures at least a minimal level of professional oversight. A recurring question is how much administrative overhead is affordable as the pressure on the long-term care dollar grows.

Medicare-certified home health agencies are required to complete an OASIS (Outcome and Assessment Information Set) form at several stages of care to track outcomes and need for care. This recording burden has proven onerous for many agencies.

Medicaid funds can be used to provide home health care to persons eligible for nursing home care. Until recently, Medicaid funds have not been widely used for home care. In fact, until 1980, one state (New York) accounted for almost 95 percent of the Medicaid moneys spent on home health care. (It is still by far the largest user of Medicaid home care.) Home care under Medicaid must have a physician's authorization, but the patient need not be homebound, and the care need not be "skilled." All agencies delivering home care under Medicaid must meet Medicare certification standards, but if no organized home health agencies exist in a region, a registered nurse may be reimbursed for the services. Home care can be provided under two auspices under Medicaid. It is a mandated service and it can be part of a waivered service package (i.e., services authorized in lieu of nursing home care). In practice, states have often modeled their Medicaid home care benefits after the medically oriented Medicare benefit and thus restricted its use. Under Medicaid, the nursing care is a required component of home health services, and the state has the option to provide physical, occupational, and speech therapy; medical social services; and personal-care services. Medicaid allows homemaking assistance on a more generous basis than does Medicare. Personal-care services must be prescribed by a physician and supervised by a registered nurse. These services may not be delivered by persons related to the patient.

Recent changes in legislation have broadened the permissible use of Medicaid moneys to support a wide variety of long-term care services in an effort to reduce nursing home costs. A number of states have received waivers to develop this broader package of services in lieu of nursing home care, but most of these waivered services are limited in the numbers of "slots" they are allowed. The waivers require some evidence of budget neutrality. The assumption is that as more care is provided in the community, fewer people will use nursing homes.

Despite the growth of home care under Medicaid and the growing numbers of alternative waiver programs, the large bulk of Medicaid long-term care funds continue to flow to nursing homes. However, the relative dominance of spending on nursing home care varies widely from state to state. An analysis of 1996 data showed that only 18 percent of Medicaid long-term care expenditures go to home and community-based services; the proportion ranges from 44 percent (Oregon) to 0.05 percent (Pennsylvania). Nationally, total monthly expenditure on home and community-based services per person age 65+ was $247, with a range from $4137 (Alaska) to $16 (Tennessee). Nursing home Medicaid expenditures per person age 65+ likewise varied widely, from $2163 in New York to $343 in Nevada, with a national average of $893 (Ladd et al., 1999).

Additional support for homemaking services comes from Title III and Title XX. Title XX provides at least four methods of payment: local public agencies can provide the service directly; they can contract with agency providers (perhaps using competitive bidding); they can purchase services from agencies at negotiated prices; or they can permit the recipient to enter into agreement with independent providers, who do not work for an agency. It is possible to have all these arrangements operating in the same community.

This provision for independent vendors has prompted controversy because maintaining standards is difficult in the absence of any supervisory system or institutional responsibility. Under Title XX, an employment category known as *chore worker* has emerged; although performing functions similar to the home health aide and the homemaker, chore workers do not need to be tightly supervised and cannot be reimbursed under Medicare or Medicaid.

Persons eligible for cash assistance from the state, and other persons with low incomes and unmet service needs, are eligible for Title XX as long as 50 percent of a state's annual federal allotment is expended on those receiving cash assistance. Fees are charged to those whose family income exceeds 80 percent of the state's median income for a family of four.

Home services are one of four priority items under Title III of the Older Americans Act. Although the dollar volume is low, this source is important because means testing (whereby eligibility is set by income) is prohibited for programs under the Older Americans Act, making it possible to target a group that cannot afford private care but is ineligible for Title XX or Medicaid. Generally speaking, the Area Agency on Aging subcontracts for home care services rather than providing them directly. The usual pattern is that Administration on Aging dollars permit existing agencies to develop or expand a home care component. Services vary from area to area but can include personal care, homemaker service, chore service, and service for heavier jobs (e.g., minor home repairs or renovations, insect eradication, gardening, and painting). The provisions for assistance under the Area Agency on Aging are sharply limited by their constrained budgets and the competing demands for programs.

The extent of services under these several programs is still limited at present, although enthusiasm for in-home care is growing. The total sum of public dollars spent on home care remains only a fraction of that devoted to nursing homes.

OTHER SERVICES

A number of other modes of care can be tapped on behalf of elderly patients. Table 15-5 lists some of these services. However, despite their growing availability, they are still not widely used. The most frequently used service in that set is the senior center, a service designed for the well elderly person.

Day care can fulfill a number of needs. Most day care programs provide some combination of recreational and restorative activity. In contrast to senior centers, which are usually sponsored by recreational departments and targeted at the well elderly, day care programs serve persons with limited functional ability. Some are for cognitively impaired persons. The programs provide supervised activities, which may improve basic ADL skills and social skills. At the very least, they provide an important respite for the primary caregiver and thus may

TABLE 15-5   EXAMPLES OF COMMUNITY LONG-TERM CARE PROGRAMS

Home care (home nursing and homemaking)	Caregiver support
Adult day care	Congregate housing
Adult foster care	Home repairs
Assisted living	Meals (congregate and
Geriatric assessment	in-home)
Hospice/terminal care	Respite care
Telephone reassurance	Emergency alarms

make the critical difference for allowing an impaired older person to remain at home. To increase efficiency, most programs serve any given client fewer than 5 days a week, usually 2 or 3 days.

Other forms of day care can include a larger medical component. Some areas have developed day hospitals for seniors, where virtually all the services of the hospital are available on an ambulatory basis. Emphasis is usually placed on rehabilitation, especially occupational and physical therapy. The adult day health center is an intermediate model, which combines day care with nursing, physical therapy, and perhaps social work. Such sites can also be used for periodic ambulatory care clinics.

A problem common to all day-care programs is transportation. It is hard to arrange, expensive, and time-consuming. Special vans are usually needed, and, to avoid excessive travel times, services are usually confined to very limited areas.

In many communities, a variety of services exist to help seniors: ombudsmen, peer counselors, mental health clinics, transportation, congregate meal sites, and meals-on-wheels—just to name a few. Availability varies greatly from place to place. Good sources of information are the social work department in a hospital and the Area Agency on Aging.

The physician cannot be expected to know all the resources available for geriatric patients and will have to rely on other professionals to make appropriate arrangements to take advantage of them. But a physician should have a good sense of what can be done in general and what needs to be done for any particular patient. Often knowing what is needed but not locally available can lead to its development, particularly if responsible professionals take an active role on behalf of their patients.

Figure 15-7 summarizes the pattern of support for long-term care services to older persons.

CASE MANAGEMENT

The growing interest in the plethora of community long-term care services has sparked some concerns about the need to control use. A frequent answer is *case management*. This term has been widely and variably used. The basic components of case management are assessment, prescription, authorization, coordination, and monitoring.

These are issues very close to activities of primary care and hence may lead to some concern about role overlap between the case manager and the primary care physician. It is possible for physicians to serve as case managers, but most do not have the interest or the resources to perform this task. It is usually more efficient to look to other disciplines to perform this function but to recognize the important role of the physician in the overall care of the long-term care patient. Where a full range of geriatric services is available, case management is usually included.

Regardless of discipline, the case manager faces some difficult tasks. There is often a discrepancy between responsibility and authority. It is very different to prescribe, authorize, or mandate.

Case managers may or may not have the purchasing authority to pay for services they feel are necessary. Case managers may easily find themselves in the same bind as physicians. Specifically, they are expected to serve simultaneously as patient advocates and gatekeepers. The two roles are incompatible. For everyone's peace of mind, it is important to clarify at the outset who is the principal client. Because many decisions involve advocating on behalf of one group over another, this distinction is critical. It is very different to work on behalf of a client to obtain all the resources you believe they need than it is to work to distribute a fixed pool of resources to those who will best use them.

Another frequently heard concern about case management is the need to affix responsibility. On the one hand, the easiest way to do this is to give the case manager a budget and expect the case manager to work within it to achieve the most possible. However, some have expressed anxieties that the person charged with authorizing services should be at arm's length from those providing them. Specific concerns are heard about hospital discharge planners' decisions as to when to refer patients to services owned or operated by the hospital. There is a real potential for client skimming. Similarly, if the case manager works for a caregiving agency, there is the risk that that agency may get a disproportionate share of the choicest clients. On the other hand, even when case managers are separated from direct care, they are not immune to pressure from the purveyors, just as the physician is pursued by the drug companies.

Case management has also become a mainstay of managed care. In this context, cases are usually identified on the basis of some risk indicators—either a record of heavy use of services or the presence of risk factors that imply such a pattern in the future. While some case management within managed care is patient-centered, operating on the premise that closer care can stave off costly problems, much of it revolves around primarily utilization controls.

Several states have begun experimenting with a program called "cash and counseling." Modeled after successful programs in California and Europe, disabled seniors can receive direct cash payments for care, which they can, in turn, use to purchase services, including from relatives. There is still some uneasiness about just how much discretion such programs should allow, many still require limited choices of vendors and evidence that the funds were used for the intended purposes. Nonetheless, these efforts represent a new direction of giving frail older clients more leeway in how to obtain services.

_____

References

AARP Public Policy Institute, and The Lewin Group: *Out-of-Pocket Health Spending by Medicare Beneficiaries Age 65 and Older: 1997 Projections.* Washington, DC, American Association of Retired Persons, 1997.

Cutler DM: Declining disability among the elderly. *Health Aff (Millwood)* 20(6):11–27, 2001.

Dey AN: *Characteristics of Elderly Nursing Home Residents: Data from the 1995 National Nursing Home Survey. Advance Data from Vital and Health Statistics.* Hyattsville, MD, National Center for Health Statistics, 1997.

Eng C, Pedulla J, Eleazer GP, et al: Program of All-inclusive Care for the Elderly (PACE): an innovative model of integrated geriatric care and financing. *J Am Geriatr Soc* 45:223–232, 1997.

Hing E, Sekscenski E, Strahan G: *The National Nursing Home Survey; 1985 Summary for the United States.* [Vital and Health Statistics Series 13, No. 97, DHHS Pub. No. (PHS) 89-1758.] Washington, DC, U.S. Public Health Service, 1989.

Hoffman C, Rice D, Sung H-Y: Persons with chronic conditions: their prevalence and costs. *JAMA* 276:1473–1479, 1996.

Institute of Medicine: *Improving the Quality of Care in Nursing Homes.* Washington, DC, National Academy Press, 1986.

Kane RA: Long-term care and a good quality of life: bringing them closer together. *Gerontologist* 41(3):293–304, 2001.

Kane RA, Kane RL, Ladd R: *The Heart of Long-term Care.* New York, Oxford University Press, 1998.

Kane RA, Wilson KB: *Assisted Living in the United States: A New Paradigm for Residential Care for Older Persons?* Washington, DC, American Association of Retired Persons, 1993.

Kane RL: Managed care as a vehicle for delivering more effective chronic care for older persons. *J Am Geriatr Soc* 46:1034–1039, 1998.

Kane RL: Setting the PACE in chronic care. *Contemp Gerontol* 6(2):47–50, 1999.

Kane RL, Chen Q, Blewett LA, et al: Do rehabilitative nursing homes improve the outcomes of care? *J Am Geriatr Soc* 44:545–554, 1996.

Kane RL, Friedman B: State variations in Medicare expenditures. *Am J Public Health* 87:1611–1619, 1997a.

Kane RL, Garrard J, Skay CL, et al: Effects of a geriatric nurse practitioner on the process and outcomes of nursing home care. *Am J Public Health* 79:1271–1277, 1989.

Kane RL, Illston LH, Miller NA. Qualitative analysis of the Program of All-inclusive Care for the Elderly (PACE). *Gerontologist* 32:771–780, 1992.

Kane RL, Kane RA: A nursing home in your future? *N Engl J Med* 324:627–629, 1991.

Kane RL, Kane RA, Finch M, et al: S/HMOs, the second generation: building on the experience of the first social health maintenance organization demonstrations. *J Am Geriatr Soc* 45(1):101–107, 1997b.

Kane RL, Kane RA, Ladd RC, et al: Variation in state spending for long-term care: factors associated with more balanced systems. *J Health Polit Policy Law* 23:363–390, 1998.

Kane RL, Keckhafer G, Flood S, et al: The effect of Evercare on hospital use. *J Am Geriatr Soc* [In press].

Kennedy J, LaPlante MP, Kaye HS: Need for assistance in the activities of daily living. *Disabil Stat Abstr* 18:1–4, 1997.

Kosecoff J, Kahn KL, Rogers WH, et al: Prospective payment system and impairment at discharge. The "quicker-and-sicker" story revisited. *JAMA* 264:1980–1983, 1990.

Kramer AM, Steiner JF, Schlenker RE, et al: Outcomes and costs after hip fracture and stroke: a comparison of rehabilitation settings. *JAMA* 277:396–404, 1997.

Ladd RC, Kane RL, Kane RA: *State LTC Profiles Report, 1996.* Minneapolis, MN, University of Minnesota School of Public Health, 1999.

Manton KG, Corder L, Stallard L: Chronic disability trends in elderly US populations: 1982–1994. *Med Sci* 94:2593–2598, 1997.

Moon M: What Medicare has meant to older Americans. *Health Care Fin Rev* 18(2):49–59, 1996.

National Center for Health Statistics: *Health, United States, 1996–1997 and Injury Chartbook.* Hyattsville, MD, NCHS, 1997.

Phillips CD, Sloane PD, Hawes C, et al: Effects of residence in Alzheimer disease special care units on functional outcomes. *JAMA* 278:1340–1344, 1997.

Rich MW, Beckham V, Wittenberg C, et al: A multidisciplinary intervention to prevent the readmission of elderly patients with congestive heart failure. *N Engl J Med* 333:1190–1195, 1995.

Scanlon WJ: *Long-Term Care: Baby Boom Generation Presents Financing Challenges* (testimony before the Special Committee on Aging. US Senate) (GAO/T-HEHS- 98-107). Washington, DC, Health Financing and Systems Issues; Health, Education, and Human Services Division, 1998.

Spence DA, Wiener JM: Nursing home length of stay patterns: results from the 1985 national nursing home survey. *Gerontologist* 30(1):16–20, 1990.

US Census Bureau: *Statistical Abstract of the United States: 1996.* Washington, DC, US Government Printing Office, 1996.

US Department of Health and Human Services, HCFA, and Office of Research and Demonstrations: *Health Care Financing Review: Statistical Supplement, Table 16.* Baltimore, MD, USDHHS, 1997a.

US Department of Health and Human Services, HCFA, and Office Research and Demonstrations: *Health Care Financing Review: Statistical Supplement, Table 88.* Baltimore, MD, USDHHS, 1997b.

Welch HG, Wennberg DE, Welch WP: The use of Medicare home health services. *N Engl J Med* 335:324–329, 1996.

Wunderlich G S, Kohler P (eds): *Improving the Quality of Long-term Care. Report of the Institute of Medicine.* Washington, DC, National Academy Press, 2001.

Zimmerman DR, Karon SL, Arling G, et al: Development and testing of nursing home quality indicators. *Health Care Fin Rev* 16(4):107–127, 1995.

Suggested Readings

Boult C, Boult L, Pacala JT: Systems of care for older populations of the future. *J Am Geriatr Soc* 46:499–505, 1998.

Lachs MS, Ruchlin HS: Is managed care good or bad for geriatric medicine? *J Am Geriatr Soc* 45:1123–1127, 1997.

Morgan RO, Virnig BA, DeVito CA, et al: The Medicare–HMO revolving door—the healthy go in and the sick go out. *N Engl J Med* 337:169–175, 1997.

Pepper Commission: *A Call for Action: The Pepper Commission U.S. Bipartisan Commission on Comprehensive Health Care*. Washington, DC, US Government Printing Office, 1990.

Silverstone B, Hyman HK: *You & Your Aging Parent*. New York, Pantheon, 1976.

Vladeck BG: *Unloving Care: The Nursing Home Tragedy*. New York, Basic Books, 1980.

CHAPTER 16

NURSING HOME CARE

The focus of this chapter is the clinical care of nursing home residents. Some of the basic demographic and economic aspects of nursing home care are discussed in Chaps. 2 and 15. The poor quality of care provided in many nursing homes has been recognized for decades (Vladek, 1980). Since the Institute of Medicine issued its critical report in 1986 (Institute of Medicine, 1986) and the mandating of the Resident Assessment Instrument in 1987, the overall quality of care has improved somewhat. A more recent Institute of Medicine report, however, indicates there is still considerable room for further improvements in care quality (Institute of Medicine, 2000).

Despite the logistic, economic, and attitudinal barriers that can foster inadequate medical care in the nursing home, many straightforward principles and strategies can lead to improvements in the quality of medical care provided to nursing home residents. Fundamental to achieving these improvements is a clear perspective on the goals of nursing home care, which are in many respects quite different from the goals of medical care in other settings and patient populations.

THE GOALS OF NURSING HOME CARE

The modern nursing home serves multiple roles. Table 16-1 lists the key goals of nursing home care. While the prevention, identification, and treatment of chronic, subacute, and acute medical conditions are important, most of these goals focus on the functional independence, autonomy, quality of life, comfort, and dignity of the residents. Physicians who care for nursing home residents must keep these goals in perspective at the same time the more traditional goals of medical care are being addressed.

The heterogeneity of the nursing home population must also be recognized in order to focus and individualize the goals of care. This heterogeneity results in a diversity of goals for nursing home care. Nursing home residents can be subgrouped into five basic types (Fig. 16-1). While it is not always possible to isolate these different types of residents geographically, and although residents often overlap or change between the types described, subgrouping nursing home residents in

TABLE 16-1   GOALS OF NURSING HOME CARE

1. Provide a safe and supportive environment for chronically ill and
   dependent people
2. Restore and maintain the highest possible level of functional
   independence
3. Preserve individual autonomy
4. Maximize quality of life, perceived well-being, and life satisfaction
5. Provide comfort and dignity for terminally ill patients and their loved
   ones
6. Stabilize and delay progression, whenever possible, of chronic medical
   conditions
7. Prevent acute medical and iatrogenic illnesses, and identify and treat
   them rapidly when they do occur

this manner will help the physician and interdisciplinary team to focus the care-planning process on the most critical and realistic goals for individual residents.

The underlying social contract implied by nursing home admission is quite different for each of these groups. In some cases, access to treatment takes precedence over the living environment; in other circumstances, the environment may be the most critical element of care. Those admitted to a nursing home with the intent of active treatment and discharge home may be willing to accept a living situation akin to that of a hospital in the expectation that the benefit they receive from treatment will offset any discomfort or inconvenience. For terminally ill persons under the hospice model, the living environment is made as flexible and supportive as possible. Efforts are directed toward making these patients comfortable and permitting them to enjoy their last days.

There is a trend to separate the cognitively impaired from those who are primarily physically impaired. There is a growing number of special care units (SCUs) for the cognitively impaired where their care can be coordinated to maximize attention to the behavioral aspects of dementia care and to minimize the use of psychoactive drugs and restraints while maintaining a safe environment. Some see SCUs as a way of achieving better results. Others view them as controlled environments in which demented residents can be treated more humanely by staff who have chosen to concentrate on such care. Still others see the primary gain from SCUs as removing otherwise disruptive patients from the environment of those still alert enough to resent the intrusion. There are no strong data, however, that demonstrate major improvements in outcomes of patients treated on these units.

Residents who are more cognitively intact may benefit from newer forms of institutional care such as assisted living (described in Chap. 15). These residents

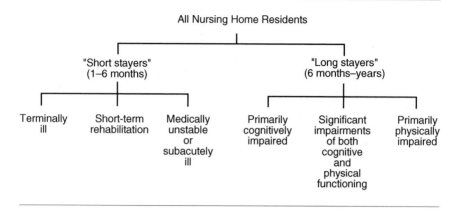

— FIGURE 16-1 —   *Basic types of nursing home patients.*

can maximize their quality of life in individual rooms that afford them privacy and a greater sense of control over their surroundings. Those residents who are, for all intents and purposes, completely out of touch with their environments (e.g., those in permanent vegetative states or advanced dementia) may be well served by simple environments designed to maintain them safely. These individuals are the subject of increasing ethical debate (see Chap. 17).

CLINICAL ASPECTS OF CARE FOR NURSING HOME RESIDENTS

In addition to the different goals for care in the nursing home, several factors make the assessment and treatment of nursing home residents different from those in other settings (Table 16-2). Many of these factors relate to the process of care and are discussed in the following section. (For a more complete discussion of medical care in the nursing home, see the suggested readings and Ouslander et al., 1997.) A fundamental difference in the nursing home is that medical evaluation and treatment must be complemented by an assessment and care-planning process involving staff from multiple disciplines. The integral involvement of nurses' aides in the development and implementation of care plans is crucial to high-quality nursing home care. Data on medical conditions and their treatment are integrated with assessments of the functional, mental, and behavioral status of the resident in order to develop a comprehensive data base and individualized plan of care.

Medical evaluation and clinical decision making for nursing home residents are complicated for several reasons. Unless the physician has cared for the resident

TABLE 16-2   FACTORS THAT MAKE ASSESSMENT AND TREATMENT IN THE
NURSING HOME DIFFERENT FROM THAT IN OTHER SETTINGS

1. The goals of care are often different (see Table 16-1)
2. Specific clinical disorders are prevalent among nursing home residents
   (see Table 16-3)
3. The approach to health maintenance and prevention differs (see Table 16-6)
4. Mental and functional status are just as important, if not more so, than
   medical diagnoses
5. Assessment must be interdisciplinary, including:
   a. Nursing
   b. Psychosocial
   c. Rehabilitation
   d. Nutritional
   e. Other (e.g., dental, pharmacy, podiatry, audiology, ophthalmology)
6. Sources of information are variable:
   a. Residents often cannot give a precise history
   b. Family members and nurses' aides with limited assessment skills
      may provide the most important information
   c. Information is often obtained over the telephone
7. Administrative procedures for record keeping in both nursing homes and
   acute care hospitals can result in inadequate and disjointed information
8. Clinical decision making is complicated for several reasons:
   a. Many diagnostic and therapeutic procedures are expensive, unavail-
      able, or difficult to obtain and involve higher risks of iatrogenic ill-
      ness and discomfort than are warranted by the potential outcome
   b. The potential long-term benefits of "tight" control of certain chronic
      illnesses (e.g., diabetes mellitus, congestive heart failure, hyperten-
      sion) may be outweighed by the risks of iatrogenic illness in many
      very old and functionally disabled residents
   c. Many residents are not capable (or are questionably capable) of par-
      ticipating in medical decision making, and their personal preferences
      based on previous decisions are often unknown (see Table 16-7)
9. The appropriate site for and intensity of treatment are often difficult
   decisions involving medical, emotional, ethical, economic, and legal
   considerations that may be in conflict with each other in the nursing
   home setting
10. Logistic considerations, resource constraints, and restrictive reimburse-
    ment policies may limit the ability of and incentives for physicians to
    carry out optimal medical care of nursing home residents

before nursing home admission, it may be difficult to obtain a comprehensive medical data base. Residents may be unable to relate their medical histories accurately or to describe their symptoms, and medical records are frequently unavailable or incomplete, especially for residents who have been transferred between nursing homes and acute-care hospitals. When acute changes in status occur, initial assessments are often performed by nursing home staff with limited skills and are transmitted to physicians by telephone. Even when the diagnoses are known or strongly suspected, many diagnostic and therapeutic procedures among nursing home residents are associated with an unacceptably high risk:benefit ratio. For example, a barium enema may cause dehydration or severe fecal impaction; nitrates and other cardiovascular drugs may precipitate syncope or disabling falls in frail ambulatory residents with baseline postural hypotension; and adequate control of blood sugar may be extremely difficult to achieve without a high risk for hypoglycemia among cognitively impaired diabetic residents with marginal or fluctuating nutritional intake who may not recognize or complain of hypoglycemic symptoms.

Further compounding these difficulties is the inability of many nursing home residents to participate effectively in important decisions regarding their medical care. Their previously expressed wishes are often not known, and an appropriate or legal surrogate decision maker has often not been appointed. These issues are discussed further on in this chapter and in Chap. 17.

Table 16-3 lists the most commonly encountered clinical disorders in the nursing home population. They represent a broad spectrum of chronic medical illnesses; neurological, psychiatric, and behavioral disorders; and problems that are especially prevalent in frail older adults (e.g., incontinence, falls, nutritional disorders, chronic pain syndromes). Although the incidence of iatrogenic illnesses has not been systematically studied in nursing homes, it is likely to be as high as or higher than that in acute-care hospitals. The management of many of the conditions listed in Table 16-3 is discussed in some detail in other chapters of this text (for specific conditions, see Table of Contents and Index).

In addition to the numerous factors already mentioned that render the medical assessment and treatment of these conditions different, the process of care in nursing homes also differs substantially from that in acute care hospitals, clinics, and home care settings.

PROCESS OF CARE IN THE NURSING HOME

The process of care in nursing homes is strongly influenced by numerous state and federal regulations, the highly interdisciplinary nature of nursing home residents' problems, and the training and skills of the staff that delivers most of the hands-on care. Federal rules and regulations contained in the Omnibus Budget Reconciliation Act of 1987 (OBRA 1987) and implemented in 1991 place heavy

TABLE 16-3   COMMON CLINICAL DISORDERS IN THE NURSING HOME
POPULATION

Medical conditions
    Chronic medical illnesses
    Congestive heart failure
    Degenerative joint disease
    Diabetes mellitus
    Obstructive lung disease
    Renal failure
    Infections
        Lower respiratory tract
        Urinary tract
        Skin (pressure sores, vascular ulcers)
        Conjunctivitis
        Gastroenteritis
    Gastrointestinal disorders
        Reflux esophagitis
        Constipation
        Diarrhea

Malignancies

Neuropsychiatric conditions
    Dementia
    Behavioral disorders associated with dementia
        Wandering
        Agitation
        Aggression
        Depression

Neurological disorders other than dementia
    Stroke
    Parkinsonism
    Multiple sclerosis
    Brain or spinal cord injury

Functional disabilities necessitating rehabilitation
    Stroke
    Hip fracture
    Joint replacement
    Amputation

TABLE 16-3   COMMON CLINICAL DISORDERS IN THE NURSING HOME
POPULATION (*Continued*)

Geriatric problems
    Delirium
    Incontinence
    Gait disturbances, instability, falls
    Malnutrition, feeding difficulties, dehydration
    Pressure sores
    Insomnia
Chronic pain: musculoskeletal conditions, neuropathies, malignancy
Iatrogenic disorders
    Adverse drug reactions
    Falls
    Nosocomial infections
    Induced disabilities
    Restraints and immobility, catheters, unnecessary help with basic
        activities of daily living
Death and dying

emphasis on assessment and care planning as a means of achieving the highest practicable level of functioning for each resident and the use of the Resident Assessment Instrument.

Physician involvement in nursing home care and the nature of medical assessment and treatment offered to nursing home residents are often limited by logistic and economic factors. Few physicians have offices based either inside the nursing home or in close proximity to the facility. Many physicians who do visit nursing homes care for relatively small numbers of residents, often in several different facilities. Many nursing homes, therefore, have numerous physicians who make rounds once or twice per month, who are not generally present to evaluate acute changes in resident status, and who attempt to assess these changes over the telephone. In some areas, practice patterns are shifting to a model of physician–nurse practitioner practices caring for large numbers of residents in several nursing homes. Many nursing homes do not have ready availability of laboratory, radiologic, and pharmacy services with the capability of rapid response, further compounding the logistics of evaluating and treating acute changes in medical status. Thus, nursing home residents are often sent to hospital emergency rooms, where they are evaluated by personnel who are generally not familiar with their baseline status and who frequently lack training and interest in the care of frail and dependent elderly patients.

Restrictive Medicare and Medicaid reimbursement policies may also dictate certain patterns of nursing home care. While physicians are required to visit nursing home residents only every 30 to 60 days, many residents require more frequent assessment and monitoring of treatment—especially with the shorter acute-care hospital stays brought about by the prospective payment system. While Medicare reimbursement for physician visits in nursing homes has improved, reimbursement for a routine visit is generally inadequate for the time that is required to provide good medical care in the nursing home, including travel to and from the facility; assessment and treatment planning for residents with multiple problems; communication with members of the interdisciplinary team and the resident's family; and proper documentation in the medical record. Activities often essential to good care in the nursing home, such as attendance at interdisciplinary conferences, family meetings, complex assessments of decision-making capacity, and counseling residents and surrogate decision makers on treatment plans in the event of terminal illness, are generally not reimbursable at all. Medicare intermediaries restrict reimbursement for rehabilitative services for residents not covered under Part A skilled care, thus limiting the treatment options for many residents. Although Medicaid programs vary considerably, many provide minimal coverage for ancillary services that are critical for optimum medical care, and may restrict reimbursement for several types of drugs that may be especially helpful for nursing home residents.

Amid these logistic and economic constraints, expectations for the care of nursing home residents are high. Table 16-4 outlines the various types of assessment generally recommended for the optimal care of nursing home residents. Physicians are responsible for completing an initial assessment within 72 hours of admission and for arranging for monthly visits thereafter for the next 90 days. Licensed nurses assess new residents as soon as they are admitted, on a daily basis, and generally summarize the status of each resident weekly. The nationally mandated Minimum Data Set (MDS) must be completed within 14 days of admission and updated when a major change in status occurs; several sections must be routinely updated on a quarterly basis.

The extent of involvement of other disciplines in the assessment and care-planning process varies depending on the residents' problems, the availability of various professionals, and state regulations. Representatives from nursing, social services, dietary management, activities, and rehabilitation therapy (physical and/or occupational) participate in an interdisciplinary care-planning meeting. Residents are generally discussed at this meeting within 2 weeks of admission and quarterly thereafter. The product of these meetings is an interdisciplinary care plan that separately lists interdisciplinary problems (e.g., restricted mobility, incontinence, wandering, diminished food intake, poor social interaction), goals for the resident related to the problem, approaches to achieving these goals, target dates for achieving the goals, and assignment of responsibilities for working toward the goals among the various disciplines. These care plans are an important force in driving nursing staff behavior and expectations and should be reviewed by the primary physician.

TABLE 16-4   IMPORTANT ASPECTS OF VARIOUS TYPES OF ASSESSMENT IN THE NURSING HOME

TYPE OF ASSESSMENT	TIMING	MAJOR OBJECTIVES	IMPORTANT ASPECTS
Medical Initial	Within 72 h of admission	Verify medical diagnoses Document baseline physical findings, mental and functional status, vital signs, and skin condition Attempt to identify potentially remediable, previously unrecognized medical conditions Get to know the resident and family (if this is a new resident) Establish goals for the admission and a medical treatment plan	A thorough review of medical records and physical examinations is necessary Relevant medical diagnoses and baseline findings should be clearly and concisely documented in the patient's record Medication lists should be carefully reviewed and only essential medications continued Request for specific types of assessment and input from other disciplines should be made A data base should be established (see example in Fig. 16-2)
Periodic	Monthly or every other month	Monitor progress of active medical conditions Update medical orders Communicate with patient and nursing home staff	Progress notes should include clinical data relevant to active medical conditions and focus on changes in status Unnecessary medications, orders for care, and laboratory tests should be discontinued

TABLE 16-4 IMPORTANT ASPECTS OF VARIOUS TYPES OF ASSESSMENT IN THE NURSING HOME (*Continued*)

TYPE OF ASSESSMENT	TIMING	MAJOR OBJECTIVES	IMPORTANT ASPECTS
			Mental, functional, and psychosocial status should be reviewed with nursing home staff and changes from baseline noted
			The medical problem list should be updated
As needed	When acute changes in status occur	Identify and treat causes of acute changes	Onsite clinical assessment by the physician (or nurse practitioner or physician's assistant), as opposed to telephone consultations, will result in more accurate diagnoses, more appropriate treatment, and fewer unnecessary emergency room visits and hospitalization
			Vital signs, food and fluid intake, and mental status often provide essential information
			Infection, dehydration, and adverse drug effects should be at the top of the differential diagnosis for acute changes in status
Major reassessment	Annual	Identify and document any significant changes in status and new potentially remediable conditions	Targeted physical examination and assessment of mental, functional, and psychosocial status and selected laboratory tests should be done (see Table 16-6)

Discipline	Timing	Tasks	Comments
Nursing	On admission, and then routinely with monitoring of daily and weekly progress; complete Minimum Data Set (MDS) within 14 days, update when major change in status occurs and annually; update selected sections quarterly	Identify biopsychosocial and functional status strengths and weaknesses Develop an individualized care plan Document baseline data for ongoing assessments	Particular attention should be given to emotional state, personal preferences, and sensory function Careful observation during the first few days of admission is important to detect effects of relocation Potential problems related to other disciplines should be recorded and communicated to appropriate members of the interdisciplinary care team
Psychosocial	Within 1-2 weeks of admission and as needed thereafter	Identify any potentially serious psychosocial signs and symptoms and refer to mental health professional if appropriate Determine past social history, family relationships, and social resources Become familiar with personal preferences regarding living arrangements	Getting to know the family and their preferences and concerns is critical to good nursing home care Relevant psychosocial data should be communicated to the interdisciplinary team
Rehabilitation (physical and occupational therapy)	Within days of admission and daily or weekly thereafter (depending on the rehabilitation program)	Determine functional status as it relates to basic activities of daily living Identify specific goals and time frame for improving specific areas of function Monitor progress toward goals	Small gains in functional status can improve chances for discharge as well as quality of life Not all residents have areas in which they can reasonably be expected to improve; strategies to maintain function should be developed for these residents

TABLE 16-4 IMPORTANT ASPECTS OF VARIOUS TYPES OF ASSESSMENT IN THE NURSING HOME (*Continued*)

TYPE OF ASSESSMENT	TIMING	MAJOR OBJECTIVES	IMPORTANT ASPECTS
		Assess progress in relation to potential discharge	Assessment of and recommendation for modifying the environment can be critically important for improving function and discharge planning
Nutritional	Within days of admission and then periodically thereafter	Determine nutritional status and needs Identify dietary preferences Plan an appropriate diet	Restrictive diets may not be medically necessary and can be unappetizing Weight loss should be identified and reported to nursing and medical staff
Interdisciplinary care plan	Within 1–2 weeks of admission and every 3 months thereafter	Identify interdisciplinary problems Establish goals and treatment plans Determine when maximum progress toward goals has been reached	Each discipline should prepare specific plans for communication to other team members based on their own assessment
Capacity for medical decision making*	Within days of admission and then whenever changes in status occur	Determine which types of medical decisions resident is capable of participating in A resident who is still capable of making decisions independently should be encouraged to identify a surrogate decision maker in the event the resident later loses this decision-making capacity	Residents with varying degrees of dementia may still be capable of participating in many decisions regarding their medical care Attention should be given to potentially reversible factors that can interfere with decision-making capacity (e.g., depression, fear, delirium, metabolic and drug effects)

Preferences regarding treatment intensity* and nursing home routines	Within days of admission and periodically thereafter	Determine residents' wishes as to the intensity of treatment they would want in the event of acute or chronic progressive illness	If the resident lacks capacity for many or all decisions, appropriate surrogate decision makers should be identified (if not already done)
			Attempt to identify specific procedures the resident would or would not want
			This assessment is often made by ascertaining the resident's prior expressed wishes (if known), or through surrogate decision makers (legal guardian, durable power of attorney for health care, family)
			Family and health professional concerns should be considered, but the resident's desires should be paramount
			The resident's capacity may fluctuate over time because of physical and emotional conditions

* See Table 16-7 and Chap. 17.

– 437 –

The MDS is intended to assist nursing home staff in identifying important clinical problems and to trigger the use of Resident Assessment Protocols (RAPs), which have been developed for 18 common clinical conditions. The MDS and the RAPs are critical tools for developing individual care plans. The interdisciplinary care-planning process serves as a cornerstone for resident management in many facilities, but is a difficult and time-consuming process that requires leadership and tremendous interdisciplinary (and interpersonal) cooperation.

Staffing limitations in relation to the amount of time and effort required makes intensive interdisciplinary care planning and teamwork unrealistic in many nursing homes. Although physicians are seldom directly involved in the care-planning meetings in most facilities, they are generally required to review and sign the care plan, and may find the team's perspective very valuable in planning subsequent medical care.

Implementation of the OBRA 1987 regulations primarily affects the activities of the nursing home staff. But some aspects of these regulations have a direct bearing on physicians who are caring for nursing home residents. Several of the RAPs require involvement of the physician in the evaluation and management of common geriatric conditions seen in nursing home residents (e.g., delirium, incontinence). The RAPs do not directly address many common medical conditions (e.g., congestive heart failure, arthritis, infections) that must be identified and managed outside the MDS/RAP paradigm. Perhaps the most direct effect on physicians relates to the specifications around the use of psychoactive medications. OBRA 1987 defines criteria for appropriate use of these medications, and requires the documentation of specific diagnoses as well as the quantitative documentation of the response of target behavioral symptoms to these drugs. Psychoactive medications can no longer be used simply as a means to control symptoms of aggressive or disruptive behavior (i.e., as "chemical restraints"), or on a continued as-needed basis. These rules have stimulated a rethinking of psychoactive drug use among nursing home residents, and there is evidence that the prescription of these drugs has changed since OBRA 1987 went into effect (Llorente et al., 1998). The appropriate use of antipsychotics for patients with dementia and psychosis must be distinguished from the use of drugs as "chemical restraints." Physician attention is also directed to the use of physical restraints. In keeping with changing attitudes about such care, the use of these restraints is generally discouraged. Restraints can be applied only upon a physician's order and only after documenting that less restrictive measures are not effective. Physical restraints can be safely removed from most residents (Evans et al., 1997). While not all residents can be free of restraints at all times, a restraint-free environment is an appropriate goal in the nursing home setting.

The general pressure for better documentation of care and assessments should provide a welcome improvement in the quality of care for nursing home residents. These rules will inevitably mean that physicians will be asked to make more detailed clinical notes, especially with respect to indicating the underlying reasons for their actions.

Although these changes may place a modest added burden on the attending physician, they do not demand a great deal of extra effort and should help to provide a better environment in which to practice.

STRATEGIES TO IMPROVE MEDICAL CARE IN NURSING HOMES

Several strategies might improve the process of medical care delivered to nursing home residents. Four strategies are briefly described: (1) the use of improved documentation practices; (2) a systematic approach to screening, health maintenance, and preventive practices for the frail, dependent nursing home population; (3) the use of nurse practitioners or physicians' assistants; and (4) use of practice guidelines and related quality improvement activities.

In addition to these strategies, strong leadership of a medical director who is appropriately trained and dedicated to improving the facilities' quality of medical care is essential in order to develop, implement, and monitor policies and procedures for medical services. The role of the medical director in nursing homes is discussed in detail elsewhere (see the suggested readings). The medical director should set standards for medical care and serve as an example to the medical staff by caring for some of the residents in the facility. The medical director should also be involved in various committees (pharmacy, infection control, quality assurance), and should involve interested medical staff in these committees, as well as in educational efforts through formal in-service presentations, teaching rounds, and appropriate documentation procedures.

The federal government's approach to improving the quality of care in nursing homes is based on the OBRA 1987 rules, and the MDS and RAPs in particular. Computerized MDS data is now used to generate selected quality indicators and to identify outlier facilities that may require targeted evaluation (Zimmerman et al., 1995). While some data suggest that various aspects of nursing home care have improved since the implementation of the OBRA 1987 rules and regulations, many caveats about these early data have been voiced (Ouslander, 1997). Other approaches to improving quality will be necessary to complement the OBRA rules and regulations (Kane, 1998).

Documentation Practices

Nursing home residents often have multiple coexisting medical problems and long previous medical histories. Residents often cannot relate their medical histories, and their previous medical records are frequently unavailable or incomplete. There is also a danger in perpetuating old diagnoses that are inaccurate. This is especially true for psychiatric diagnoses, but may also occur for other medical diagnoses such as congestive heart failure and stroke. Thus, it is difficult and sometimes impossible to obtain a comprehensive medical data base. The effort should, however, be invested and not wasted. Critical aspects of the medical data base should be recorded on one page or face sheet of the medical record. Figure 16-2 shows an example of a format for a face sheet. Additional standardized documentation should contain social information, such as individuals to contact at critical times and information about the resident's treatment status in the event of acute illness. These data are essential to the care of the resident and should be readily available in one place in the record, so that when emergencies arise, when medical consultants see the resident, or when members of the interdisciplinary team need an overall perspective, they are easy to locate. The face sheet should be copied and sent to the hospital or other health care facilities to which the resident might be transferred. Time and effort is required in order to keep the face sheet updated. For facilities with access to computers and/or word processing, incorporating the face sheet into a database should be relatively easy and facilitate its rapid completion and periodic updating.

Medical documentation in progress notes for routine visits and assessments of acute changes is frequently scanty and/or illegible. Statements such as "stable" or "no change" are too frequently the only documentation for routine visits. While time constraints may preclude extensive notes, certain standard information should be documented. The SOAP (*s*ubjective, *o*bjective, *a*ssessment, *p*lan) format for charting routine notes is especially appropriate for nursing home residents (Table 16-5). Simple forms, flow sheets, or databases with word-processing capabilities can be used to enable physicians to efficiently produce legible, concise, yet comprehensive progress notes. Another tool for documenting change in residents over time is the benchmark approach using flow sheets (see Chap 4).

Another area in which medical documentation is often inadequate relates to the residents' decision-making capacity and treatment preferences. These issues are discussed briefly at the end of this chapter as well as in Chap. 17. In addition to placing critical information in a standardized format in readily accessible locations, it is essential that physicians thoroughly and legibly document all discussions they have had with the resident, family, or legal guardians; they must also document any durable power of attorney for health care about these issues. Failure to do so may result not only in poor communication and inappropriate treatment, but also in substantial legal liability. Notes about these issues should not be removed from the medical record and are probably best kept on a separate page behind the face sheet.

Screening, Health Maintenance, and Preventive Practices

A second approach to improving medical care in nursing homes is the development and implementation of selected screening, health maintenance, and preventive practices. Table 16-6 lists examples of such practices. With few exceptions, the efficacy of these practices has not been well studied in the nursing home setting. In addition, not all the practices listed in Table 16-6 are relevant for every nursing home resident. For example, some of the annual screening examinations are inappropriate for short-stayers or for many long-staying residents with end-stage dementia (see Fig. 16-1). Thus, the practices outlined in Table 16-6 must be tailored to the specific nursing home population, as well as for the individual resident, and must be creatively incorporated into routine care procedures as much as possible in order to be time-efficient, cost-effective, and reimbursable by Medicare.

Nurse Practitioners and Physician Assistants

A third strategy that may help to improve medical care in nursing homes is the use of nurse practitioners and physician assistants. This approach appears to be cost-effective in both managed care and fee-for-service settings (Burl et al., 1998; Ackerman and Kemle, 1998), and these health professionals may be especially helpful in carrying out specific functions in the nursing home setting. Physician assistants and nurse practitioners can bill for services under fee-for-service Medicare; moreover, several states will reimburse their services, and individual facilities and/or physician groups can hire them on a salaried basis. Evercare is a managed care program for long-stay nursing home residents that uses a nurse practitioner-based model of care and is available in several states. Nurse practitioners may have an especially helpful perspective in interacting with nursing staff about the nonmedical aspects of care for nursing home residents. Nurse practitioners and physician's assistants can be very helpful in implementing some of the screening, monitoring, and preventive practices outlined in Table 16- 6, and in communicating with interdisciplinary staff, families, and residents at times when the physician is not in the facility. One of the most appropriate roles for nurse practitioners and physicians' assistants is in the initial assessment of acute or subacute changes in resident status. They can perform a focused history and physical examination, and can order appropriate diagnostic studies. Several algorithms have been developed for this purpose, one of which is shown in Fig. 16-3. This strategy enables the onsite assessment of acute change, the detection and treatment of new problems early in their course, more appropriate utilization of acute care hospital emergency rooms, and the rapid identification of residents who need to be hospitalized.

Clinical Practice Guidelines and Quality Improvement Activities

Several clinical practice guidelines relevant to nursing home care have been developed by the American Medical Directors Association (AMDA). In addition,

MEDICAL FACE SHEET

ACTIVE MEDICAL PROBLEMS

1. _____
2. _____
3. _____
4. _____
5. _____
6. _____
7. _____
8. _____

PAST HISTORY

A. Acute hospitalizations since admission to JHA

Diagnoses   Month/Year

1. _____   ___/___
2. _____   ___/___
3. _____   ___/___
4. _____   ___/___

NEUROPSYCHIATRIC STATUS

A. Dementia   ___ Absent   ___ Present

   If present:

   ___ Alzheimer's   ___ Mixed
   ___ Multi-infarct   ___ Uncertain/Other

B. Psychiatric/behavioral disorders

1. _____
2. _____

C. Usual mental status

   ___ Alert, oriented, follows simple instructions
   ___ Alert, disoriented, but can follow simple directions
   ___ Alert, disoriented, cannot follow simple directions
   ___ Not alert (lethargic, comatose)

D. Most recent Mini Mental State Score

   ___/30 (Date ___/___/___)

FUNCTIONAL STATUS

B. Major surgical procedures *before* admission to JHA

Procedure   Year

1. _____ _____

2. _____ _____

3. _____ _____

4. _____ _____

C. Allergies

1. _____

2. _____

A. Ambulation
— Unassisted
— With cane
— With walker
— Unable
— Transfer:___ Ind ___ Dep

B. Continence

	Cont	Inc
Urine	—	—
Stool	—	—

C. Basic ADL

	Ind	Dep
Bathing	—	—
Dressing	—	—
Grooming	—	—
Feeding	—	—

D. Vision
— Adequate for regular print
— Impaired-can see large print
— Highly impaired-but can get around
— Severely impaired-has difficulty getting around

E. Hearing
— Adequate
— Minimal difficulty
— Hears only w/amplifier
— Highly impaired-no useful hearing

TREATMENT STATUS   (See treatment Status Sheet Note Date ___ / ___ / ___)

— Full code   — DNR   — DNR, do no hospitalize   — No tube feeding

This form completed by _____ Date ___ / ___ / ___

— FIGURE 16-2 — *Example of a face sheet for a nursing home record.*

TABLE 16-5   SOAP FORMAT FOR MEDICAL PROGRESS NOTES ON NURSING HOME RESIDENTS

Subjective	New complaints
	Symptoms related to active medical conditions
Objective	General appearance and mood
	Weight
	Vital signs
	Physical findings relevant to new complaints and active medical conditions
	Laboratory data
	Reports from nursing staff
	Progress in rehabilitative therapy (if applicable)
	Reports of other interdisciplinary team members
	Consultant reports
Assessment	Presumptive diagnosis(es) for new complaints or changes in status
	Stability of active medical conditions
	Responses to psychotropic medications (if applicable)
Plans	Changes in medications or diet
	Nursing interventions (e.g., monitoring of vital signs, skin care)
	Assessments by other disciplines
	Consultants
	Laboratory studies
	Discharge planning (if relevant)

the 18 RAPs contain basic approaches to common conditions among nursing home residents. While these guidelines are largely based on expert opinion rather than on controlled clinical trials, they are helpful as a basis for standards of practice that will improve care. Implementation and maintenance of practice guidelines can be difficult in nursing homes, as it is in other practice settings (Schnelle et al., 1997).

Clinical practice guidelines can be useful tools in an overall quality improvement program. Nursing homes are required to have an ongoing quality assurance committee. The most effective approaches are probably those ones based on principles of total quality management (TQM) or continuous quality improvement (CQI) (Schnelle et al., 1993). These approaches use front-line staff to monitor objective outcomes (such as the frequency of falls, severity of incontinence, adverse drug reactions, and skin problems) and to identify work processes that can

TABLE 16-6   SCREENING, HEALTH MAINTENANCE, AND PREVENTIVE PRACTICES IN THE NURSING HOME

Practice	Recommended Frequency*	Comment
		SCREENING
History and physical examination	Yearly	Focused exam including rectal, breast, and, in some women, pelvic exam
Weight	Monthly	Generally required Persistent weight loss should prompt a search for treatable medical, psychiatric, and functional conditions
Functional status assessment, including gait and mental status testing and screening for depression†	Yearly	Functional status assessed periodically by nursing staff using the Minimum Data Set (MDS) Systematic global functional assessment done at least yearly using MDS to detect potentially treatable conditions (or prevent complications) such as early dementia, depression, gait disturbances, urinary incontinence
Visual screening	Yearly	Assess acuity, intraocular pressure, identify correctable problems
Auditory	Yearly	Identify correctable problems
Dental	Yearly	Assess status of any remaining teeth, fit of dentures, and identify any pathology
Podiatry	Yearly	More frequently in diabetics and residents with peripheral vascular disease Identify correctable problems and ensure appropriateness of shoes

TABLE 16-6 SCREENING, HEALTH MAINTENANCE, AND PREVENTIVE PRACTICES IN THE NURSING HOME (*Continued*)

Practice	Recommended frequency*	Comment
		Screening
Tuberculosis	On admission and yearly	All residents and staff should be tested
		Booster testing recommended for nursing home residents (see text)
Laboratory tests	Yearly	These tests have reasonable yield in the nursing home population
Stool for occult blood		
Complete blood count		
Fasting glucose		
Electrolytes		
Renal function tests		
Albumin, calcium, phosphorus		
Thyroid function tests (including thyroid-stimulating hormone level)		

MONITORING IN SELECTED RESIDENTS

All residents Vital signs, including weight	Monthly	More often if unstable or subacutely ill
Diabetes Fasting and postprandial glucose, glycosylated hemoglobin	Every 1-2 months when stable	Fingerstick tests may be useful if staff can perform reliably
Residents on diuretics or with renal insufficiency [creatinine >2 or blood urea nitrogen (BUN) >35]: electrolytes, BUN, creatinine	Every 2-3 months	Nursing home residents are more prone to dehydration, azotemia, hyponatremia, and hypokalemia
Anemic residents who are on iron replacement or who have hemoglobin <10: hemoglobin/hematocrit	Monthly until stable, then every 2-3 months	Iron replacement should be discontinued once hemoglobin value stablizes
Blood level of drug for residents on specific drugs, for example: Carbamazepine Digoxin Dilantin Lithium Theophylline Nortriptyline	Every 3-6 months	More frequently if drug treatment has just been initiated

TABLE 16-6 SCREENING, HEALTH MAINTENANCE, AND PREVENTIVE PRACTICES IN THE NURSING HOME (*Continued*)

PRACTICE	RECOMMENDED FREQUENCY*	COMMENT
		PREVENTION
Influenza vaccine	Yearly	All residents and staff with close resident contact should be vaccinated
Amantadine	Within 24–48 h of outbreak of suspected influenza A	Dose should be reduced to 100 mg/d in older adults; further reduction if renal failure present Unvaccinated residents and staff should be treated throughout outbreak; vaccinated can be treated until their symptoms resolve
Pneumococcal/pneumonia bacteremia Pneumococcal vaccine	Once	
Tetanus booster	Every 10 years, or every 5 years with tetanus-prone wounds	Many older people have not received primary vaccinations; they require tetanus toxoid, 250–500 units of tetanus immune globulin, and completion of the immunization series with toxoid injection 4–6 weeks later and then 6–12 months after the second injection
Tuberculosis Isoniazid 300 mg/d for 9–12 months	Skin-test conversion in selected residents	Residents with abnormal chest film (more than granuloma), diabetes, end-stage renal disease, hematological malignancies, steroid or immunosuppressive therapy, or malnutrition should be treated

Antimicrobial prophylaxis for residents at risk‡	Generally recommended for dental procedures, genitourinary procedures, and most operative procedures	Chronically catheterized residents should not be treated with continuous prophylaxis (see Chap. 8)
Body positioning and range of motion for immobile residents	Ongoing	Frequent turning of very immobile residents is necessary to prevent pressure sores Semiupright position is necessary for residents with swallowing disorders or enteral feeding to help prevent aspiration Range of motion to immobile limbs and joints is necessary to prevent contractures
Infection-control procedures and surveillance	Ongoing	Policies and protocols should be in effect in all nursing homes Surveillance of all infections should be continuous to identify outbreaks and resistance patterns
Environmental safety	Ongoing	Appropriate lighting, colors, and the removal of hazards for falling are essential in order to prevent accidents Routine monitoring of potential safety hazards and accidents may lead to alterations that may prevent further accidents

* Frequency may vary depending on resident's condition.
† The MDS can be supplemented by various standardized tools (see Chap. 3).
‡ See Chap. 3.

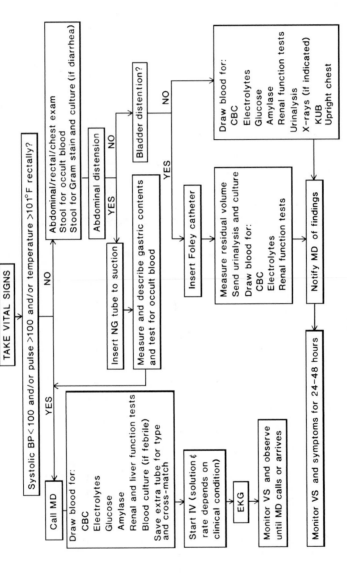

— FIGURE 16-3 — *Example of an algorithm protocol for the management of acute abdominal pain in the nursing home by a nurse practitioner or physician's assistant. CBC = complete blood cell count; EKG = electrocardiogram; IV = intravenous; KUB = kidneys, ureters, bladder; MD = medical doctor; NG = nasogastric; VS = vital signs.*

be modified to continuously improve these outcomes. Effective CQI activities will require the further development of software such as that which is used for incontinence care (Schnelle et al., 1995). Nursing home administrators, directors of nursing, and medical directors must create an environment that provides incentives for ongoing CQI activities in order to maintain these programs over time.

SUBACUTE CARE AND THE NURSING HOME— ACUTE-CARE HOSPITAL INTERFACE

The need for high levels of skilled postacute care will continue to place increased demands on nursing homes. Medicare risk health maintenance organizations (HMOs) commonly admit patients with acute but relatively stable conditions (e.g., deep vein thrombosis, cellulitis) directly to nursing homes without an acute hospital stay. As a result, nursing homes are providing more and more high-level skilled care. The term *subacute care* has many connotations; for the purposes of this chapter, it refers to skilled care reimbursed by Medicare Part A (or by a capitated system) in a free-standing nursing home. Subacute care is also discussed in Chap. 15, and more detail is provided in the suggested readings.

Caring for subacutely ill patients in a free-standing nursing home intensifies many of the challenges already alluded to in this chapter (see Table 16-2). This level of care requires greater involvement of physicians, nurse practitioners, and physician assistants; nursing staff trained for more acute patients; ready availability of ancillary services such as lab, x-ray, physical, and respiratory therapy; and more intensive discharge planning. Moreover, Medicare reimbursement for Part A services is being "bundled," so that nursing homes will be at financial risk for services that are ordered by medical staff, including drugs, laboratory tests, x-rays, and therapies. This reimbursement structure requires unprecedented cooperation between physicians and nursing home administrators in order to make this form of subacute care economically viable.

As a result of the increasing acuity and frailty of the nursing home resident population, transfer back and forth between the nursing home and one or more acute care hospitals is common. The major reasons for transfer include infection and the need for parenteral antimicrobials and hydration as well as acute cardiovascular conditions and hip fractures. Transfer to an acute care hospital is often a disruptive process for a chronically or subacutely ill nursing home resident. In addition to the effects of the acute illness, nursing home residents are subject to acute mental status changes and a myriad of potential iatrogenic problems (see Chap. 5). Probably the most prevalent of these iatrogenic problems are related to immobility, including deconditioning, difficulty regaining ambulation and/or transfer capabilities, and the development of pressure sores.

Because of the risks of acute care hospitalization, the decision to transfer a resident to the emergency room or hospitalize a resident must carefully balance a number of factors. A variety of medical, administrative, logistic, economic, and ethical issues can influence decisions to hospitalize nursing home residents. Decisions regarding hospitalization often boil down to the capabilities of the physician and the nursing home staff to provide services in the nursing home, the preferences of the resident and the family, and the logistic and administrative arrangements for acute hospital care. If, for example, the nursing home staff has been trained and has the personnel to institute intravenous therapy without detracting from the care of the other residents, or if it has arranged for an outside agency to oversee intravenous therapy and there is a nurse practitioner or physician's assistant to perform follow-up assessments, the resident with an acute infection who is otherwise medically stable may best be managed in the nursing home.

ETHICAL ISSUES IN NURSING HOME CARE

Ethical issues arise as much or more in the day-to-day care of nursing home residents as in the care of patients in any other setting. Table 16-7 outlines several common ethical dilemmas that occur in the nursing home. Although most attention has been directed toward those marginally able to express their preferences, important daily ethical dilemmas also face those who are capable of decision making. These more subtle problems are easily overlooked. Physicians, nurse practitioners, and physicians' assistants providing primary care must serve as strong advocates for the autonomy and quality of life for nursing homes residents.

Nursing homes do care for an extraordinarily high concentration of individuals who are unable or are questionably capable of participating in decisions concerning their current and future health care. Among these same individuals severe functional disabilities and terminal illnesses are prevalent. Thus, questions regarding individual autonomy, decision-making capacity, surrogate decision makers, and the intensity of treatment that should be given at the end of life arise on a daily basis. These questions are both troublesome and complex but must be dealt with in a straightforward and systematic manner in order to provide optimal medical care to nursing home residents within the context of ethical principles and state and federal laws. Nursing homes should be encouraged to develop their own ethics committees or to participate in a local existing committee in another facility. Ethics committees can be helpful in educating staff; developing, implementing, and monitoring policies and procedures; and in providing consultation in difficult cases. Some practical methods of approaching ethical issues are discussed in Chap. 17.

References

Ackerman RJ, Kemle KA: The effect of a physician assistant on the hospitalization of nursing home residents. *J Am Geriatr Soc* 46:610–614, 1998.

TABLE 16-7   COMMON ETHICAL ISSUES IN THE NURSING HOME*

ETHICAL ISSUE	EXAMPLES
Preservation of autonomy	Choices in many areas are limited in most nursing homes (e.g., mealtimes, sleeping hours) Families, physicians, and nursing home staff tend to be paternalistic
Decision-making capacity	Many nursing home residents are incapable or are questionably capable of participating in decisions about their care There are no standard methods of assessing decision-making capacity in this population
Surrogate decision making	Many nursing home residents have not clearly stated their preferences or appointed a surrogate before becoming unable to decide for themselves Family members may be in conflict, have hidden agendas, or be incapable of or unwilling to make decisions
Quality of life	This concept is often entered into decision making, but it is difficult to measure, especially among those with dementia Ageist biases can influence perceptions of nursing home residents' quality of life
Intensity of treatment	A range of options must be considered, including cardiopulmonary resuscitation and mechanical ventilation, hospitalization, treatment of specific conditions (e.g., infection) in the nursing home without hospitalization, enteral feeding, comfort or supportive care only

* See also Chap. 17.

Burl JB, Bonner A, Rao M, Khan AM: Geriatric nurse practitioners in long-term care: demonstration of effectiveness in managed care. *J Am Geriatr Soc* 46:506–510, 1998.

Evans LK, Strumpf NE, Allen-Taylor SL, et al: A clinical trial to reduce restraints in nursing homes. *J Am Geriatr Soc* 45:675–681, 1997.

Institute of Medicine: *Improving the Quality of Care in Nursing Homes.* Washington, DC, National Academy Press, 1986.

Institute of Medicine: *Improving the Quality of Nursing Home Care.* Washington, DC, National Academy Press, 2000.

Kane RL: Assuring quality in nursing home care. *J Am Geriatr Soc* 46:232–237, 1998.

Kramer AJ, Steiner JF, Schlenker RE, et al: Outcomes and costs after hip fracture and stroke: a comparison of rehabilitation settings. *JAMA* 277(5):396–404, 1997.

Llorente MD, Olsen EJ, Leyva O, et al: Use of antipsychotic drugs in nursing homes: current compliance with OBRA regulations. *J Am Geriatr Soc* 46:198–201, 1998.

Ouslander JG: The Resident Assessment Instrument (RAI): promise and pitfalls. *J Am Geriatr Soc* 45:975–976, 1997.

Schnelle J, Ouslander JG, Cruise PA, et al.: Policy with technology: a barrier to improving nursing home care. *The Gerontologist* 37(4):527–532, 1997.

Schnelle JF, McNees P, Crook V, et al: The use of a computer-based model to implement an incontinence management program. *Gerontologist* 36:656–665, 1995.

Schnelle JF, Ouslander JG, Osterweil D, Blumenthal S: Total quality management: administrative and clinical applications in nursing homes. *J Am Geriatr Soc* 41:1259–1266, 1993.

Vladek B: *Unloving Care: The Nursing Home Tragedy.* New York, Basic Books, 1980.

Zimmerman DR, Karon SL, et al: Development and testing of nursing home quality indicators. *Health Care Fin Rev* 16(4):107–127, 1995.

Suggested Readings

Nursing Home Care (General)

Harvell J: Subacute care: its role and the assurance of quality. *Annu Rev Gerontol Geriatr* 16:37–59, 1996.

Levenson SA (ed.): *Medical Direction in Long-term Care: A Guidebook for the Future,* 2d ed. Durham, NC, Carolina Academic Press, 1993.

Levenson SA: *Subacute and Transitional Care Handbook.* St. Louis, Beverly Cracom, 1996.

Ouslander J, Osterweil D: Physician evaluation and management of nursing home residents. *Ann Intern Med* 121:584–592, 1994.

Ouslander J, Osterweil D, Morley J: *Medical Care in the Nursing Home,* 2d ed. New York, McGraw-Hill, 1996.

Smith RL, Osterweil D: The medical director in hospital-based transitional care units. *Med Dir Long-term Care* 11:373–389, 1995.

ETHICAL ISSUES IN THE CARE OF OLDER PERSONS

Ethics is a fundamental part of geriatrics. Some people would go so far as to describe geriatrics as end-of-life care. Issues around medical futility play a central role. The big question, of course, is defining what is futile. Ageism can play a strong role.

While ethical dilemmas are central to the practice of medicine itself, the dependent nature of the geriatric patient raises special concerns. Discussions of ethics and aging seem to focus on the roles of autonomy and rationing. In many instances, the former may be used as basis for the latter. Ironically, the greatest ethical attention is focused on the group who are least able to express a preference: those in some form of vegetative state.

There has been great pressure (including federal regulations) to encourage older persons to indicate their preferences in advance for how they would wish to be treated in the event that they are too incapacitated to express their wishes. This advocacy has been viewed as sparing unnecessary suffering. However, it is also conveniently directed at cost control. Thus, there is a danger that compassion can be used to disguise economy. Despite a growing enthusiasm for these advance directives among many health professionals and policy makers, recent studies raise serious questions about older patients' enthusiasm for curtailing efforts to prolong their lives (Tsevat et al., 1998). This report is consistent with earlier findings that people's fears of developing a given chronic illness are much greater than the enthusiasm of those with such illnesses to get rid of the same problem (Torrance, 1987).

The issues that tend to attract the greatest attention are those affecting life-and-death decisions: Should one withhold or withdraw treatment? Do you resuscitate? What about tube feeding? These are each important and taxing questions posed in the context of real people. However, they arise much less often than do the less-heralded ethical dilemmas that confront us each day as we decide about discharge from hospital, arrange placement in a nursing home, or recommend therapies. Consideration of the ethics of geriatric care must address the full spectrum of these issues.

AUTONOMY AND BENEFICENCE

Table 17-1 provides a framework for discussing ethical issues. Two principal components to ethical discussions are the concepts of autonomy and beneficence. *Autonomy* refers to one's right to control one's destiny, that is, to exert one's will. Obviously there are limits to how freely such control can be expressed, but for geriatric purposes the principal issue revolves around whether the patient is able to assess the situation and make a rational decision independently. This raises the second concept. *Beneficence* refers to the duty to do good for others, to help them directly and in avoiding harm. This idea comes very close to paternalism, where one becomes the agent of another in order to make decisions as a father might do for a child. Such action directly conflicts with the principle of autonomy.

Physicians face a difficult set of choices in practice when they seek to walk these often fine lines. As Meier and Cassel (1986) note:

> Although the medical community has frequently been attacked for its paternalistic attitude toward patients, it is usually conceded that paternalism can be justified if certain criteria are met: if the dangers averted or benefits gained for the person outweigh the loss of autonomy resulting from the intervention; if the person is too ill to choose freely; and if other persons in similar circumstances would likely choose the same intervention.

The challenge then comes down to several fundamental issues:

1. Is the patient capable of understanding the dilemma?
2. Is the patient able to express a preference?
3. Has the patient received accurate information about the benefits and risks?
4. Are there clear options? Have they been made clear?
5. What happens when the patient's preferences are contrary to the physician's or the patient's family's?

COMPETENCE AND INFORMED CONSENT

In the case of elderly persons, much of the concern is directed toward the issue of understanding and expressing opinions. The two most extreme cases are the comatose patient, who clearly cannot communicate, and the aphasic patient, who may be unable to communicate effectively. In the former case, we must look for other ways to preserve autonomy. In the latter, we must be very careful to assess and separate areas of communication from reasoning.

TABLE 17-1   MAJOR ETHICAL PRINCIPLES

Beneficence
   The obligation to do good
Nonmaleficence
   The obligation to avoid harm
Autonomy
   Duty to respect persons and their right to independent self-determination
   regarding the course of their lives and issues concerning the integrity of
   their bodies and minds
Justice
   Nondiscrimination: duty to treat individuals fairly; not to discriminate on
   the basis of irrelevant characteristics
   Distribution: duty to distribute resources fairly, nonarbitrarily, and
   noncapriciously
Fidelity
   Duty to keep promises

There is an important difference between the concepts of competence and decision-making capability. The former is a legal term that refers to a person's ability to act reasonably after understanding the nature of the situation being faced. Someone not competent to act on his or her own behalf requires an agent to act *for* them.

In the case of dementia, persons may or may not be capable of understanding and interpreting complex situations and of making a rational decision. Intellectual deficits are spotty. A person may get lost easily or forget things but still be able to make decisions. A good example is the classic absent-minded professor. The presence of a formal diagnosis of dementia, even by type, may not be a sufficient indicator of the individual's ability to comprehend and express a meaningful preference. Just as it is wrong to infantilize such patients by directing questions to others more quick to respond, so, too, might it be inappropriate to prejudge their ability to participate in decisions about their own care.

Determining cognitive ability and decision-making capacity is not easy. One must distinguish memory from understanding. Physicians' judgments about patients' capacity to consent were much better for cognitively intact patients than for mildly demented patients. It is important to separate executive intellectual function from simple verbal recall ability (Marson et al., 1997). Two studies considered these issues. In one, younger age and more education were predictors of understanding informed consents, but simplifying the form did not consistently improve understanding (Taub et al., 1986). In the second study, varying the mode of presentation of information was not very helpful (Tymchuk et al., 1986). However, major deficits in short-term memory or verbal knowledge were associated with reduced understanding. Neither study attempted any form assistance such as reminders or prompts. Patients with memory deficits may need special help in recalling the components of the issue, but once reminded, they can often express a clear, sensible opinion.

One criterion for decision making, often presented with regard to informed consent, is the confirmation of the decision after a period of time during which the patient can consider the issues at hand. Clearly, memory is an important ingredient in such an approach. Its feasibility will vary greatly with circumstances. The pressures of contemporary funding sadly prohibit such a reasonable approach to many crucial decisions. Contrast the situation for deciding about posthospital placement with that about discontinuing treatment or pursuing a high-risk treatment. The former decision is typically made under great duress, with utilization review looming. Choices are frequently poorly described and the consequences of the alternatives, when such are even presented, are not well defined.

The other side of the coin is the question of how information is presented. To make a rational decision, we all need a clear sense of the alternatives, including their benefits and risks. Ideally, a person making a care decision would have complete information about the full range of options and the risks and benefits associated with each option. The decision-making process would be structured to allow the individual (and perhaps the family) to identify which outcomes (from a large menu) they are most keen to assure. The physician is a major source of this information. More often than not, the range of alternatives is foreshortened to emphasize those deemed most appropriate. Rarely are patients given the full description of the benefits and risks. In some instances, this is appropriate, because the entire list of all possible risks may be excessive and a discussion of very serious yet very rare conditions may inappropriately frighten a patient.

When decisions about nursing home entry are made, they are not given the same level of serious attention accorded those about surgery. In many cases, physicians may not know all the risks and benefits, but they never will until they are forced to address them. When patients face decisions about entering a nursing home, for example, they need to understand the options at several levels. First, is a nursing home the best answer? What are the trade-offs between safety, privacy, and loss of autonomy? What other service configurations might work? At what cost, financial and otherwise? Second, they need to choose among nursing homes. Which one offers the social environment that suits their lifestyles as well as having available resources to meet their physical needs? In too many cases, patients do not get to choose in either category. Decisions, especially decisions made in hospitals, are made under great time pressure.

ADVANCE DIRECTIVES AND END-OF-LIFE CARE

It is important to distinguish between advance directives and decisions at the end of life. The former asks people to make decisions about how they believe they would wish to be cared for were they in some hypothetical situation of severe impairment. The latter addresses much more real issues. Unfortunately, the debate on end-of-life care confuses these two quite distinct decisions.

Advance Directives

One way of trying to deal with the situation when the patient cannot express a preference is to encourage the development of advance directives, in which persons indicate what they want done under such circumstances. Federal law requires that all persons entering a hospital or a nursing home be offered the opportunity to indicate advance directives. Too often this exercise means that older persons are confronted with long lists of possible procedures and asked to choose which ones they would want to have if the occasion arose. Done poorly, the experience can provoke unnecessary anxiety and lead to poor decisions that may be regretted later. The two most common forms of these advance directives are living wills and durable powers of attorney. The former indicates in as much detail as possible what actions should or should not be taken under specific circumstances.

These living wills have been criticized as being too vague or too specific, and some research shows that a person's intentions and preferences change with circumstances. People usually are more anxious to avoid a bad condition than to get rid of it once it occurs. Similarly, it is difficult to know for certain how you would feel if you were faced with a certain life-threatening choice.

Living wills most often address the issue of extraordinary actions to sustain life, generally the question of resuscitation, but they can also cover such things as hospitalization, use of life-sustaining therapies including parenteral and tube feeding, and even the use of antibiotics. They provide a means to indicate whether the patient prefers that heroic measures not be undertaken. In one sense, the more specific such orders are, the better. Under what conditions? What constitutes a heroic measure? Another class of extraordinary measures is the use of artificial life supports. Again there is a need for specificity. Is a feeding tube the equivalent of a respirator? Some would argue that it is (Steinbrook and Lo, 1988).

Forgoing heroic measures need not mean abrogating all interest in surviving. One terrible anecdote is told about a nursing home staff that allowed a patient to choke to death on aspirated food because he had signed a "do not resuscitate" (DNR) request. Does not wanting cardiopulmonary resuscitation mean that the patient does not want to have his or her pneumonia treated? DNR is not synonymous with "do not care." Although there is a desire for specificity, both ethical and practical considerations enter into the picture. Few persons are prepared to sit down with a list of circumstances and actions to indicate in a calm, rational way that if this occurs, this is what I want done or not done. At best, one may get a sense of a person's priorities and feelings about active efforts. Despite the requirement that advance directives be solicited whenever an older person is admitted to a health care institution, some suggest that it is unrealistic to expect that persons can make clear, thoughtful determinations at such a time of high stress.

The danger of not building the decision into the admission routine, or at least the admission data-collection process, is that it goes unattended. If the decision is best postponed until a calmer time after a period of adjustment, it should not be forgotten. There are standard forms available to guide you in making choices and indicating preferences, but filling out such a list may be disconcerting. More than two-thirds of the states have some form of living will legislation, but the precise nature of those laws varies greatly in terms of what must be specified and under what conditions the delineated preferences can be followed.

An alternative to the living will approach of prior specification is the designation of a proxy, who is authorized to act on the patient's behalf if that person is unable to communicate. This designation can be done by using a durable power of attorney, previously used to transfer control of property. States must specifically extend their durable power of attorney statutes to cover medical decisions. Under this approach one can specify both the person one wishes to act as agent and the conditions under which such a proxy should be exercised. Table 17-2 shows the components of a durable power of attorney for health care.

With both the living will and the durable power of attorney, there is some potential for misuse. Decisions once made can be difficult to revoke. What is the test of mental competence that allows one to change one's mind about a decision to not use life-support systems? Stories are told about families who followed the patient's instructions even when the patient appeared to have a change of mind.

In the absence of any specification of actions or agents, someone must be identified to act for a person who is unable to act on his or her own behalf. There are legal procedures to accomplish this, which vary from state to state. In general, the two major classes of legally empowered agents are conservators and guardians. The latter usually have greater powers. A formal legal decision is needed to establish such a condition.

A critical question is, who is best qualified to assume that responsibility? Common wisdom suggests that it is the next of kin, but some argue that it should be the person most familiar with the patient's preferences, the person who can most closely estimate what the patient would have wanted. A rarely seen relative might know much less about the patient's wishes or lifestyle than might a close friend, clergyman, or even the attending physician.

The choice should rest on the level of knowledge possessed. Where there are multiple contenders for the role, the courts may have to decide who is best

TABLE 17-2 COMPONENTS OF A DURABLE POWER OF ATTORNEY FOR HEALTH CARE*

Creation of durable power of attorney for health care
Statement that gives intention and refers to statute(s) authorizing such

Designation of health care agent
Statement naming and facilitating access to (address, telephone number) agent; state laws will vary as to who may serve as agent—some states preclude providers of health care or employees of institutions where care is given; person designated as agent should have agreed to assume this role

General statement of authority granted
Statement about circumstances under which the agent is granted power and indications of the power the agent will have in that event (usually a general statement about right to consent or refuse or withdraw consent for care, treatment, service or procedure, or release of information subject to any specific provisions and limitations indicated)

Statement of desires, special provisions, and limitations
Opportunity to indicate general preferences (e.g., wish not to have life prolonged if burdens outweigh benefits; wish for life-sustaining treatment unless in coma that physicians believe to be irreversible, then no such efforts; wish for all possible efforts regardless of prognosis); opportunity for specific types of things wanted done or not done and indications for such actions

Signatures
Individual dated signature
Witnesses (better notarized): witnesses cannot be those named as agents, providers of health care, or employees of facilities giving such care

Conditions
Form should have place where person signing indicates awareness of rights, including the right to revoke the document and the conditions under which the document comes into force; some states require a mandatory maximum period such a document can be valid without renewal

*Many state medical associations can provide a copy of a basic form of a durable power of attorney for health care.

positioned to know the patient's preferences. In cases where there is no one appropriate, the court may appoint a public guardian.

Agents, whether designated by durable power of attorney or chosen as the best available person, are vulnerable to pursuing their own interests rather than the patient's. At best, they must make inferences about the patient's wishes from their knowledge of the patient or the choice indicated in the durable power document. Surrogates' decisions may not be congruent with the wishes of the individuals they represent. They can be sincerely torn between acting in what they perceive to be the individual's wishes and best interests, two different perspectives on the issue.

Court decisions suggest that families and physicians may not have the last word in decisions about the care of incompetent persons. In the case of a demented woman with a legal guardian, the court ordered that a state ombudsman had to become involved in the decision to prevent premature discontinuation of tube feeding (Lo and Dornbrand, 1986).

Substantial controversy surrounds end-of-life care. On the one side are those who argue that in our effort to avoid confronting the reality of death, we engage in a great deal of futile and expensive care (Lynn, 1986). Others counter that much of the claims for substantial potential savings from eliminating such care are spurious (Emanuel and Emanuel, 1994; Emanuel, 1996).

End-Of-Life Care

Advance directives provide a basis for making end-of-life decisions for those persons who are incapable of expressing their preferences at the time; but many people are capable of making these decisions. For them, the decision making is quite different. They are faced with difficult choices that are based in current experience. In contrast to hypothetical imaginings of what it would be like to be in a given state, these people are experiencing that state or something quite close to it.

End-of-life decisions can be based on beliefs about both quantitative and qualitative futility. The former refers to an expectation that death is highly likely and that further efforts to postpone it are not likely to succeed. The latter addresses the quality of life if the patient survives. Will it be a life worth living?

A study looking at a large group of older patients thought to be in terminal condition who were receiving intensive care has raised a number of questions about how the health professionals handle end-of-life situations. The original goal of the study was to make care teams more comfortable with such care and encourage them to forgo dramatic and traumatic therapeutic interventions where they seemed futile. Despite active training efforts the study team achieved only modest changes in clinician behavior (SUPPORT Principal Investigators, 1995). They interpreted this lack of effect as a treatment failure but an alternative interpretation would suggest that the absence of a response was because the clinicians were not comfortable terminating care. This behavior is supported by a study from the same effort that indicated that many frail older persons were not anxious to give up years of life even if it meant becoming disease free (Tsevat et al., 1998). Indeed many patients and their families are not anxious to forgo intensive care, even if the hopes of success are modest (Danis et al., 1988).

These findings raise serious questions about the ethical basis for the prevalent enthusiasm for advance directives. Some observers see this effort as a means of implementing rationing sub rosa. When prominent ethicists called for overt rationing on the basis of age (Callahan, 1987), gerontologists rose up to cry "ageism." However, some of these same defenders of older persons' rights see in advance directives an opportunity for autonomy.

Managing the end of patient's life is a serious undertaking. In addition to facilitating decisions about the extent of heroic measures to be tried, much can be done to make that period as peaceful and unpleasant as possible. First-order issues involve the relief of unnecessary symptoms, such as pain, itching, nausea, and shortness of breath. Palliative care, which began with the hospice movement (see Chap. 15), has made great strides in bringing care not only into the hospital but also into patients' homes. In addition to avoiding inappropriate prolongation of dying, other end-of-life tasks include helping the patient to achieve a sense of control, relieving burdens, and strengthening relationships with loved ones (Singer et al., 1999). Although physicians, patients, and family members may share many beliefs about what is important in end-of-life care, they do not always agree. Table 17-3 lists attributes that were held in common by all three parties in a national survey, but there were several areas where dying patients placed substantially more emphasis than their physicians (Steinhauser et al., 2000):

- Being mentally aware
- Not being a burden to family or society
- Be able to help others
- Feel one's life is complete
- Be at peace with God
- Have funeral arrangements planned

Determining when further care is futile is difficult. The American Medical Association (AMA) has outlined an approach to make this determination (Council on Ethical and Judicial Affairs, AMA, 1999). Some people would argue that there are circumstances when it is justifiable to go beyond providing palliative care to facilitate the process of dying (Quill et al., 1999).

The decision to withdraw life support can be emotionally painful. Clinicians have a vital role to play in providing timely clinical and prognostic information as well as emotional and social support to families. They can make it easier to accept the dying if they provide aggressive symptom control (Prendergast and Puntillo, 2002).

TABLE 17-3   AREAS OF GENERAL AGREEMENT AMONG PATIENTS, PHYSICIANS, AND FAMILY MEMBERS ABOUT END-OF-LIFE CARE

Be kept clean	Have physical touch
Name a decision maker	Know that one's physician is comfortable talking about death and dying
Have a nurse with whom one feels comfortable	
Know what to expect about one's physical condition	Have physician who knows one as a whole person
Have someone who will listen	Share time with close friends
Maintain one's dignity	Believe family is prepared for one's death
Trust one's physician	
Have financial affairs in order	Feel prepared to die
Be free of pain	Presence of family
Maintain a sense of humor	Treatment preferences in writing
Say goodbye to important people	Not die alone
Be free of shortness of breath	Remember personal accomplishments
Be free of anxiety	
Have physician with whom one can discuss fears	Receive care from personal physician
Resolve unfinished business with family or friends	

Source: Steinhauser et al., 2000

THE PHYSICIAN'S ROLE

A physician may feel under great pressure in facilitating end-of-life decisions. The physician is at once the patient's advocate, an agent of society, and a person in his or her own right. At times, the physician's preferences will differ from those of the patient or the patient's agent.

Nor are there only two poles to work between. Especially in the care of dependent older persons, family may exert strong influences to pursue what they perceive as the best interests of the patient or for other reasons. The physician must keep in mind who is the client.

An important issue is how actively should physician preferences be voiced. Physicians have an obligation to provide patients with a full set of information:

the alternatives and the risks and benefits associated with each option, and to be sure that the patient appreciates that information. It is difficult to be fully objective in many instances.

Few physicians have enough information to discuss the range of options and their associated risks and benefits; even fewer are capable of estimating the effects of competing risks from other conditions if the immediate problem is alleviated (Welch et al., 1996). Values may unconsciously distort the way options are portrayed; risks may be minimized or even overlooked. Some physicians prefer to think of themselves simply as conduits of information, whereas others believe strongly that their opinions should be counted, arguing that the physician is often the most knowledgeable person involved and has a duty to guide, or at least suggest, a course of therapy. In some cases, patients may specifically ask for advice or even indicate that they want the doctor to make the decision. Despite efforts to maintain a shared decision-making relationship, physicians will often find themselves unequal partners because of their authoritarian position. This deference is especially true with the current group of geriatric patients who were raised with a much more respectful set of beliefs about physicians than is currently the case among younger generations. The contemporary geriatrician must struggle hard to encourage the maximum autonomy from patients.

In an era of litigation, many physicians are understandably wary of taking charge. Fearful of being held responsible, they may wash their hands of the decision. Physicians find themselves smack in the middle of the pulls between autonomy and beneficence.

Physicians who want to do what is best for their patients will offer their opinions and give their reasons. But in the end, they cannot override the patient. If they find themselves in strong disagreement, they can assist patients to find new sources of care, but they cannot abandon a patient because of a difference of opinion. Physicians and hospitals facing patients who want to act in a way different from their convictions have often worked very hard to transfer the locus of care, but until that transfer is accomplished, they are stuck with dealing with patients on their terms or going to court. A recent court decision affirmed that "competent patients have the right to decline life-prolonging treatment, even if physicians disagree because of conscience or ethics." Moreover, the hospitals and physicians involved would not be criminally or civilly liable if they carried out the patient's wishes in these matters.

A difficult problem for most physicians is when to introduce the topic of the patient's need to consider some form of advance directive. Speaking about such topics may seem like conceding defeat, but it represents a significant service to the patient, who needs to plan for the future appropriately. A legal vehicle designating who has legal responsibility can save much heartache later, even when it may not be legally binding.

The physician's role has come under special scrutiny with regard to end-of-life care because of the actions of certain physicians who have openly practiced assisted suicide (Sachs et al., 1995). In a 1996 national survey of physicians, 11 percent of respondents said that they would be willing to prescribe medications to hasten a patient's death and 7 percent would use lethal injections. These proportions rose to 36 percent and 24 percent, respectively, if such practices were to be made legal (Meier et al., 1998). The appropriate role of physicians in participating in this activity is a topic of active debate. Many physicians and ethicists hold that a physician cannot and should not be responsible for fostering both life and death (Bachman et al., 1996). A few states have passed legislation permitting such physician-assisted suicides, but even in those places many physicians are reluctant to participate for fear of reprisal.

A committee of the American College of Physicians and the American Society of Internal Medicine has identified seven legal myths about end-of-life care that may prevent adequate care: (Meisel et al., 2000)

1. Forgoing life-sustaining treatment for patients without decision-making capacity requires evidence that this was the patient's actual wish.
2. Withholding or withdrawing artificial fluids and nutrition from terminally ill or permanently unconscious patients is illegal.
3. Risk-management personnel must be consulted before life-sustaining treatment can be terminated.
4. Advance directives must comply with specific forms, are not transferable across states, and govern all future treatment decisions; oral advance directives are unenforceable.
5. If a physician prescribes or administers high doses of medication to relieve pain or discomfort in a terminally ill patient, which results in death, the physician will be criminally prosecuted.
6. When a terminally ill patient's suffering is overwhelming despite palliative care, and the patient requests a hastened death, there are no legally permissible options to ease suffering.
7. The 1997 US Supreme Court decisions outlawed physician-assisted suicide.

Similarly, many patients are not aware of their rights (Silveira et al., 2000).

SPECIAL PROBLEMS WITH NURSING HOME RESIDENTS

Nursing home residents present some special problems. Patients are usually admitted to nursing homes because of a reduced capacity to cope. Many suffer from some degree of cognitive impairment. In one sense they are subject to a cruel paradox: because the quality of their daily lives may be so miserable, their lives are seen to have less value. It is easier to justify inattention or withholding extensive care.

Table 17-4 lists four areas where clinical decisions in treating long-term-care patients may pose the greatest ethical dilemmas. As noted in Chap. 16, beyond the usually considered question of resuscitation, the physician faces

TABLE 17-4   MAJOR TOPICS FOR CLINICAL ETHICAL DECISIONS ABOUT
NURSING HOME RESIDENTS

Resuscitation
Transfer to more intensive level of care
Treatment of infections and other intercurrent physiological derangements
Nutrition and hydration
Source: Lynn, 1986.

difficult decisions in determining when it is appropriate to transfer a patient
from a nursing home to a hospital or when to intervene aggressively to treat
changes in physiologic status from fluid imbalance or infection. Perhaps one
of the most perplexing areas is when to pursue heroic measures to maintain
nutritional supports.

Especially with the tremendous growth in technology for establishing effective but expensive nutritional regimens in persons incapable of eating on their
own for sustained periods, this issue is faced with increasing frequency. Artificial
feeding decisions seem to arouse more controversy than other life-sustaining
treatment issues. The growing consensus seems to favor the view that tube and
intravenous feedings are more akin to a medical intervention than to routine nursing care or comfort care (Steinbrook and Lo, 1988).

Physicians must be diligent in working to preserve the patient's personhood.
Essentially nursing home residents should not lose any of their rights as people just
because they enter a nursing home. They should be eligible to participate in a full
range of activities and to make choices about their lives and their health care. They
should be the first ones consulted about changes in their condition or therapy. Visits
to a nursing home should be more like home calls or office visits than hospital visits.

In practice, this freedom is often not allowed. One set of arguments for con-
straining nursing home resident choice is the limitations imposed by any institution. Just as college students must eat at certain times and choose from a menu,
so, too, must nursing home residents. But the similarity breaks down when one
appreciates the limited options available to the residents. They cannot easily order
in a pizza or go out for a beer. Again part of the restriction is imposed by their
medical status. Pizza and beer may be prohibited from their diet.

Often this medicalization represents its own set of ethical dilemmas. When is
dietary control a greater good than culinary pleasure? But too often medical
orders become excuses for not individualizing regimens. Few conditions are
aggravated by different hours of going to bed. In fact, sleeping medications might
be prescribed less often if there were more flexibility in bedtimes. Similarly, participation in activities or the right to privacy become major issues in a world

shrunk to nursing home proportions. How much say should a resident have in the choice of a roommate? Some would argue that single rooms should be the norm. The same people who would not deign to share a hotel room with a stranger for a single night seem to have no problem committing nursing home residents to roommates for years. An often repressed subject is the nursing home resident's rights to sexual privacy. Neither age nor dependency means a need to abrogate all rights to a sexual life. Sexual intimacy requires privacy. Too often nursing home staffs are insensitive and intolerant to these needs (McCartney et al., 1987).

There is a danger that the physician will treat the staff's needs rather than the patient's needs. Care should be exercised to avoid prescribing "as-needed" restraints or sedatives to offer easy ways for staff to deal with behaviors they find disruptive. Too available recourse to such orders strips the patient of personhood and makes the patient simply an object to be controlled.

Decisions about advance directives take on special meaning in the nursing home context. Because the likelihood of survival is quite low, the value of cardiopulmonary resuscitation (CPR) must be carefully evaluated (Applebaum et al., 1990; Wanzer et al., 1989; Murphy, 1988). However, one cannot assume that all nursing residents have elected to forego active care (O'Brien et al., 1995).

Because nursing home residents are vulnerable, special care is needed to protect their rights. Uhlmann and colleagues have developed an excellent set of principles and practices for this purpose (Uhlmann et al., 1987). The general goal is to maximize the resident's autonomy in making decisions about treatment. Several ombudsman groups have created a parallel set of concerns in the form of a resident's bill of rights, which outlines the choices that should be available and the protections that can be sought. The Institute of Medicine study of nursing home quality took special pains to emphasize the need to integrate quality-of-life considerations with quality of care (Institute of Medicine, 1986).

The Nursing Home Reform Act of 1987 [part of the Omnibus Budget Reconciliation Act of 1987 (OBRA 1987)] created major reforms in the way nursing home residents are managed. The prescriptions for avoiding physical restraints led to dramatic reductions in their use (Kane et al., 1993). Likewise, requirements for closer attention to the use of psychoactive medications greatly reduced their use as well.

One useful approach to buffer the relations between the nursing home, outside investigators and practitioners, and the residents is to establish an ethics committee composed of persons within and without the home (Glasser et al., 1988). Traditionally such committees began with the major charge of overseeing research activities, but they have increasingly begun to take responsibility for reviewing and facilitating standards for other aspects of the institution's activities and for serving as resources to establish guidelines for managing decision making around ethically difficult areas. Such committees are especially useful when they operate in a proactive manner, exploring issues in advance rather than assessing actions already taken. In many instances, they offer a disinterested forum where these very sensitive matters can be discussed with maximum dispassion and all sides of an issue aired.

SPECIAL CASE OF DEMENTIA

The wishes of patients with dementia may be ignored or undervalued. Although a diagnosis of dementia does not necessarily imply an inability to state preferences (Freedman et al., 1991), as noted earlier, physicians have more difficulty assessing competence to make decisions among such patients. Because dementia effectively robs individuals of personality as well as memory, it can be very difficult to assess the quality of lives and hence the extent of effort appropriate to prolong them (Lynn, 1986; Callahan, 1995). As already noted, the loss of cognitive function makes patient participation in decision making very difficult. Those left to act as agents for the demented patient must struggle with the difficult issue of when the loss of self-awareness and ability to maintain relationships constitutes substantial suffering. The loss of intellect is perhaps the most serious loss experienced by people. In one effort to explore the value of alternative outcomes among nursing home residents, if the resident was described as having loss of cognitive ability, all outcomes were rated substantially lower by a variety of persons, including care providers, family, policy makers, and the general public (Kane et al., 1986).

The management of demented patients poses additional problems. Demented persons are frequently intrusive. They threaten the privacy of those cognitively intact residents who must live with them. It does not seem right to diminish the quality of life for the latter in the name of efficiency, or in some hope that they will stimulate the demented. Separate programs or units seem much more humane and sensible. Some have expressed concern about the burden on staff, but this anxiety does not seem to be borne out by experience. The separation allows more appropriate programming and facility design.

In fact, the basic plans for facilities for the physically impaired and the cognitively impaired are also diametrically opposed. The former need ready access to nursing stations and short distances to walk, whereas the latter are best left to wander unimpeded in an eventually enclosed area with as much space as possible. In the continuum of special care facilities for the demented, we are now seeing the extension of the principles of hospice care to this group and their families (Volicer et al., 1986).

POLICY ISSUES

Older people are prime targets for rationing efforts because they consume disproportionately large amounts of medical care and because they are seen as having already lived their lives. They have less to offer future generations. Given the difficulty of launching a frontal attack to curtail spending on older people, more devious approaches have been used. Some of these are cloaked in ethical concepts. At a more subtle level, measures of program effectiveness tend to use something equivalent to the quality-adjusted life year (QALY). This term implies that valuable life is that lived free of dependency. Gerontological researchers have called it *active life expectancy* (Katz et al., 1983). Such proxies for program effectiveness incorporate ethical components subtly. We have not established the base on which to put a value on life lived at some level of dependency. To assume that it has no value, as is implied by active life years, appears to contradict the very purpose for geriatrics, which treats primarily dependent older people. Many older people would actively challenge the tenet that disability implies an absence of quality of life. Severely disabled persons at various ages can continue to enjoy pleasant and productive lives. As advocates for their patients, geriatricians must be extremely vigilant to how such terms are used both in everyday speech and in analyses. It is important to bear in mind that any measure that uses life expectancy will tend to be biased against the elderly. One that relies on dependency as the primary outcome implies that those who are dependent no longer count; by such logic disability is equivalent to death. At a time when there is an effort to pit one generation against another, care must be taken to avoid setting the terms of the debate such that the outcome is inevitable.

An important ethical issue closely linked to long-term care policy concerns the appropriate role of caregivers. In Chap. 15, we noted the central role played by informal caregivers, who constitute the backbone of long-term care. The question then is, how much of such care should they be expected to provide? What is the nature of the obligation of one generation to another, or even to spouses and siblings from the same generation? A substantial portion of informal care is undoubtedly provided out of love and compassion. This approach works well when it is left up to the family to decide how much care they can give, but what happens when such care becomes mandated? Pressure to control public costs of long-term care could easily lead to demands to require care from families or to require that families pay directly for a certain amount of that care. Concerns have already been expressed about the possibility that older persons are manipulating their assets to become unfairly eligible for Medicaid coverage. Although there is little substantiation for these claims of divestiture, advertisements for seminars on how to do it create an image of exploitation. Policies of familial responsibility would undoubtedly create a new demand for private long-term care insurance, because preservation of older persons' assets primarily benefits the heirs.

Much has been made about the money spent in the last year of life. Approximately 28 percent of the Medicare budget goes to the 5 percent of Medicare patients who die each year (Lubitz and Riley, 1993). Moreover, costs increase as death approaches; the costs during the last month of life represent approximately 40 percent of the total costs for the last year of life (Emanuel, 1996). However, hospice care has not been shown to provide substantial cost savings because most of the costs have been incurred before hospice care is initiated. Perhaps because physicians and patients are reluctant to admit defeat, the hospice alternative is used only very late in the course of terminal illness. Likewise, DNR orders are often given only late in a hospital stay (Bedell et al., 1986).

The emergence of managed care as a major health care force affecting older persons raises its own set of ethical issues. Here, too, the goal of rationing care may be played out in a different arena. Whereas managed care offers older persons some attractive advantages, its propensity to reduce access to care can be a major threat.

By hiding behind a complex bureaucracy, managed care companies can effectively thwart consumer feedback while claiming that the majority of their older customers are satisfied with the care they receive. Sometimes only dogged efforts, even to the point of litigation, are needed to generate a systemic response to a complaint. Medicare has determined that the benefits and costs will be set in the context of those for fee for service. In effect, the consumer has been removed from the loop until the time of enrollment.

SUMMARY

Ethical issues around care of older people are played out at all levels.

Policy issues largely address questions of access and coverage, but these can be influenced by an individual clinician's beliefs about what elements of care are "appropriate" for older people. These beliefs, in turn, can reflect stereotypes. Microethical issues occur at the bedside when decisions about initiating or continuing treatment are made.

These decisions, too, are based on beliefs about appropriateness, including who should have the ultimate word about how much and what kind of care is rendered. Some of these decisions are couched as ethical issues because the requisite facts are not known. Once evidence is presented about the efficacy of a therapy for older persons, the tenor of the discussion changes. Often other factors than age are much better predictors of who will likely benefit from a given type of treatment. Great care must be taken to avoid couching rationing decisions as ethical dilemmas. Measures that discount older or frail people will inevitably lead to decisions against treating older persons.

Elderly patients should not lose their rights to full consideration of options and participation in the decisions that affect their care. The principles of autonomy and beneficence, which form a central part of the ethics of medicine in general, are strained with dependent older persons because the temptation toward paternalism is greater in the presence of the tendency to infantilize frail elderly patients, especially when they cannot readily communicate. Concerns about how to make decisions for persons unable to express their own preferences are often couched in terms of fear of litigation, but the growing body of experience suggests that carefully pursued efforts to establish agency and act accordingly will not put physicians or institutions at great risk of lawsuits. Finally, it is important to recognize that the life of dependent older persons, especially those in nursing homes, is composed of many little incidents. The daily loss of dignity, privacy, and self-respect may be too readily ignored. To be truly the patient's advocate, the physician must be vigilant to these small but critical ethical insults. It would be the greatest irony if geriatric patients were daily abused while living, only to become the subject of profound ethical analysis about dying. This is precisely the kind of behavior geriatrics is in business to prevent.

References

Applebaum GE, King JE, Finucane TE: The outcome of CPR initiated in nursing homes. *J Am Geriatr Soc* 38:197–200, 1990.

Bachman JG, Alcser KH, Doukas DJ, et al: Attitudes of Michigan physicians and the public toward legalizing physician-assisted suicide and voluntary euthanasia. *N Engl J Med* 334:303–309, 1996.

Bedell SE, Pelle D, Maher PL, Cleary P: Do-Not-Resuscitate orders for critically ill patients in hospital. *JAMA* 256:233–237, 1986.

Callahan D: *Setting Limits: Medical Goals in an Aging Society.* New York, Simon and Schuster, 1987.

Callahan D: Terminating life-sustaining treatment of the demented. *Hastings Center Rep* 25(6):25–31, 1995.

Council on Ethical and Judicial Affairs, AMA: Medical futility in end-of-life care. *JAMA* 282:937–941, 1999.

Danis M, Patrick DL, Southerland LI, Green ML: Patients' and families' preferences for medical intensive care. *JAMA* 260:797–802, 1988.

Emanuel EJ: Cost savings at the end of life. *JAMA* 275:1907–1914, 1996.

Emanuel EJ, Emanuel LL: The economics of dying: The illusion of cost savings at the end of life. *N Engl J Med* 330:540–544, 1994.

Freedman M, Stuss DT, Gordon M: Assessment of competency: the role of neurobehavioral deficits. *Ann Intern Med* 15:203–208, 1991.

Glasser G, Zweibel NR, Cassel CK: The ethics committee in the nursing home: results of a national survey. *J Am Geriatr Soc* 36:150–156, 1988.

Institute of Medicine: *Improving the Quality of Care in Nursing Homes.* Washington, DC, National Academy Press, 1986.

Kane RL, Bell RM, Riegler SZ: Value preferences for nursing-home outcomes. *Gerontologist* 26:303–308, 1986.

Kane RL, Williams CC, Williams TF, et al: Restraining restraints: changes in a standard of care. *Annu Rev Public Health* 14:545–584, 1993.

Katz K, Branch LG, Branson MH, et al: Active life expectancy. *N Engl J Med* 309:1218–1224, 1983.

Lo B, Dornbrand L: The case of Claire Conroy: will administrative review safeguard incompetent patients? *Ann Intern Med* 106:869–873, 1986.

Lubitz JD, Riley GF: Trends in Medicare payments in the last year of life. *N Engl J Med* 328:1092–1096, 1993.

Lynn J: Dying and dementia. *JAMA* 256:2210–2213, 1986.

Marson DC, Hawkins L, McInturff B, et al. Cognitive models that predict physician judgments of capacity to consent in mild Alzheimer's disease. *J Am Geriatr Soc* 45:458–464, 1998.

Marson DC, McInturff B, Hawkins L, et al: Consistency of physician judgments of capacity to consent in mild Alzheimer's disease. *J Am Geriatr Soc* 45:453–457, 1997.

McCartney JR, Izeman H, Rogers D, et al: Sexuality and the institutionalized elderly. *J Am Geriatr Soc* 35:331–333, 1987.

Meier DE, Cassel CK: Nursing home placement and the demented patient: a case presentation and ethical analysis. *Ann Intern Med* 104:98–105, 1986.

Meier DE, Emmons CA, Wallenstein S, et al: A national survey of physician-assisted suicide and euthanasia in the United States. *N Engl J Med* 338:1193–1201, 1998.

Meisel A, Snyder L, Quill T: Seven legal barriers to end-of-life care. *JAMA* 284:2495–2501, 2000.

Murphy DJ: Do-not-resuscitate orders: time for reappraisal in long-term care institutions. *JAMA* 260:2098–2101, 1988.

O'Brien LA, Grisso JA, Maislin G, et al: Nursing home residents' preferences for life-sustaining treatments. *JAMA* 274:1775–1779, 1995.

Prendergast TJ, Puntillo KA: Withdrawal of life support: intensive caring at the end of life. *JAMA* 288:2732–2740, 2002.

Quill T, Lo B, Brock DW: Palliative options of last resort. *JAMA* 278:2099–2104, 1999.

Sachs GA, Ahronheim JC, Rhymes JA, et al: Good care of dying patients: the alternative to physician-assisted suicide and euthanasia. *J Am Geriatr Soc* 43:577–578, 1995.

Silveira MJ, DiPiero A, Gerrity MS, Feudtner C: Patients' knowledge of options at the end of life. *JAMA* 284:2483–2488, 2000.

Singer PA, Martin DK, Kelner M: Quality end-of-life care. *JAMA* 281:163–168, 1999.

Steinbrook R, Lo B: Artificial feeding—solid ground, not a slippery slope. *N Engl J Med* 318:286–290, 1988.

Steinhauser KE, Christakis NA, Clipp EC, McNeilly M, McIntyre L, Tulsky JA: Factors considered important at the end of life by patients, family, physicians and other care providers. *JAMA* 284:2476–2482, 2000.

SUPPORT Principal Investigators: A controlled trial to improve care for seriously ill hospitalized patients: the study to understand prognoses and preferences for outcomes and risks of treatments (SUPPORT). *JAMA* 274:1591–1598, 1995.

Taub HA, Baker MT, Sturr JF: Informed consent for research: Effects of readability, patient age, and education. *J Am Geriatr Soc* 34:601–606, 1986.

Torrance GW: Utility approach to measuring health-related quality of life. *J Chronic Dis* 40:593–600, 1987.

Tsevat J, Dawson NV, Wu AW, et al: Health values of hospitalized patients 80 years or older. *JAMA* 279:371–375, 1998.

Tymchuk AJ, Ouslander JG, Rader N: Informing the elderly: a comparison of four methods. *J Am Geriatr Soc* 34:818–822, 1986.

Uhlmann RF, Clark H, Pearlman RA: Medical management decisions in nursing home patients. *Ann Intern Med* 106:879–885, 1987.

Volicer L, Rheaume Y, Brown J, et al: Hospice approach to the treatment of patients with advanced dementia of the Alzheimer type. *JAMA* 256:2244–2245, 1986.

Wanzer SH, Federman DD, Adelstein SJ, et al: The physician's responsibility toward hopelessly ill patients. A second look. *N Engl J Med* 320:844–849, 1989.

Welch HG, Albertsen PC, Nease RF, et al: Estimating treatment benefits for the elderly: the effect of competing risks. *Ann Intern Med* 124:577–584, 1996.

Suggested Readings

Barrett-Connor E, Stuenkel CA: Questions of life and death in old age. *JAMA* 279:622–623, 1999.

Beauchamp TL, Childress JF: *Principles of Biomedical Ethics.* New York, Oxford University Press, 1979.

Buckwalter KC (ed): End-of-life research: focus on older populations. *Gerontologist,* Special Issue III, vol 42, 2002.

Cooper-Kazaz R, Friedlander Y, Steinberg A, Sonnenblick M: Longitudinal changes in attitudes of offspring concerning life-sustaining measures for their terminally ill patients. *J Am Geriatr Soc* 47:1337–1341, 1999.

Grant MD, Rudberg MA, Brody JA: Gastrostomy placement and mortality among hospitalized Medicare beneficiaries. *JAMA* 279:1973–1976, 1998.

Lynn J: Measuring quality of care at the end of life: a statement of principles. *J Am Geriatr Soc* 45:526–527, 1997.

Meier DE, Morrison RS, Cassel CK: Improving palliative care. *Ann Intern Med* 127:225–230, 1997.

Quill TE: Initiating end-of-life discussions with seriously ill patients. *JAMA* 284:2502–2507, 2000.

SUGGESTED GERIATRIC MEDICAL FORMS

KATZ INDEX OF INDEPENDENCE IN ACTIVITIES OF DAILY LIVING (ADL)

The index of independence in activities of daily living is based on an evaluation of the functional independence or dependence of patients in bathing, dressing, going to the toilet, transferring, continence, and feeding. Specific definitions of functional independence and dependence appear below the index.

A. Independent in feeding, continence, transferring, toileting, dressing, and bathing
B. Independent in all but one of these functions
C. Independent in all but bathing and one additional function
D. Independent in all but bathing, dressing, and one additional function
E. Independent in all but bathing, dressing, toileting, and one additional function
F. Independent in all but bathing, dressing, toileting, transferring, and one additional function
G. Dependent in all six functions
Other   Dependent in at least two functions, but not classifiable as C, D, E, or F. Independence means without supervision, direction, or active personal assistance, except as specifically noted below. This is based on actual status and not on ability. Patients who refuse to perform a function are considered as not performing the funtion, even though they are deemed able.

Bathing (sponge, shower, or tub)
Independent: needs assistance only in bathing a single part (as back or disabled extremity) or bathes self completely
Dependent: needs assistance in bathing more than one part of the body and in getting in or out of tub or does not bathe self

Transfer
Independent: moves in and out of bed independently and moves in and out of chair independently (may or may not be using mechanical supports)
Dependent: assistance in moving in or out of bed and/or chair; does not perform one or more transfers

Dressing

Independent: gets clothes from closets and drawers; puts on clothes, outer garments, braces; manages fasteners; act of tying shoes excluded

Dependent: does not dress self or remains partly undressed

Toileting

Independent: gets to toilet; gets on and off toilet; arranges clothes; cleans organs of excretion (may manage own bedpan used at night only and may not be using mechanical supports)

Dependent: uses bedpan or commode or receives assistance in getting to and using toilet

Continence

Independent: urination and defecation entirely self-controlled

Dependent: partial or total incontinence in urination or defecation; partial or total control by enemas, catheters, or regulated use of urinals and/or bedpans

Independent: gets food from plate or its equivalent into mouth (precutting of meat and preparation of food, as buttering bread, are excluded from evaluation)

Dependent: assistance in act of feeding (see above); does not eat all or parenteral feeding

LAWTON/BRODY INSTRUMENTAL ACTIVITIES OF DAILY LIVING SCALE

Action	Score
Ability to Use Telephone	
Operates telephone on own inititiatve—looks up and dials numbers, etc.	1
Dials a few well-known numbers	1
Answers telephone but does not dial	1
Does not use telephone at all	0
Shopping	
Takes care of all shopping needs independently	1
Shops independently for small purchases	0
Needs to be accompanied on any shopping trip	0
Completely unable to shop	0
Food Preparation	
Plans, prepares, and serves adequate meals independently	1
Prepares adequate meals if supplied with ingredients	0
Heats and serves prepared meals, or prepares meals but does not maintain adequate diet	0
Needs to have meals prepared and served	0
Housekeeping	
Maintains house alone or with occasional assistance (e.g., "heavy work-domestic help")	1
Performs light daily tasks such as dishwashing, bedmaking	1
Performs light daily tasks but cannot maintain acceptable level of cleanliness	1
Needs help with all home maintenance tasks	1
Does not participate in any housekeeping tasks	0
Laundry	
Does personal laundry completely	1
Launders small items—rinses socks, stockings, etc.	1
All laundry must be done by others	0
Mode of Transportation	
Travels independently on public transportation or drives own car	1
Arranges own travel via taxi, but does not otherwise use public transportation	1
Travels on public transportation when assisted or accompanied by another	1
Travel limited to taxi or automobile with assistance of another	0
Does not travel at all	0

Action	Score
Responsibility for Own Medications	
Is responsible for taking medication in correct dosages at correct times	1
Takes responsibility if medication is prepared in advance in separate dosages	0
Is not capable of dispensing own medication	0
Ability to Handle Finanaces	
Manages financial matters independently (budgets, write checks, pays rent, bills, goes to bank), collects and keeps track of income	1
Manages day-to-day purchases, but needs help with banking, major purchases, etc.	1
Incapable of handling money	0

(From Lawton, MP, Brody, E: Assessment of older people: self-maitaining and instrumental activities of daily living. *Gerontologist* 9:181, 1969. Reprinted with permission.)

MAIN COMPONENTS OF THE TINETTI FALL RISK SCALE

Balance Assessment
- Sitting balance (in a hard, straight-backed chair)
- Arising from chair
- Immediate standing balance (first 3–5 seconds)
- Standing balance
- Balance with eyes closed (with feet as close together as possible)
- Turning balance (360 degrees)
- Nudge on sternum (patient standing with feet as close together as possible, examiner pushes with light even pressure over sternum 3 times; reflects ability to withstand displacement)
- Neck turning (patient asked to turn head sideways and look up while standing with feet as close together as possible)
- One leg standing balance
- Back extension (ask patient to lean back as far as possible, without holding onto object if possible)
- Reaching up (have patient attempt to remove an object from a shelf high enough to require stretching or standing on toes)
- Bending down (patient is asked to pick up small objects, such as a pen, from the floor)

Gait Assessment (Patient stands with examiner at end of obstacle-free hallway. Patient uses usual walking aid. Examiner asks patient to walk down hallway at usual pace. Examiner observes one component of gait at a time. For some components the examiner walks behind the patient; for other components, the examiner walks next to the patient. May require several trips to complete.)

- Initiation of gait (patient is asked to begin walking down hallway)
- Step height (begin observing after first few steps; observe one foot, then the other; observe from side)
- Step length (observe distance between toe of stance foot and heel of swing foot; observe from side; do not judge first few or last few steps; observe one side at a time)
- Step symmetry (observe the middle part of the patch, not the first or last steps; observe from side; observe distance between heel of each swing foot and toe of each stance)
- Step continuity
- Path deviation [observe from behind; observe one foot over several strides; observe in relation to line on floor (e.g., tiles) if possible; difficult to assess if patient uses walker]
- Trunk stability (observe from behind; side to side motion of trunk may be a normal gait pattern, need to differentiate this from instability)
- Walk stance (observe from behind)
- Turning while walking

Source: Tinetti ME: Performance-oriented assessment of mobility problems in elderly patients. *J Am Geriatr Soc* 34:119–126, 1986.

REUBEN'S PHYSICAL PERFORMANCE TEST

	Time, seconds*	Scoring	Score
1. Write a sentence (The whale lives in the blue ocean)	___	$\leq$10 s = 4 10.5–5 s = 3 15.5– 20 s = 2 >20 s = 1 Unable = 0	___
2. Simulate eating	___	$\leq$10 s = 4 10.5–5 s = 3 15.5– 20 s = 2 >20 s = 1 Unable 0	___
3. Lift a book and put it on a shelf	___	$\leq$2 s = 4 2.5–4 s = 3 4.5–6 s = 2 Unable = 0	___
4. Put on and remove a jacket	___	$\leq$10 s = 4 10.5–5 s = 3 15.0– 20 s = 3 >20 s = 1	___
5. Pick up penny from floor	___	$\leq$2 s = 4 2.5–4 s = 3 4.5–6 s = 2 Unable = 0	___

6. Turn 360°   Discontinuous steps   0
Continuous steps   2
Unsteady (grabs, staggers)   0
Steady   2

6. Turn 360°	Discontinuous steps	0
	Continuous steps	2
	Unsteady (grabs, staggers)	0
	Steady	2
7. 50-ft-walk test	_____	$\leq$15 s = 4
		15.5–20 s = 3
		20.5–25 s = 2
		>25 s = 1
		Unable = 0
8. Climb one flight of stairs[†]	_____	$\leq$5 s = 4
		5.5–10 s = 3
		10.5–15 s = 2
		>15 s = 1
		Unable = 0
9. Climb stairs[†]	Number of flights of stairs up and down (maximum four)	_____

TOTAL SCORE (maximum 36 for 9-item test, 28 for 7-item test)   ____9 items   ____7 items

* Round time off to nearest 0.5 seconds.
† Omit for 7-item test.
Note: For details of administering the test, see Reuben DB, Siu AL: An objective measure of physical function of elderly persons: the physical performance test. *J Am Geriatr Soc* 38: 1105–1112, 1990.

MINI-MENTAL STATE EXAM (MMSE)

Maximum Score

Orienation

5   What is the (year) (date) (day) (month) (season)?

5   Where are we (state) (county) (town) (hospital) (floor)?

Registration

3   Name 3 objects: 1 second to say each. Then ask the patient all 3 after you have said them. Give 1 point for each correct answer. Then repeat them until he or she learns all 3. Count trial and record.
Trials

Attention and calculation

5   Serial 7s: 1 point for each correct. Stop after 5 answers. Alternately, spell "world" backwards.

Recall

3   Ask for 3 objects repeated above. Give 1 point for each correct answer.

Language

2   Name a pencil and watch (2 points)

1   Repeat the following: "no ifs, ands, or buts" (1 point)

3   Follow a 3-stage command: "Take a paper in your right hand, fold it in half, and put it on the floor." (3 points)

1   Read and obey the following: "Close your eyes." (1 point)

1   Write a sentence. Must contain subject and verb and be sensible. (1 point)

Visual-motor integrity

1   Copy design (2 intersecting pentagons. All 10 angles must be present and 2 must intersect.) (1 point)

Total score_____

30

Source: Folstein MF, Folstein S, McHugh PR: Mini-mental state: a practical method for grading the cognitive state of patients for the clinician. *Psychiatr Res* 12, 189-198, 1975.

THE GERIATRIC DEPRESSION SCALE

Choose the best answer for how you felt the past week:

1. Are you basically satisfied with your life?	Yes	No*
2. Have you dropped many of your activities and interests?	Yes*	No
3. Do you feel that your life is empty?	Yes*	No
4. Do you often get bored?	Yes*	No
5. Are you hopeful about the future?	Yes	No*
6. Are you bothered by thoughts you can't get out of our head?	Yes*	No
7. Are you in good spirits most of the time?	Yes	No*
8. Are you afraid that something bad is going to happen to you?	Yes*	No
9. Do you feel happy most of the time?	Yes	No*
10. Do you often feel helpless?	Yes*	No
11. Do you often get restless and fidgety?	Yes*	No
12. Do you prefer to stay at home rather than going out and doing new things?	Yes*	No
13. Do you frequently worry about the future?	Yes*	No
14. Do you feel you have more problems with memory than most?	Yes*	No
15. Do you think it is wonderful to be alive now?	Yes	No*
16. Do you often feel downhearted and blue?	Yes*	No
17. Do you feel pretty worthless the way you are now?	Yes*	No
18. Do you worry a lot about the past?	Yes*	No
19. Do you find life very exciting?	Yes	No*
20. Is it hard for you to get started on new projects?	Yes*	No
21. Do you feel full of energy?	Yes	No*
22. Do you feel that your situation is hopeless?	Yes*	No
23. Do you think that most people are better off than you are?	Yes*	No
24. Do you frequently get upset over little things?	Yes*	No
25. Do you frequently feel like crying?	Yes*	No
26. Do you have trouble concentrating?	Yes*	No
27. Do you enjoy getting up in the morning?	Yes	No*
28. Do you prefer to avoid social gatherings?	Yes*	No
29. Is it easy for you to make decisions?	Yes	No*
30. Is your mind as clear as it used to be?	Yes	No*

Note: Each answer indicated by an asterisk counts 1 point. Scores between 15 and 22 suggest mild depression; scores above 22 suggest severe depression. The 15-item short form includes questions 1–4, 7–10, 12, 14, 15, 17, and 21–23. On the short form, scores between 5 and 9 suggest depression; scores above 9 generally indicate depression.

Source: Yesavage JA, Brink TL: Development and validation of a geriatric screening scale: a preliminary report. *J Psychiatr Res* 17 (1), 37–49, 1983.

KEY COMPONENTS OF A COMPREHENSIVE GERIATRIC ASSESSMENT: THE MEDICAL HISTORY AND PHYSICAL EXAM

A. Medical History

1. Patient's major complaint(s) (in patient's own or caregiver's language)

_____

_____

2. Prior surgery

Date   Surgical procedure

_____/_____/_____   _____

_____/_____/_____   _____

3. Other hospitalizations

Date   Hospital   Diagnoses

_____/_____/_____   _____   _____

_____/_____/_____   _____   _____

4. Health maintenance

   a. TB test status _____

   b. Immunization status _____

      1. Pneumococcal _____

      2. Tetanus _____

      3. Influenza _____

   c. Last dental visit _____

   d. Last Papanicolaou (Pap) test _____

   e. Last mammogram _____

5. Allergies: _____

6. Habits   No   Yes

   a. Smoking   _____   _____

b. Alcohol consumption

If yes, specify amount and duration _____

c. Diet _____

d. Exercise _____

7. Current medications

Prescribed drugs   Dosage and frequency

_____   _____

_____   _____

_____   _____

Over-the-counter drugs   Dosage and frequency

_____   _____

_____   _____

_____   _____

_____   _____

8. Symptom review

a. Patient's overall rating of own health

_____ Excellent _____ Very good _____ Good _____ Fair _____ Poor

b. Selected symptom review (enter C for chronic, N for new).

If positive, describe briefly.

_____ Anorexia

_____ Fatigue

_____ Weight loss (10 lb in 6 months)

_____ Insomnia

_____ Pain (describe)

_____ Headache

_____ Visual impairment

_____ Hearing impairment

_____ Dental/ denture discomfort

_____ Cough or wheezing

A. Medical History (*Continued*)

___ Dyspnea
___ Exertional chest discomfort
___ Orthopnea
___ Edema
___ Claudication
___ Dizziness/ unsteadiness
___ Falls
___ Syncope
___ Dysphagia
___ Abdominal pain
___ Change in bowel habit or constipation
___ Blood in stool
___ Urinary frequency and/ or urgency
___ Nocturia
___ Hesitancy, straining, or intermittent stream
___ Incontinence
___ Foot problems
___ Focal weakness or sensory loss
___ Transient visual disturbance
___ Forgetfulness
___ Depression
___ Disruptive behavior/ wandering

9. Depression screen

For the following question, which description comes closest to the way you have been feeling during the past month ?

	All the time	Most of the time	Some of the time	A little of the time	None of the time

How much of the time, during the past month, have you felt downhearted and blue?

Answer of " all the time" or " most of the time" should raise suspicion of depression, and a full depression scale should be administered.

10. Functional status

a. Instrumental and basic activities of daily living

	Fully independent	Needs some human assistance (including supervision)	Totally independent
IADLs			
Preparing meals	____	____	____
Managing money	____	____	____
Managing medications	____	____	____
Using telephone	____	____	____
BADLs			
Bathing	____	____	____
Ambulation	____	____	____
Transfer	____	____	____
Dressing	____	____	____
Personal grooming	____	____	____
Toileting	____	____	____
Eating	____	____	____

b. Functional limitations

For how long (if at all) has your health limited you in each of the following activities? (Check the category which is the best description.)

	Limited for more than 3 months	Limited for 3 months or less	Not limited at all
The kinds or amounts of *vigorous* activities you can do, like lifting heavy objects, running, or participating in strenuous sports	____	____	____
The kinds or amounts of *moderate* activities you can do, like moving a table or carrying groceries	____	____	____
The kinds of work or housework you can do around your home	____	____	____
Working at a job	____	____	____
Walking uphill or climbing stairs	____	____	____
Bending, lifting, or stooping	____	____	____

A. Medical History (*Continued*)

Walking one block ___ ___

Eating, dressing, bathing, or using the toilet ___ ___

B. Physical Examination

1. Vital signs

	Supine	Sitting	Standing
Blood pressure	___ / ___	___ / ___	___ / ___
Pulse (per minute)	___	___	___

Respiratory rate (per minute) ___

Weight (lb) ___ Height ___

Weight last examination (lb) ___

(date of last examination ___ / ___ / ___)

2. Skin

___ Excessive dryness

___ Rash (Describe:

___ Lesions— suspected malignant (Location: ___

___ Pressure sores

Location	Size (cm)	Stage (I– IV)
_____	___	___
_____	___	___
_____	___	___

3. Hearing

___ Hears normal voice

___ Hears whispered voice

___ Hears 1024-Hz tuning fork

___ Impaired

___ Wears hearing aid

___ Cerumen impacted in ear canals

___ Frequency threshold at 40 dB ___

4. Vision

Able to read newsprint _____ With corrective lenses _____ Without corrective lenses _____

Visual acuity

	Reading	Distance
Right	_____ / _____	_____ / _____
Left	_____ / _____	_____ / _____

Cataract present: _____ Right _____ Left

Funduscopic findings

Normal	Abnormal (describe)	Unable to visualize
Right _____	_____	_____
Left _____	_____	_____

5. Mouth

_____ Poor oral hygiene

Dentures

_____ None _____ Good fit _____ Poor fit

_____ Sores under dentures _____ Other lesion (describe)

6. Neck

Range of motion	Normal _____	Abnormal _____
Thyroid	_____	_____

_____ Thyroid scar

_____ Mass (describe)

7. Lymph nodes

_____ No lymphadenopathy

_____ Enlarged nodes (Describe: _____)

8. Breasts

Mass present? _____ Yes _____ No

If yes: _____ Right _____ Left (Describe: _____)

Other abnormality _____

B. Physical Examination (*Continued*)

9. Lungs

	No	Yes		No	Yes
Crackles	___	___	Bronchospasm	___	___
Rhonchi	___	___	Other (specify)	___	___

If yes, describe: _____

10. Cardiovascular

a. Heart

	No	Yes
Irregular rhythm	___	___
Murmur	___	___
S_3	___	___
S_4	___	___
Other (specify)	___	___

If yes, describe: _____

b. Bruits

	None	Right	Left
Carotid		___ Right	___ Left
Femoral		___ Right	___ Left

c. Distal pulses

	Present	Absent
Right dorsalis pedis	___	___
Right posterior tibial	___	___
Left dorsalis pedis	___	___
Left posterior tibial	___	___

d. Edema

	None	1+	2+	3+	4+
Pedal	___	___	___	___	___
Tibial	___	___	___	___	___
Sacral	___	___	___	___	___

11. Abdomen

Liver size _____ cm

Abdominal masses _____ None _____ Pulsatile _____ Other

Bruits _____ Yes _____ No

Tenderness _____ Yes _____ No

Describe positive findings:

12. Rectal

_____ Diminished/ absent sphincter tone

_____ Enlarged prostate (Describe: _____)

_____ Prostate mass

_____ Rectal mass

_____ Fecal impaction

Occult blood _____ Negative _____ Positive

13. Genital/ pelvic

a. Men

_____ Normal

_____ Abnormal (Describe: _____)

b. Women

_____ Normal

_____ Abnormal (Describe: _____)

_____ Vaginal atrophy _____ Mass

_____ Atrophic vaginitis _____ Tenderness

_____ Pelvic prolapse _____ Other

Pap test done _____ Yes _____ No

14. Musculoskeletal

	None	Spine	Shoulders	Elbows	Hands	Hips	Knees	Feet
Deformity	___	___	___	___	___	___	___	___
Limited range of motion	___	___	___	___	___	___	___	___
Tenderness	___	___	___	___	___	___	___	___
Prominent swelling or inflammation	___	___	___	___	___	___	___	___

Description of deformity or limited range of motion: _____

B. Physical Examination (*Continued*)

15. Neurologic

a. Mental status

	Intact	Impaired
Orientation		
Person	_____	_____
Place	_____	_____
Time	_____	_____
Situation	_____	_____
Memory		
Remote	_____	_____
Recent	_____	_____
Object recall after 5 min	_____	_____
Immediate (repetition)	_____	_____

(If dementia is suspected, further assessment should be undertaken. See "Dementia Assessment" on the following pages.)

b. Mood/affect:

_____ Appropriate   _____ Labile   _____ Depressed
_____ Agitated   _____ Anxious

c. General

	Normal	Abnormal (describe)
Cranial nerves	_____	_____
Motor		
Strength	_____	_____
Tone	_____	_____
Sensation		
Pin	_____	_____
Touch	_____	_____
Vibration	_____	_____
Reflexes	_____	_____
Cerebellar		
Finger to nose	_____	_____

Heel to shin _____
Romberg _____
Gait _____
Description of abnormal findings: _____

	Absent	Present (describe)
d. Other signs		
Resting tremor	___	
Cogwheel rigidity	___	
Bradykinesia	___	
Intention tremor	___	
Involuntary movements	___	
Pathologic reflexes	___	

Description of findings present: _____

C. Laboratory Data

Test/ procedure	Date	Normal	Abnormal (describe)
_____	___/___/___	_____	_____
_____	___/___/___	_____	_____
_____	___/___/___	_____	_____

D. Problem List

Medical problems _____

Functional status problems _____

Psychosocial problems _____

DEMENTIA ASSESSMENT

A. History

1. Active medical conditions

_____

_____

2. Medications

_____

_____

3. History of (describe):
_____ Hypertension
_____ Stroke
_____ Transient ischemic attack
_____ Depression
_____ Other psychiatric disorder

4. Current symptoms (complaints of patient or family)
_____ Memory loss
_____ Forgets recent events
_____ Forgets things just said
_____ Forgets names of people
_____ Forgets words
_____ Gets lost
_____ Asks questions or tells stories repeatedly
_____ Confused about date or place

_____ Can't do simple calculations
_____ Can't understand what is read or said
_____ Impairment of other cognitive functions
_____ Anxiety/agitation
_____ Paranoia
_____ Delusions/hallucination
_____ Wandering
_____ Disruptive behavior
_____ Incontinence

5. Onset of symptoms
_____ Recent (days to few weeks)
_____ Longer duration (months)
_____ Uncertain

6. Progression of symptoms
_____ Rapid
_____ Gradual
_____ Stepwise (irregular, stuttering deteriorations)
_____ Uncertain

7. Activities of daily living (ADL)
Does the impairment of cognitive function interfere with instrumental ADL?
_____ Yes _____ No
If yes, which ones? _____
Basic ADL? _____ Yes _____ No
If yes, which ones? _____

B. Physical Examination

1. General appearance
_____ Normal
_____ Abnormal (Describe: _____)

– 495 –

B. Physical Examination (*Continued*)

	Normal	Abnormal
2. Blood pressure		
Right arm ____/____		
Left arm ____/____		
3. Hearing	Normal	Abnormal
Normal voice	____	____
Audioscopic screening	No	Yes
4. Orientation		
Person	____	____
Place	____	____
Time	____	____
Situation	____	____
5. Memory function	Normal	Impaired
Remote	____	____
Recent (object recall after 5 min)	____	____
Immediate (digit repetition)	____	____
6. Mini-Mental State Exam Score	____/30	
7. Other cognitive functions	Normal	Impaired
General fund of knowledge	____	____
Simple calculations	____	____
Ability to write name	____	____
Interpretations of proverbs	____	____
Naming common objects	____	____
Name animals (12 in 1 min is normal)	____	____
Insight	____	____
Judgment	____	____
Ability to follow simple verbal commands (e.g., "Touch your left ear with your right hand")	____	____

8. Thought content
   _____ Normal
   _____ Delusions
   _____ Paranoid ideation
   _____ Other (Describe: _____)
9. Mood/affect (standardized screening tests are available)
   _____ Appropriate _____ Depressed _____ Labile _____ Agitated
   _____ Other (Describe: _____)
10. Behavior during examinations   Yes   No
    Good attention and concentration   _____   _____
    Good effort to answer questions and perform tasks   _____   _____
    Many "don't know" answers   _____   _____
11. Remainder of neurologic examination
    _____ Focal neurologic signs (Describe: _____

    _____ Signs of parkinsonism (Describe: _____
    Pathological reflexes:
    _____ Babinski
    _____ Hoffman
    _____ Grasp
    _____ Palmomental
    Gait:
    _____ Normal
    _____ Abnormal (Describe: _____
    _____ Other abnormality (Describe: _____
    Sensory examination:
    _____ Normal
    _____ Abnormal (Describe: _____

B. Physical Examination (*Continued*)

12. Hachinski ischemia score

Characteristic	Point score
Abrupt onset	2
Stepwise deterioration	1
Somatic complaints	1
Emotional incontinence	1
History or presence of hypertension	1
History of strokes	2
Focal neurologic symptoms	2
Focal neurologic signs	2

Total score: _____

(Score of 4 or more suggests multi-infarct dementia.)

C. Diagnostic Studies

	Normal	Abnormal
Blood:		
CBC	_____	_____
Sedimentation rate	_____	_____
Glucose	_____	_____
BUN	_____	_____
Electrolytes	_____	_____
Calcium	_____	_____
Liver function tests	_____	_____
Free thyroxine index	_____	_____
TSH	_____	_____
VDRL	_____	_____
Vitamin B_{12}	_____	_____
Folate	_____	_____

Radiographic:

    Chest film | |

    CT or MRI scan | |

Other:

    Urinalysis | |

    ECG | |

    EEG | |

D. Clinical Diagnosis

_____ Probable primary degenerative dementia (Alzheimer's type)

_____ Multi-infarct dementia

_____ Dementia with Lewy bodies

_____ Mixed

_____ Uncertain

_____ Depression

_____ Other potentially reversible cause of dementia (describe)

INCONTINENCE ASSESSMENT

I. Assessment of Acute Incontinence and Reversible Factors

_____ If incontinence is of recent onset (within a few days) and/ or associated with an acute illness, check for any of the following:

_____ Acute urinary tract infection

_____ Fecal impaction

_____ Acute confusion (delirium)

_____ Immobility

_____ Drug effects (e.g., excessive sedation, polyuria caused by diuretics, urinary retention, other autonomic effects)

_____ Metabolic abnormality with polyuria (e.g., hyperglycemia, hypercalcemia)

If incontinence persists despite management of any of these conditions and/or resolution of an acute illness, further assessment (as shown in Part II) should be pursued.

II. Assessment of Persistent Incontinence

A. History

1. Do you ever leak urine when you don't want to? _____ No, never _____ Yes

2. Do you ever have trouble getting to the toilet on time or have accidents getting your clothes or bed wet? _____ No, never _____ Yes

Do you every wear any pads to protect yourself from leakage? _____ No, never _____ Yes

3. How long have you had a problem with urinary leakage?

_____ Less than 1 week

_____ 1 to 4 weeks

_____ 1 to 3 months

_____ 4 to 12 months

_____ 1 to 5 years

_____ Longer than 5 years

4. How often do you leak urine?

_____ Less than once per week

_____ More than once per week, but less than once per day

_____ About once per day
_____ More than once per day
_____ Continual leakage
_____ Variable

5. Does the leakage occur
_____ Mainly during the day
_____ Mainly at night
_____ Both night and day

6. When you leak urine, how much leaks?
_____ Just a few drops
_____ More than a few drops but less than a cupful
_____ More than a cupful (enough to wet clothes and/or bed linens)
_____ Variable
_____ Unknown

7. Do any of the following cause you to leak urine?
_____ Coughing
_____ Laughing
_____ Exercise or other forms of straining
_____ Inability to get to the toilet in time

8. How often do you normally urinate?
_____ Every 6 to 8 h or less often
_____ About every 3 to 5 h
_____ About every 1 to 2 h
_____ At least every hour or more often
_____ Frequency varies
_____ Unknown

9. Do you wake up at night to urinate?
_____ Never or rarely
_____ Yes, usually once

A. History (*Continued*)

_____ Yes, two or three times per night
_____ Yes, four or more times per night
_____ Yes, but frequency varies

10. Once your bladder feels full, how long can you hold your urine?
_____ As long as you want (several minutes at least)
_____ Just a few minutes
_____ Less than a minute or two
_____ Not at all
_____ Cannot tell when bladder is full

11. Do you have any of the following when you urinate?
_____ Difficulty in getting the urine started
_____ Very slow stream or dribbling
_____ Straining to finish
_____ Discomfort or pain
_____ Burning
_____ Blood in the urine

12. Have you had any previous evaluation or treatment for the incontinence?
_____ No
_____ Yes (Describe: _____)

13. Are you currently using any of the following to help with the urinary leakage?
_____ Bed or furniture pads
_____ Sanitary napkins
_____ Other types of pads in your underwear
_____ Special undergarments
_____ Medication
_____ Bedside commode
_____ Urinal
_____ Other (Describe: _____)

14. Is the urinary leakage enough of a problem that you consider surgery for it?

_____ Yes _____ Possibly _____ No

15. Are you constipated?

_____ No _____ Yes _____ Average # BM/ week

16. Do you ever have uncontrolled loss of stool?

_____ No, never _____ Yes

17. Relevant medical history

_____ Stroke
_____ Dementia
_____ Parkinson's disease
_____ Prior CNS trauma/ surgery
_____ Other neurologic disorder
_____ Diabetes
_____ Congestive heart failure
_____ (Specify: _____)

18. Prior genitourinary history

_____ Multiple vaginal deliveries
_____ Cesarean section(s)
_____ Abdominal hysterectomy
_____ Vaginal hysterectomy
_____ Bladder suspension or sling
_____ Periuretral injection
_____ TURP (transurethral prostatectomy)
_____ Suprapubic prostatectomy
_____ Urethral stricture/dilatation
_____ Bladder tumor
_____ Pelvic irradiation
_____ Recurrent urinary tract infections

A. History (*Continued*)

19. Medications

    Diuretic _____

    Antihypertensive _____

    Other drugs that affect the autonomic nervous system _____

    Psychotropics _____

    Estrogen _____

    Other _____

20. Fluid intake

    _____ Caffeinated beverages (number per day)

    _____ Other fluids

B. Physical Examination

1. Mental status

    _____ Normal

    _____ Mild/moderate cognitive impairment

    _____ Severe cognitive impairment (unaware of toileting needs)

2. Mobility

    _____ Ambulates independently, with adequate speed

    _____ Ambulates independently, but slowly (so that ability to get to a toilet is impaired)

    _____ Not independently ambulatory, but able to use urinal, bedpan, or bedside commode independently

    _____ Chair- or bed-bound, but able to use urinal or bedpan independently

    _____ Dependent on others for toileting

3. Abdominal examination

    _____ Bladder enlarged and palpable

    _____ Bladder not palpable

    _____ Suprapubic tenderness

4. Neurologic examination of lower extremities

    _____ Normal

_____ Evidence of upper motor neuron lesion
_____ Evidence of lower motor neuron lesion
_____ Peripheral neuropathy

5. Rectal examination
_____ Decreased resting rectal sphincter tone
_____ Decreased perianal sensation
_____ Absent bulbocavernosus reflex
_____ Prostate enlarged
_____ Prostate cancer suspected

6. Voluntary contraction of rectal sphincter
_____ Good
_____ Fair
_____ Poor
_____ Unable

7. External genitalia
_____ Skin irritation
_____ Diminished sensation
_____ Abnormal (Describe: _____)

8. Vaginal examination
_____ Atrophic vaginitis
_____ Mild prolapse
_____ Moderate/ severe prolapse
_____ Rectocele
_____ Adenexal or uterine mass
_____ Stress incontinence (supine)

C. Diagnostic Studies

1. Cough test with full bladder for stress incontinence (standing)
_____ No leakage
_____ Leakage, small amount

C. Diagnostic Studies (*Continued*)

_____ Leakage, large amount
_____ Delayed leakage

2. Voided volume
_____ Unable _____ mL

3. Postvoid residual
_____ mL (or volume in bladder _____ mL)

4. Urinalysis
_____ Normal
_____ Hematuria (or positive heme and dipstick)
_____ Pyuria (or positive leukocyte esterase)
_____ Bacteriuria (or positive nitrite)

D. Management

_____ Treatment reversible factors (describe)
_____ Treat for urge incontinence
_____ Treat for stress incontinence
_____ Treat for mixed incontinence
_____ Manage supportively
_____ Refer for further evaluation
_____ Reason:

Specific treatment program

_____

_____

_____

_____

_____

ASSESSMENT FOR PATIENTS WHO FALL

1. Current medical problems

_____
_____
_____
_____

2. Medications

_____
_____
_____

3. Is there a previous history of falls?
   _____ Yes   _____ No
   If yes:
   Number of previous falls _____
   Is there a pattern?
   Frequency

   _____

   Time of day

   _____

   Position

   _____

   Activity

   _____

   Circumstances

   _____

4. Circumstances surrounding current fall
   Time of day

   _____

   Location

   _____

   Relationship to specific activities (e.g., toileting, climbing or descending stairs, exercise, turning head)

   _____
   _____
   _____

   Witness(es) reports

   _____
   _____
   _____

Environmental hazards (e.g., poor lighting, loose rug, uneven floor, other obstacles)

_____

_____

_____

5. Patient's description of and reasons for the fall (in patient's words)

_____

_____

_____

_____

6. Questions to the patient (and/or witness)
   a. Did you know you were going to fall?
      _____ Yes   _____ No
   b. After you fell, did you know what happened?
      _____ Yes   _____ No
   c. Did you lose consciousness (pass out)?
      _____ Yes   _____ No
      If yes, how long were you unconscious? _____ minutes
      Were you aware of what happened after you awoke?
      _____ Yes   _____ No
      Had you lost control of your bowel or bladder?
      _____ Yes   _____ No
   d. Were you able to get up right away?
      _____ Yes   _____ No
   e. Did you have any pain or injury after the fall?
      _____ Yes   _____ No
   f. Did you do any of the following just before the fall?
      _____ Trip
      _____ Slip
      _____ Stand up quickly
      _____ Turn your head suddenly
      _____ Cough
      _____ Urinate
      _____ Have a bowel movement
      _____ Eat a large meal
   g. Did you have any of the following symptoms just before you fell?
      _____ Lightheadedness
      _____ Vertigo (spinning around the room or vice versa)
      _____ Palpitations
      _____ Shortness of breath
      _____ Weakness or numbness on one side of the body
      _____ Sudden weakness of both legs
      _____ Slurred speech
      _____ Difficulty saying what you wanted to say
      _____ Strange smells
      _____ Flashing lights (scotomata)

7. Physical assessment
  a. Postural vital signs

	Supine	Sitting	Standing
Blood pressure	_____ / _____	_____ / _____	_____ / _____
Pulse	_____	_____	_____
Blood pressure other arm		_____ / _____	

  b. Skin
    _____ Bruises
    _____ Diminished turgor
  c. Vision
    _____ Adequate for independent ambulation
    _____ Limits mobility, but still independent
    _____ Inadequate for independent ambulation
  d. Neck
    _____ Supple
    _____ Full range of motion
    _____ Symptoms with rotation
  e. Cardiovascular
    _____ Arrhythmia
    _____ Murmur suggestive of aortic stenosis
    _____ Signs of heart failure (Describe: _____
    _____)
    _____ Cartoid bruit(s)
  f. Musculoskeletal
    _____ Trauma and/or suspected fracture
    _____ Deformity
    _____ Limited range of motion
    _____ Joint inflammation
  g. Podiatric
    Are any of the following impairing ambulation?
    _____ Callouses
    _____ Bunions
    _____ Nail deformity
    _____ Ulceration
    _____ Poorly fitted or otherwise inadequate shoes
  h. Neurological
    _____ Abnormal mental status
    _____ Focal neurological sign(s)
    _____ Muscular weakness
    _____ Bradykinesia
    _____ Resting tremor
    _____ Peripheral neuropathy
    _____ Ataxia, finger to nose
    _____ Ataxia, heel to shin
    Describe positive findings: _____
    _____

  i. Mobility
      _____ Ambulates independently
      _____ Uses aid
             _____ Cane
             _____ Quad-cane
             _____ Walker
      _____ Wheelchair, able to transfer independently
      _____ Wheelchair, needs help to transfer
  j. Stability and gait

	Normal	Abnormal
Sitting balance	_____	_____
Rising from sitting to standing	_____	_____
Standing balance with eyes open	_____	_____
Standing balance with eyes closed		
(Romberg test)	_____	_____
Initiation of walking	_____	_____
Length of stride	_____	_____
Distance feet apart	_____	_____
Turning	_____	_____
Sitting down	_____	_____

      Describe positive fidings: _____
      _____
      _____

8. Diagnostic studies

Test/procedure	Result
_____	_____
_____	_____
_____	_____
_____	_____
_____	_____
_____	_____
_____	_____
_____	_____
_____	_____

SELECTED INTERNET RESOURCES ON GERIATRICS

These resources were last verified in April, 2003.

ORGANIZATIONS

Administration on Aging	http://www.aoa.gov/
AgeNet Eldercare Network	http://www.caregivers.com/
Alzheimer's Association	http://www.alz.org/
Alzheimer's Disease Education & Referral Center	http://www.alzheimers.org/
American Academy of Pain Medicine	http://www.painmed.org
American Association of Homes and Services for the Aging	http://www.aahsa.org
American Association of Retired Persons	http://www.aarp.org/
American Geriatrics Society	http://www.americangeriatrics.org/
American Geriatrics Society Foundation for Health in Aging	http://www.healthinaging.org/
American Health Care Association	http://www.ahca.org/
American Medical Directors Association	http://www.amda.com/
American Pain Foundation	http://www.painfoundation.org/
American Pain Society	http://www.ampainsoc.org/
American Parkinson Disease Association	http://www.apdaparkinson.org/

American Society of Consultant
  Pharmacists   http://www.ascp.com/

American Society on Aging   http://www.asaging.org/

Arthritis Foundation   http://www.arthritis.org/

Center to Advance Palliative Care   http://www.capc.org

Centers for Disease Control and
  Prevention   http://www.cdc.gov/

Gerontological Society of America   http://www.geron.org/

Medicare   http://www.medicare.gov/

National Association for Continence   http://www.nafc.org/

National Association of Area
  Agencies on Aging (N4A)   http://www.n4a.org

National Association of Directors of   http://www.nadona.org/
  Nursing Administration/Long
  Term Care

National Association of Nutrition and   http://www.nanasp.org
  Aging Services Programs

National Council on the Aging   http://www.ncoa.org

National Institute on Aging   http://www.nih.gov/nia

National Parkinson Foundation   http://www.parkinson.org/

CLINICAL TOPICS – FOR PROFESSIONALS

Pain Management

"Chronic Pain Management in the   http://www.amda.com/info/cpg/
  Long-Term Care Setting"   chronicpain.htm

"The Management of Chronic Pain in   http://www.americangeriatrics.org/
  Older Persons"   products/chronic_pain.pdf

Control of pain in patients with cancer.   http://www.guidelines.gov/
  A national clinical guideline.   FRAMESETS/guideline_fs.asp?
                                                 guideline=002136&sSearch_string=
                                                 cancer+ pain+management

"Treatment of Pain at the End of Life"   http://www.ampainsoc.org/advocacy
                                                 /treatment.htm

American Society of Pain   http://www.aspmn.org
  Management Nurses

Urinary Incontinence

Evidence-based clinical practice guideline. Continence for women.	http://www.guideline.gov/ FRAMESETS/guideline_fs.asp? guideline=002151&sSearch_string= visual+impairment+in+the+elderly
National Association for Continence	http://www.nafc.org/
Making a Difference in Senior Care: A Focus on Bladder Control Problems	http://www.seniorcaremeds.com/

Alzheimer's Disease

"Dementia" (Clinical Practice Guideline)	http://www.amda.com/info/cpg/ dementia.htm
"Progress Report on Alzheimer's Disease 2000"	http://www.alzheimers.org/pubs/ prog00.htm

Depression

"Detection of Depression in the Cognitively Intact Older Adult"	http://www.guideline.gov/VIEWS/ summary.asp?guideline=729& summary_type=brief_summary&vie w=brief_summary&sSearch_string=
"Pharmacotherapy Companion to Depression"	http://www.amda.com/info/cpg/ depressiontherapy.htm

Medications

American Society of Consultant Pharmacists	http://www.ascp.com/

Low Vision

Age-related macular degeneration: Clinical guidelines	http://www.guideline.gov/ FRAMESETS/guideline_fs.asp? guideline=002314&sSearch_string= macular+degeneration
American Academy of Ophthalmology	http://www.aao.org/

American Glaucoma Society	http://www.glaucomaweb.org/
Care of the patient with age-related macular degeneration	http://www.guideline.gov/ FRAMESETS/guideline_fs.asp? guideline=001215&sSearch_string= macular+degeneration
Macular Degeneration Foundation	http://www.es.org
Macular Degeneration International	http://www.maculardegeneration.org
Macular Degeneration Network	http://www.macular-degeneration.org
Macular Degeneration Partnership	http://www.macd.net
"Screening for Visual Impairment in the Elderly" and "Primary Open-Angle Glaucoma Suspect" (Clinical Practice Guideline) and Primary	http://www.guideline.gov/body_ home.asp

Hearing Impairment

American Academy of Audiology	http://www.audiology.org
Clinical Advisory: NIDCD/VA Clinical Trial Finding Can Benefit Millions with Hearing Loss	http://www.nlm.nih.gov/databases/ alerts/hearing.html
Guidelines for Provision of Hearing Aids for VA Patients	http://www.va.gov/visns/visn02/ network/policies/10n2-98-00.doc
Hearing Loss	http://www.merck.com/pubs/ mmanual/section7/chapter82/82b.htm
Hearing Loss Clinical Resources: Geriatrics	http://fsumed-dl.slis.ua.edu/clinical/ otorhinolaryngology/ear/inner-ear/ hearing-loss.htm#Geriatrics

Parkinson's Disease

| American Parkinson's Disease Association – Free brochures for patients and caregivers | http://www.apdaparkinson.org/ |

CLINICAL TOPICS – FOR PATIENTS

General

A Consumer's Guide to Nursing Facilities	http://www.ahca.org/forms/ consumer_request.html
American Geriatrics Society Foundation for Health in Aging	http://www.healthinaging.org/
5 Wishes	http://www.agingwithdignity.org/ 5wishes.html
Nursing Home Compare	http://www.medicare.gov/ nhcompare/home.asp
"Nursing Home Checklist"/ "Eldercare Checklist"	http://www.caregivers.com/
Retirement & Elder Care	http://www.nolo.com/category/ ret_home.html
"10 Legal Myths About Advance Directives"	http://www.abanet.org/elderly/ myths.html

Pain Management

"Chronic Pain"	http://www.painfoundation.org/page. asp?file=documents/doc_037.htm
"Managing Cancer Pain"	http://www.painfoundation.org/ page.asp?file=documents/ doc_012.htm
Pain (PDQ): Supportive Care-Patients	http://www.cancernet.nci.nih.gov/
"Questions and Answers about Arthritis Pain"	http://www.niams.nih.gov/hi/topics/ arthritis/arthpain.htm

Urinary Incontinence

About the Overactive Bladder Campaign	http://www.afud.org/oab/general/ campaign.html
Bladder Control for Women	http://www.niddk.nih.gov/health/ urolog/uibcw/bcw/bcw.htm

Overactive Bladder: The Facts	http://www.ncoa.org/content.cfm?sectionID=109&detail=163
Your Medicine and Bladder Control	http://www.niddk.nih.gov/health/urolog/uibcw/medicine/medicine.htm

▓ Alzheimer's Disease

"About Alzheimer's"	http://search.alz.org/AboutAD/overview.htm
"Alzheimer's Disease Fact Sheet"	http://www.alzheimers.org/pubs/adfact.html
"Family Caregivers"	http://search.alz.org/FamCare/overview.asp
National Alzheimer's Disease Centers Program Directory	http://www.alzheimers.org/pubs/adcdir.html

▓ Depression

"Depression in Later Life"	http://www.nmha.org/ccd/support/older.cfm
"If You're Over 65 and Feeling Depressed: Treatment Brings New Hope"	http://www.nimh.nih.gov/publicat/over65.cfm
National Depressive and Manic-Depressive Association	http://www.ndmda.org/

▓ Medications

ASCP's Prescription for Quality Care" Preventing Medication-Related Problems Among Older Americans	http://www.ascp.com/public/ga/quality
"Top Ten Dangerous Drug Interactions in Long-Term Care"	http://www.scoup.net/M3Project/topten/

▓ Low Vision

American Macular Degeneration Foundation	http://www.macular.org/

Facts about Age-Related Macular Degeneration	http://www.nei.nih.gov/health/ maculardegen/armd_facts.htm
"Learn about Glaucoma"	http://www.glaucoma.org/learn/
"Living with Glaucoma"	http://www.eyesight.org
Macular Degeneration International	http://www.maculardegeneration.org
Macular Degeneration Network	http://www.macular-degeneration.org
Macular Degeneration Partnership	http://www.macd.net
"Understanding and Living with Glaucoma"	http://www.glaucoma.org/script/ books.php
What You Should Know about Low Vision"	http://www.nei.nih.gov/nehep/what.htm

▓ Hearing Impairment

Healthy Hearing	http://www.healthyhearing.com
Hearing Aid Help	http://www.hearingaidhelp.com/
Hearing Loss	http://www.quickfactscenter.com/ qfcArticle.cfm?topic=17
Sound Advice on Hearing Aids	http://www.ftc.gov/bcp/conline/pubs/ health/hearing.htm

▓ Parkinson's Disease

"Basic Information About Parkinson's Disease"	http://www.apdaparkinson.org/ basicin.html
"Frequent Questions About Parkinson Disease"	http://www.parkinson.org/nfaq.htm
"NINDS Parkinson's Disease Information Page"	http://www.ninds.nih.gov/health_and_ medical/disorders/parkinsons_ disease.htm
"Parkinson's Disease-Hope Through Research"	http://www.ninds.nih.gov/health_and_ medical/pubs/parkinson_disease_ htr.htm

INDEX

Note: Page numbers followed by "t" indicate tables; page numbers followed by "f" indicate figures.